RESET OR RENAISSANCE

RESET OR RENAISSANCE

Life, Liberty, and the Quest for Enlightenment in a Post-Covid World

Volume I

TWO ROADS

An American Scholar's Covid Chronicle

Daniel Joseph Polikoff, PhD

Portal books ≈ 2024

2024
Portalbooks
An imprint of SteinerBooks/Anthroposophic Press, Inc.
834 Main Street, PO Box 358
Spencertown, New York 12165
www.SteinerBooks.org

Library of Congress Control Number: 2024932575

ISBN: 978-1-938685-51-4

Printed in the United States of America
by Integrated Books International

CONTENTS

PART II: INCREASING F(R)ICTION

PART III: INFLECTION POINT

PART IV: ENDGAMES

PART V: POST-MORTEM

PART VI: POSTSCRIPT I

PART VII: POSTSCRIPT II

PART VIII: CODA

ACKNOWLEDGMENTS

First, I would like to thank my wife Monika for her love and support through difficult times and for waking me up to realities I was initially not inclined to acknowledge. I would also like to thank John Scott Legg at SteinerBooks for stepping into the breach and providing *Reset or Renaissance* a foothold in the world and standing behind its aim of seeking a new vision of what once was called the New World.

I owe Daniel Mackler, Neil Martinson, and Alexander Polikoff a debt of gratitude for their help in editing the book. I would also like to thank my father Alexander for his lifelong example of unselfish dedication to the commonweal, tireless service to the cause of justice and truth in the public sphere and keen analytic and legal acumen, some thread of which, I hope, remains woven into the fabric of *Two Roads.*

In a similar vein, I would like to thank the courageous and caring individuals—physicians, nurses, researchers, journalists, and many others—who stood (and still stand) for truth and integrity in the midst of a hurricane of contrary opinion.

Lastly, I would like to acknowledge the courage and sacrifice of all those who suffered through the dark night of the pandemic, especially those who have tragically lost love ones, borne the burden of job loss, or suffered the travail of personal injury to themselves or someone close to them. Many have persevered with a grace (and now continuing as before) and fortitude exemplary of the nobility of human being in times seemingly intent on crushing or burying that pearl of great price forever.

I will stand here for humanity, and though I would make it kind,
I would make it true.

—Ralph Waldo Emerson, *Self-Reliance*

The welfare of humanity is always the alibi of tyrants.

—Albert Camus, *Homage to an Exile*

PREFACE

In late summer of 2021, Covid dominated the headlines of newspapers across the globe. Fifteen months after its spectacular entrance onto the stage of world history, fear of the SARS-CoV-2 virus remained intense, palpable, and all-pervasive. The highly touted Covid-19 vaccines had only just been rolled out, and governments pushed policies of mass vaccination with religious zeal. To the political volatility already generated by lockdowns, social distancing, masking, and other elements of official Covid policy was now superadded the explosive issue (*beyond* controversy for some; the very *essence* of controversy for others) of the safety and efficacy of the new Operation Warp Speed-manufactured, EUA-sanctioned[1] mRNA vaccines.

For many, distribution of the Covid-19 vaccines augured the end of the worst of times. Countless persons had lost loved ones to Covid or (whether they knew it or not) to faulty treatment protocols. Countless others who had been spared that tragic fate nonetheless suffered the consequences of economically as well as psychologically devastating restrictions. No wonder the rollout of the Covid-19 vaccines, the newest and sexiest brainchild of the scientific genius that humankind had come to entrust with the holy mantle of Truth and sovereign Power, was met with all the enthusiasm displayed by crowds gathered along the road to Jerusalem to spread palms at the feet of a prophet some two thousand years ago.

Such glad emotion, however, did not characterize every person's Covid-19 vaccine story. In the aftermath of the rollout, many other individuals were about to confront what for them were entirely unprecedented forms of social condemnation and exclusion. Others, still less fortunate, were soon to be suffering debilitating physical affliction: injury unacknowledged and indeed flatly denied by the medical establishment as well as the public at large.

For these persons, those *worst of times* were just beginning.

I borrow that phrase, of course, from Charles Dickens. In the first paragraph of his *A Tale of Two Cities,* a novel set at the onset of the French Revolution, the author employs it in provocative conjunction with its opposite:

> It was the best of times, it was the worst of times, it was the age of wisdom, it was the age of foolishness, it was the epoch of belief, it was the epoch

of incredulity, it was the season of Light, it was the season of Darkness, it was the spring of hope, it was the winter of despair.[2]

It is easy to understand why the Covid moment in history might be viewed as the worst of times. It may be more challenging to imagine a good reason why it might also be viewed as the best of times, or at least the prelude or dawn of such, "the spring of hope" in Dickens' apt phrase. A very few rich persons, including Big Tech and Big Pharma moguls, might well regard it in that light insofar as their already unfathomable net worth multiplied fantastically as life went off-site and online and governments poured unheard-of amounts of money into vaccine development and distribution.

That, however, is *not* the sort of reasoning I have in mind.

I am concerned here not with the financial munificence of a few but with the common fortune of the many; assets counted not in bytes and billions but in dollars and cents and, more important, the priceless rights and freedoms that comprise the treasured inheritance of the modern human being and the spiritual estate of every man and woman. It is with regard to the struggle to preserve—and ever more solidly to secure—the fundamental liberties that constitute the dignity of persons and the foundation of democratic society, that we may look to the still unfolding Covid moment as cause for seeing great good as well as enormous evil; increasing light as well as advancing darkness; the real possibility of a new birth or renaissance—a spring of hope and wisdom in the world—even as the dark powers of winter threaten to draw a curtain of ignorance and illusion over the face of the earth, spread wide a blizzard of despair, and blind all vision of truth and grace.

I wish to be clear, from the first, as to my own allegiances as I pursue these urgent, Covid-prompted questions of good and evil, science and politics, truth and its undoing. I do not write as a Democrat or a Republican, except insofar as I do honor the original idea signified by each of those terms. I write as no attaché of any political party but as an independent, self-reliant American and world citizen, a partisan committed to the cause of Truth, Justice, and Mercy.

In consonance with that commitment, this book represents a fit mutation of one I had already begun to write in the first months of 2021, an opus on the philosophy of Ralph Waldo Emerson. I thus stand and write on the platform of Emerson's "American Scholar."

Readers may be surprised to hear the name of Emerson featured in a volume addressing our contemporary Covid World, even if the title of the larger literary project it initiates bears the signature of the movement spearheaded by the Sage of Concord and generally known as *The American Renaissance.* Yet the very incongruity of the notion that a cultural movement inaugurated almost two hundred years ago might make a critical contribution to the public debate stirred by Covid controversies bequeaths the opus as a whole its title: *Reset or Renaissance.*

That title poses a question that doubles as a kind of challenge—one that can, like gauntlets thrown down in earlier times, lead to a fatal denouement. Nor should there be any question about the stakes involved in the larger discussion pursued in these pages. We are dealing here not only with life and death issues of public health but with questions pertaining to the constitution of our humanity and our kind's appointed destiny. Those who know anything of Emerson will recognize that such larger-than-life matters are integral to his philosophy. Emerson, visionary that he was, strove always to fathom the big picture—to see not only the innumerable small reasons that might lead from one fact to another but the "grand and immovable"[3] reasons that underlie and set the course of history.

It is the premise of this book that we find ourselves today in the midst of a conflict raging not only over the soul of the nation usually called America but over the fate of the free world. Whether conscious of the fact or not, people find themselves involved in a pitched battle between the disciples of enlightenment and those of might. By the former I mean forces conducive to the maturation of the true genius of humankind and thus progress toward wiser and more compassionate governance of the world; by the latter, I refer to those forces that deny any objective reality to the True, the Good, and the Beautiful, preferring to worship at the altar of technological mastery and an all-too-human Will to Power.

For it is not only Emerson and his American Renaissance compatriots that endeavor to give shape to future history but also many less salutary forces at work in the world today—global forces that likewise endorse a program for tomorrow and promote a vision of a transhumanist future under the aegis of what has been called (by proponents and foes alike) *The Great Reset.* If you have not heard that term or are only vaguely aware of all that it implies, you are sitting on the sidelines of history and relegating yourself to the part of a pawn in a contest of kings and queens.

Read on, then, so as to promote your own knowledge and agency. This first volume, *Two Roads: An American Scholar's Covid Chronicle*, sets the historic scene by way of a real-time chronicle of events unfolding during the heated core of the Covid pandemic: the latter half of 2021, shortly after the rollout of the Covid vaccines. *Two Roads* is no dull factual affair but an impassioned critical engagement, distinctly literary in style, with the riptide of history. Combining documentary poetics with rigorous analysis of the flood of Covid (mis?) information, *Two Roads* records one American citizen's concerted attempt to make intellectual and moral sense of a tumultuous time that shook the foundations of the world.

To enhance its currency, *Two Roads* includes two substantial postscripts. The first brings its critical review of Covid-related affairs up to date as of late August, 2023. The second analyses the intellectual and moral ground of the vaccine-centric posture that counts as a key feature of the ideology underlying official Covid policy. In so doing, it aims to translate knowledge of the past into a vision of the future guided by truth rather illusion, perspicacity rather than prejudice and conscience rather than calumny.

In the course of writing *Two Roads*, the inexorable Covid tide eventually pulled the author into deeper consideration of the *historic* sources of the ethical and political conflicts ignited by the pandemic. Volume 2, *Covid and the Apocalypse of the Modern Mind,* interrogates ideological currents that flow from deeper fathoms of intellectual history, currents now crystallized into forms of social and political power that threaten democracy in America. After laying some factual groundwork, *Apocalypse* interprets the *mindset* underlying the Great Reset agenda in light of the critical theory expounded in Adorno and Horkheimer's *The Dialectic of Enlightenment*[4] and Patrick Deneen's *Why Liberalism Failed.*[5] That analysis soon widens into a broader investigation of the foundations—spiritual, intellectual, and political—of liberalism and indeed modernity itself.

Complementing inquiry into the destructive lines of force inherent in the machinery of modernity, I aim, with equal urgency, to recover the constructive forces at work in the liberal impulses birthed in the revolutionary era. *The Apocalypse of the Modern Mind* thus strives to identify and elucidate *the dual legacy of the Enlightenment:* the genuine spiritual radiance that shines forth in the *Age of Reason* and the dark shadows cast by its brilliance. The book revolves around the riddle posed by that duplicity; endeavors to understand how the *same* historic movement responsible for many of the ideas that founded modern liberal democracy (including our operative notion of "liberty" itself) simultaneously prepares the ground for the technocratic (proto-)totalitarianism that features as the dark underside of Covid World.

It is just this task of critical discernment that Covid World prompts by exposing, in the glare of day, the deep fissures unsettling the foundations of the free world. As its title implies, *Two Roads* suggests that we find ourselves today at an historic juncture with a fateful choice to make—one that will determine whether America (and indeed humanity at large) will proceed further down the path of subjection to autocratic forms of technocratic rule or, alternatively, will find within itself sources of liberating intellectual, spiritual, and political renewal. It is the argument of this project that choice of the latter course necessarily entails rediscovery and reclamation of the seminal ideas inherent in not only the founding of the nation but animating, too, the movement of cultural and intellectual independence inspired by Ralph Waldo Emerson.

At the time of the writing of this preface, I have almost finished the first two volumes of *Reset or Renaissance.* These suffice to initiate a philosophically grounded critique of the ideology underwriting Covid World technocracy and some of the principal measures representing its practical implementation. Anyone who reads the present volume will come to know, in no uncertain terms, where this author stands on issues such as technologically enabled state control of media and mandatory vaccination and—against the background of the principles informing the founding of this country—*why* he stands there.

In order, however, to achieve real understanding of the root causes of the ideological fault lines fragmenting America today, I found it necessary to dive still deeper into intellectual history. Thus the impetus to plumb the depths of the ancient origins of the religious and scientific worldviews that continue to condition every aspect of thought and culture today (including those forms of contemporary "liberal" thought that ostensibly repudiate the canon of Western civilization). Accordingly, *Reset or Renaissance* will eventually include a third volume investigating signal aspects of ancient Hebrew, Greek, and Christian culture. Inspired by Robert Bellah's analysis of the axial age in his magisterial *Religion in Human Evolution,*[6] my treatment focuses on the crucial and ever-changing patterns of relationship between religious or spiritual and political power.

Such groundwork not only aids understanding of matters central to pressing contemporary concerns (the evolving relations, for instance, between science, church, and state), but it coincidently constitutes critical preparation for any coherent revisioning of Emersonian transcendentalism and the American Renaissance. After the third volume has been completed, *Reset or Renaissance* will conclude with a volume (or volumes) transmitting the author's attempt at just such revisioning: a systematic exposition of the (yet unspoken) philosophy and religion announced in *Nature* and underwriting Emerson's seminal texts. If even partially successful, that effort may shed new light on many of the fundamental issues challenging America and the world community today and assist all persons of good will—whether of liberal or conservative bent—better to respond to the spirit of the times that is the agent of true change in the self as well as in society.

The attainment of that end, however, is hardly guaranteed, lying, as it does, far down one of two roads open to the soul of humankind.

Let me conclude with a last word regarding the office of the American Scholar. Emerson, if he stands for anything, stands *against* modes of thinking and doing that speciously divide material from spiritual concerns, severing science, technology, and politics from history, philosophy, literature, religion, and ethics. In Emerson's book, it cannot be any special immunological expertise that will crack the Covid code, no new vaccine or other biotechnological invention, but rather minds able and willing to attempt to comprehend the whole historic complex of human concern of which Covid is but sign and symptom. "The true," declared Hegel, "is the whole," and that whole is, *à la* Emerson, the province not of the specialist or health expert but of the scholar, who takes the body, soul, and spirit of the human being as his first and last subject.

As World Economic Forum founder Klaus Schwab declares in his book *Covid-19: The Great Reset*,[7] the Covid crisis provides occasion for reexamination and conscious transfiguration of our very idea of the nature of humanity. This opus is my attempt to get a word in edgewise on that matter and to do all I possibly can to tip the balance of history toward the best rather than the worst of times.

A Note on the Genesis of the Text

Two Roads is a book I never intended to write. In late June 2021, I had just completed the first chapter of a long-in-the-making opus on Emerson, when, fearful of losing my job teaching literature and psychology at Pacifica Graduate Institute near Santa Barbara, California, I began a letter to the Institute's president, hoping to discourage him from imposing vaccine mandates at Pacifica.

The rest, as they say, is history.

Once I began committing my view of what I call Covid World to paper, I—like some poor sorcerer's apprentice—possessed little power to stem the flood that followed. Over the course of the next seven weeks, that initial letter morphed into writing that covered the essential bases of Covid World as I saw—and still see—it: pandemonium, fear, and suffering; lockdowns, social distancing, and masking; the dream of a saving vaccine and the no-holds-barred drive to realize it; the politicization and consequent compromise of science; the medical anomaly of the (mis)treatment of Covid-19 in both inpatient and outpatient settings; the outsized influence of pharmaceutical companies and the regulatory capture of government agency; the polarization of debate and the suppression of dissent under the aegis of misinformation and conspiracy theory; the plight of the vaccine-injured; and more—the whole gamut of critical concerns ignited by the pandemic. That is the purview of what ultimately became part one ("The Opening Setup") of the present volume.

My desire to draw a line in the sand and get back to other involvements (that original Emerson book!) notwithstanding, the current of Covid affairs continued to sweep me up in the floodtide of contemporary occasion. I continued both to document and critically analyze current Covid affairs up until Thanksgiving of 2021, when the tsunami of news that broke over the globe in the wake of Omicron's emergence swamped that enterprise. By that time, however, my explorations had brought me to the verge of a preliminary *theoretical* understanding of Covid World. Adorno and Horkheimer's *Dialectic of Enlightenment*—a classic of critical theory—provided a key to my evolving conceptualization of the Covid moment. Written in response to the political situation in the authors' native Germany before and during World War II (which forced them both to emigrate), *Dialectic of Enlightenment* furnishes a critical framework that can help facilitate understanding of crucial dynamics underlying Covid World in America and indeed across much of the globe.

The section titled "The Great Reset and the Dialectic of Enlightenment," was *supposed* to be the climax of what had rapidly grown into a full-length book.[8] Instead, as my inquiry into the *ideological* roots of Covid World continued to expand, it ended up serving as the beginning of a second volume. Both *Two Roads* and the forthcoming *Apocalypse* take as their premise the belief that Covid is by no means a local or circumscribed affair, just little more than the outbreak of a viral illness that disturbed the ground of the world for a while but will ultimately prove a mere wrinkle in time.

If you are one of those persons who consciously recognize the world-transformative force of Covid (by which I mean the potent effect of ideological and sociopolitical dynamics *already at work before* Covid; spectacularly *intensifying* and *manifesting* with Covid, and *continuing to operate powerfully* in our nominally "post-Covid" present), then this book will, I hope, help you understand the profound undercurrents pulling, with unsuspected power, at the kicking legs of our human race. If, on the other hand, you are one of those who acknowledge that Covid transformed the world for a while but—now that the worst is over—represents an episode that can and should largely be left behind, I hope this book will convince you otherwise. Indeed, I hope it will persuade you that *any morally committed reckoning with the practical and spiritual forces at work in the world today*, and so *any viable vision of our human future*, can—perhaps *must*—begin with an in-depth understanding of the historic significance of the Covid moment.

Building upon the narrative ground provided by *Two Roads, Covid and the Apocalypse of the Modern Mind* continues to stretch my understanding of current affairs both backward and forward in time: *back* toward the early modern origins of our STEM-dominated contemporary culture and *forward* toward alternative visions of the kind of future we, by virtue of our collective response to the Covid moment, may freely choose to welcome—or resist.

Volume I

TWO ROADS

AN AMERICAN SCHOLAR'S COVID CHRONICLE

INTRODUCTION

Note: Written toward the end of 2022 when the pandemic was still of urgent concern, this introduction employs the present tense in some contexts the current reader may imagine past.

Anyone venturing to write anything involving Covid confronts head-on the issue of audience. While no writer can lift a finger without some notion of intended readership, the temperature surrounding this topic remains so high that one can hardly approach it without risk of fever. Even now, more than two-and-a-half years after the initial Covid-19 outbreak in the spring of 2020, it is difficult to say much of real consequence without eliciting summary, often angry, dismissal from one side or the other. "Polarization" commonly describes America's political landscape today and the hurdle to be cleared in order to communicate across the aisle of ideological allegiance is historically high, so much so that an author aspiring to that end had perhaps better exchange his pen for a pole vault.

That said, the sociopolitical tension associated with the pandemic noticeably diminished in the course of 2022. In the long, uneven wake of Omicron's unstoppable yet relatively mild-mannered spread, hospitalizations and deaths have dropped, precipitating a like dive in the prevailing level of fear. Indeed, the air has cleared so much that the Covid commentator wishing to take stock of the lay of the land can identify three classes of persons comprising his prospective audience. Recognition of the general profile of each can perhaps help prepare both myself, as writer, and you, as reader, to better comprehend where we stand vis-à-vis one another.

I am not a believer in the officially authorized account of Covid World, which I like to call "the controlling narrative." Most everyone is familiar with the main lines of this story, even if that story (and how we are supposed to understand it) keeps changing. The story goes more or less as follows: Covid presents a clear and present danger to everyone's health (children and healthy young persons not excepted); measures to minimize contact with both the virus and each other (lockdowns, social distancing, masking, hand-sanitizing) are appropriate and constructive means of risk mitigation; and the Covid vaccines are safe and effective and represent the surest—indeed, the indispensable—means of combatting the disease, especially as few if any other safe and effective measures are available.

Not long ago, one could still confidently designate this official orthodoxy as the mainstream account of Covid. Over the course of the last year or so, however, its hold on the popular imagination has weakened and indeed, in the mind of many persons, broken down altogether. In the wake of vaccines (or, more properly titled, gene therapies), the deficiency of which is increasingly evident to citizens and scientists alike, public confessions of flawed performance by high-ranking officials, and the general amelioration of the severity of the disease, fewer individuals remain willing to credit the notion that the health experts setting official Covid policy know what they are doing at least as well as anyone else and certainly far better than the irresponsible actors disseminating "misinformation." Correlatively, questions arise as to whether these officials are, as a rule, discharging their responsibilities with due caution, with an acceptable degree of transparency, and in good faith. "In good faith" here means: with public health and welfare foremost in mind and thus in a manner *not* unduly influenced by corporate and other special interests.

"Fewer" persons, to be sure; nonetheless, those still ready and willing to go along with the controlling narrative continue to comprise a large class of persons, including the lion's share of medical professionals. This group that *respects, defends, and willingly enacts* official Covid policy constitutes my *first* class of readers. If you yourself fall into this category, let me express, first, my real gratitude that you have, one way or another, found your way to this page; second, my fervent hope that you will continue reading and so allow me to share with you my perspective on Covid World; and, third, that I regard the opportunity to do so as a privilege, one that I sincerely hope nothing said here will in any way abuse.

Given the way the politics of Covid have evolved in this country, most of the persons that fall into this first class are of a generally liberal persuasion. In and of itself, that fact strikes me as a profound—and profoundly disturbing—paradox. As one who himself identifies as liberally minded, and so a child of the Enlightenment, I confess that it was my own keen sense of personal and political betrayal that ignited the writing of this book. What is the ground of that betrayal?

I consider official Covid policy as *antithetical* to any enlightened regard for fact and reason, the tenets of classical liberalism, and compassionate regard for the other. In short, I regard that policy and the means of its execution as violative of the spiritual as well as political foundations of democratic society.

Why and how I believe this to be the case constitutes the real subject of this book. A tracing of multiple paths that have led to that conclusion comprise its content. Documentation and elaboration of my perspective—presentation of the relevant facts, reasoning, and (most importantly) *human stories*—defines its rather unorthodox form. Generically speaking, the latter may roughly be described as a hybrid of historical chronicle, journalistic exposé, personal essay, and philosophical investigation.

For my first class of readers, much of the information conveyed in this book may be both startling and disturbing. That is largely because authorities have sought to systemically suppress or discredit all discourse that calls the official account of Covid World into question irrespective of the quality of the critique or the integrity of its source, and have pressed both legacy and social media outlets into service in that regard. Consequently, the stories one reads if one avails oneself only of mainstream sources can be characterized, at the very best, as one-sided. I therefore hope that a reading of this book will go some ways toward providing my first class of readers a more multidimensional view of the whole Covid World picture.

The book includes an implicit defense of the credibility of the sources it cites by calling attention to the ulterior motives inscribed in the system of power that aims to delegitimize if not destroy these sources, as well as the integrated array of mechanisms by which that end is pursued. To deny the clear evidence of these forces invites ignorance of critical dysfunctions afflicting democracy in America today. That is a blindness to which I myself have been all too prone. *Two Roads* records, step by step, chapter by chapter, my own personal discovery of the frightening fact that in many respects directly affecting the very ground of my individual existence, the sociopolitical world in which I live bears little resemblance to the America I thought I knew. Indeed, the vortex of power that emerges in these pages does not begin or end at America's borders but represents both a global and globalist reality. The reader will find more on the technocratic agenda associated with the so-called *Great Reset* in volume 2, including the sociopolitical profile of its machinery as well as discussion of both the reach and limits of its formidable power.

My *second* class of reader stands opposite the first. This class comprises what may be called the Covid-dissident community. Most persons in this group long ago discovered a kind of alternative universe as far as Covid is concerned—a whole host of reasons why the official Covid narrative calls not for willing acceptance and ready compliance but for ongoing scrutiny and conscientious critique. These "second class" citizens have, perforce, availed themselves of sources of information marginalized and often censored by the mainstream. As a rule (to which there are, of course, notable exceptions), they trust not in any official stamp of approval or nominally "expert" opinion but in their own evaluation of evidence, naturally taking into account the quality of relevant information as well as the ethical and intellectual integrity of those providing it.

This class of reader will find much that is objectively familiar in *Two Roads*. Even so, I trust this reader will nonetheless profit from reading the first as well as the second volume of this opus, because (despite the familiarity of any number of the facts cited or points made) my rendering of the *other* side of the *whole integrated complex of concerns comprising the Covid saga* is original both in its style and in its analyses of crucial features of the official Covid response (see, for instance, the chapters "Losing Strategy" and "Biodynamics versus Vaccine-Distance" in Part IV). Those analyses, moreover, remain vitally pertinent to questions of how to think about future pandemics or public health crises from a sociopolitical as well as scientific point of view. *Two Roads* thus has much to say about the lessons taught by Covid-19, not only with respect to how humanity might best respond to one or another virus but—more pointedly—how an alert and educated public may critically prepare itself to regard the *framing of* and *planning for* future health emergencies on the part of national and international health experts.

That leaves my *third* class of reader. This class, in betwixt and between the other two, consists of persons who harbor real questions about the whole Covid matter but have not executed the dive into the alternative universe of Covid concern performed by the second class. For these readers, I hope this book will provide not only a new, more comprehensive view of Covid World but an entrance into a realm of independent thinking that engages many of the powerful crosscurrents beating on the shore of human society today.

Let me share a word, too, as to the temporal scope of *Two Roads: An American Scholar's Covid Chronicle*. The bulk of the book (the whole, minus the Postscripts) was written in the second half of 2021. A great deal of water has flowed under the bridge since that time, and some readers might reasonably question the pertinence of information and arguments based upon an earlier stage of the pandemic. While it is true that certain analyses undertaken in the body of the book no longer represent the latest word on a given topic or controversy, most all remain, in their own right, nonetheless relevant and valid, and almost without exception stake out positions confirmed rather than contradicted by subsequent developments in science and society.

The substantial Postscripts verify and amplify that claim, albeit in different ways. Postscript I ("Covid World, August 2023") updates the reader on many of the major developments on crucial Covid fronts (the origin of the virus; treatment options; vaccine efficacy and safety; censorship and free speech concerns, and more) that have unfolded over the course of 2022 and 2023. The title of Postscript II ("The Kennedy Candidacy and the Anatomy of Pro-Vax Prejudice") aptly describes the gist of that more forward-looking critical contribution. In many respects, both these Postscripts (written, respectively, in August and November, 2023) confront a sociopolitical landscape dramatically different from that characterizing the latter half of 2021. In a surprising number of other respects, however, little if anything essential has changed, and patterns and policies put in place in 2021 remain not only intact but also solidified and entrenched. The two Postscripts consequently furnish—not only a historical update—but, too, a concluding argument that sums and distills the critical agency of the whole text.

Let me, though, add one further comment on the persistent relevance of the main (pre-postscripts) text of *Two Roads*.

I began writing the book at a particularly pivotal moment in Covid history—a time when the initial results of the Covid-19 vaccine rollout were first beginning to register and the associated debate was heating up. Consequently, *all* the most important Covid issues were on the table at that time. That includes questions dating back to the earlier stages of the pandemic, such as the level of mortality risk posed by Covid, the accuracy of PCR tests, and the more general issue of the manipulation of data and the integrity of Covid-related science, the efficacy of lockdowns, masking, and social distancing, and the safety and efficacy of various treatment methods (including hydroxychloroquine [HCQ] and ivermectin). The misinformation and disinformation debate (along with its associated freedom of speech and censorship issues) was also very much on the table. Nor could one neglect the issue of the corruption of federal regulatory agencies—including the CDC, NIH, and FDA—on account of undue corporate/pharmaceutical company influence, and also the sway of international organizations (such as the WHO and WEF) over national and local policy. On top of all of the above, the whole host of vaccine-related questions (the safety and efficacy of the vaccines, the quality of their testing, the adequacy of regulatory oversight and safety monitoring, the legitimacy of their Emergency Use Authorization (EUA), the propriety of mandates, and the character of the financial contracts between government and pharmaceutical companies) began to swirl around and sting the American body politic like a disturbed nest of hornets. *Two Roads* was thus written at a time when it was possible to address all of these issues as well as to assess, in the eye of the storm, how the Covid-19 vaccines figured into the scientific and social dilemmas that preoccupied the country and the world.

Few if any of the aforementioned issues are wholly outdated, especially in their more general import. On the contrary, the dawn of Covid World helped bring to consciousness multiple profound concerns (such as the way the enmeshment of science and politics can drastically corrupt both; the problems inherent in the centralization and bureaucratization of healthcare and indeed government in general; the use and abuse of emergency declarations and the meaning of freedom of speech in a digital age purportedly threatened by misinformation) that Americans must confront head-on if we are to preserve any semblance of a functioning democracy. That is an urgent task for the present and foreseeable future. *It also is one that cannot be intelligently pursued without a clear-sighted and in-depth understanding of the recent as well as more distant past.*

As the book's Postscripts detail, heated controversy continues to characterize debate on many fronts. Our government has pushed ahead with its vaccine agenda, giving the go-ahead for Covid vaccines to be placed on the childhood schedule even as many states pass laws prohibiting schools from mandating the vaccine. An unprecedented number of athletes, and professionals, as well as amateurs, continue to collapse on the field, and whether or not they may be victims of vaccine-induced myocarditis compels significant public attention. Legal battles proliferate on multiple fronts, from fired workers of all stripes seeking reinstatement and restitution to the attorneys general of Missouri and Alabama challenging, in court, the federal government's pressuring of social media companies to censor disfavored Covid content in the name of "misinformation." Various forces are conspiring to award the WHO unchecked power to declare and coordinate the response to any new pandemic, overriding national sovereignty in the process. Robert F. Kennedy Jr.'s stance on Covid in particular and vaccines in general remains a matter of intense controversy, and—especially in light of his presidential candidacy—continues to magnetize the debate. The list of momentous Covid-related matters seems endless.

All these instances of concrete controversy feature as nodes of a much larger saga, an ideological conflict that encompasses them all. As the historic drama continues to unfold, I hope this book can help readers gain a broader and deeper understanding of the scientific, sociopolitical, and spiritual dimensions of the Covid moment, one that I have no doubt will long be regarded—for better or for worse—as a watershed in time.

PART I

THE OPENING SETUP

Chapter 1

MARCH SNOW STORM

When Covid-19 first burst upon the world, the novel disease inspired boundless dread in the hearts and minds of millions. Little was known as to how contagious or lethal the SARS-CoV-2 virus might be. Despite an initial stutter, most responsible authorities across the globe soon pushed the panic button. People were encouraged to fear the worst and to act accordingly.

In early March, 2020, campus officials at the University of Colorado at Boulder, where our son was finishing his freshman year, issued reassurances that—Covid notwithstanding—campus life would (for the time being, at least) proceed normally. Less than a week later, our son was driving through a snow storm in the Sierrras on his way home. University officials had changed their tune, and campus had been closed—and emptied—virtually overnight.

In retrospect, that level of alarm may well be regarded as disproportionate. While Covid has in fact materialized as a plague that continues to cost far too many lives, it need be acknowledged that—soon after the advent of Covid-19—responsible researchers recognized that its fatal or debilitating effect was largely concentrated in certain high-risk demographics. Much of the population (children and youth, and indeed all persons not suffering from preexisting health problems) display strong resilience in the face of the disease, and fatality rates among this sector of the human community remain extremely low.

Many knowledgeable persons consequently question the appropriateness of measures—such as wholesale lockdowns—that do not differentiate between high- and low-risk individuals, thus denying everyone access both to the outdoors and to the social intercourse so necessary for physical and mental health. Critical review of such policies, however, remains marginalized by a mainstream narrative wed to a narrow, fear-driven frame of mind aggressively resistant to any questioning of official decision-making.

Yet anyone who imagines that the salient Covid facts have been made transparently clear need to look and think again. On the front page of the *San Francisco Chronicle,* you will find case and death counts reported daily, but those big, bold numbers hide a wilderness of ambiguity. I will not here go into all the questions surrounding the notorious unreliability of tests (such as the

PCR) that were not even originally designed for diagnosis; dubious statistical methods and models; or changes in death certificate protocol (instituted, rather enigmatically, shortly before the onset of Covid-19) that most likely mean that Covid-19 played a negligible role in countless deaths nonetheless officially attributed to it.

Covid politics are deeply shaped by perception of the degree of mortal danger—the sense, felt in the gut, of existential threat any given individual faces. Consequently, careful review as to what really has been and is going on should neither be taboo nor a matter of political partisanship. On the contrary, the task of separating Covid fact from Covid fiction should be a society-wide endeavor led—though not dictated—by *impartial* science and marked by openness and objectivity.

Many persons, however, resist the critical drift of such ruminations. Pointing to the evident tragedy of countless of lives lost, such individuals maintain that quibbling about details is naught but dangerous obfuscation, imagining that *no* degree of caution should be considered excessive in the face of the deadly, invisible adversary capable of striking down anyone at any time. The evident truth remains (so such thinking goes) that our best and indeed only saving course continues to be to remain cognizant that—no matter how young or old, fit or unfit, one may be—the touch or breath of another human being may sign your death warrant. This has been and will be the case until we are saved from this predicament by our own, and everybody else's, successful vaccination.

In California, this kind of full-court press has been constantly on from the get-go. Yet the superabundance of caution associated with it has cast its own tragic shadow, one not entirely unrecognized and yet never seeming to counterbalance the dread that continues to fuel the mainstream narrative. Kids out of school, economic deprivation and loss of livelihood, social isolation, marked increases in mental health crises, suicides and homicides: occasionally we see some numbers pertaining to these dark matters (which disproportionately affect less affluent communities without the economic and technological resources available to others), but they remain largely overshadowed by the specter of death that looms like a giant scarecrow over the Covid-darkened landscape. Anybody, moreover, who dares seriously question the *core* of the calculus written into the mainstream narrative—the idea that mass vaccination represents the solution to the Covid problem—risks, to this day, serious reprisal.

Once the Covid vaccines became available for general use in spring 2021, most American citizens were anxious to get with the program. A significant minority, however, were not. Initially, no one had spoken of *compelling* cooperation by means of mandates. That, however, soon changed.

Like CU Boulder and other institutions of higher learning, Pacifica Graduate Institute closed its campus in March 2020. In June, I received a letter from the president of Pacifica intimating that—when campus reopened at some as yet uncertain date in the future—the Institute might well institute a mandate requiring vaccination of all staff and students who wished to set foot on campus.

As one of those persons who harbored grave doubts as to the safety and efficacy of the vaccine, I naturally saw gathering storm clouds threatening my future at Pacifica. Given the Covid climate in California, I knew the odds were stacked against me. Rather than passively awaiting my fate, I opted for a more proactive course, a sort of preemptive epistolary strike.

Here, for the record, is the long beginning of that letter:

June 29, 2021

Dear President Cambray:

I write in response to your June 25th update regarding campus reopening. I am disappointed that Pacifica education will remain exclusively online for the fall 2021 quarter, and while I look forward to resuming in-person instruction in the first (winter) quarter of 2022, I must take particular note of Pacifica's strong encouragement that all community members vaccinate, and, still more, your letter's covert indication that Pacifica might consider mandating vaccination for its staff and students upon the full—rather than emergency—FDA authorization of Covid vaccines. As a professor who deeply values the opportunity to be a part of Pacifica's unique educational mission, I write to strongly discourage Pacifica Graduate Institute from taking such a step, one that seems to me contrary to the very foundation of that mission. Please allow me to describe, in some detail, why I believe this to be so, as the matter is of great consequence, not only for myself personally but for the wider Pacifica community.

As poets, mythographers, and depth psychologicists, we should find it insufficient—indeed, even a dereliction of duty—to begin and end with what seems to many the self-evident truth: namely, that Covid represents a serious threat to our collective welfare, and that all socially conscientious persons should consent, without delay, to the "safe and effective" vaccines finally available to us. The corollary of this popular opinion is the reverse side of the same coin: if one does not wish so to consent, one must be an irrational, uncaring creature, an immoral Covidiot deserving vilification and exile—the kind of punishment reserved for criminals and social code breakers in humanity's tribal past.

Does not history teach, again and again, that notions which many regard as incontrovertible truths (the superiority, for instance, of a given race, class, or gender) all too often function as the taproot of evil?

So it is, I am afraid, with the plague of Covid-19 and the vaccines that most see as our principal means of deliverance. I do not impute wrong to the choice to undergo vaccination on the part of individual persons, but rather to the whole supposedly authoritative Covid narrative (one in which those vaccines play a leading role) and the belief that it is reprehensible even to *question* that narrative, so that those who do so are deemed worthy of scorn and social retribution. Down that intolerant road—the road more and more traveled by—lies the erosion of the intellectual and spiritual freedom essential to science, democratic society, and indeed the vibrant life of soul itself.

What is that narrative, the story of Covid-19 as told to us by government officials, health experts, and approved media outlets? All are familiar with it. Covid-19 is a viral disease that originated zoonotically (passing from an animal to human population) in or near Wuhan, China in 2019 and quickly spread by way of infectious contagion to the better part of the world, including the United States. Because it is a potentially debilitating disease capable of rapidly inflicting unimaginable harm, drastic and indeed unprecedented measures—lockdowns, masking, and social distancing—were (and still, in certain places, are) justified and indeed necessary to limit its spread. Meanwhile, on the medical front, as no effective treatments were or are at hand, suffering humanity has had no recourse but to await the development of lifesaving vaccines. Now that heroic scientific effort has made such available, and these have proved safe and effective, it is incumbent upon all right-minded persons to vaccinate and so do their part to end Covid-19's reign of terror and cast off the shadow of death and fear that have too long darkened the world.

While most persons accept this narrative, most every aspect of it can and has been questioned, including the precise nature of the disease itself, the mode of its origination, the actual prevalence of the disease and number of fatalities attributable to it, the necessity and efficacy of given preventative measures, the availability (or lack thereof) of effective treatment protocols, and the safety and efficacy of the vaccines. Unfortunately, in the run-up to the 2020 election, virtually *all* questions related to Covid became embroiled in the feverish political temper of the times, and turned into fodder for intense political partisanship. The associated polarization remains very much in effect, and continues to charge the atmosphere in a manner that makes clear, objective inquiry into key issues difficult, if not impossible. From a depth psychological perspective, this fact alone should alert the analytic mind to the presence of volatile affective and ideological complexes that should not pass without critical examination. While I can hardly review the entire field of Covid concern, I do wish to identify a number of salient matters which I, as a concerned citizen, have standing to address, and which I hold deeply relevant to the pressing matter at hand: whether or not Pacifica, or indeed *any* institution or organization, should mandate vaccination.

Let me state from the outset that I am not here in the business of contending that Covid is a hoax, or denying that the illness associated with it has exacted a real toll here at home and abroad. At the same time, summarily discrediting, or proscribing, any and all questioning of the controlling narrative as "conspiracy theory" or the peddling of "misinformation or dis-information" represents a dangerously negligent answer to many pressing questions; an uncritical blanket response that surrenders rather than upholds individual responsibility and conscientious citizenry. My own chief concerns may be enumerated as follows:

1. Key elements of the mainstream narrative are open to serious question, and consideration of these questions demand not merely blind obeisance to select authorities and their presentation of the "facts" of the case, but open, impartial, and robust inquiry and debate in both scientific and lay communities.

2. In point of fact, however, the framing of the narrative as a whole has been, if not indeed *designed*, powerfully and continuously *shaped* by vested interests acting on their own behalf rather than that of public health and welfare.

3. The upholding of the controlling narrative, has—on account of both the intense fear and political partisanship associated with it—entailed a brutal suppression of freedom of speech and expression in the private as well as public and professional sectors. With respect to the latter, this censorship has by no means been limited to repudiation of inexpert ideas or opinions, but has been systematically directed—often with violent effect—upon highly credentialed and conscientious persons and organizations.

4. This point is a reprise of my first (a questioning of the facts and logic informing the prevailing Covid narrative) but here focused sharply upon the centerpiece of that narrative: the safety and efficacy of the novel mRNA technology characteristic of the leading Covid-19 vaccines.

5. The final point recapitulates and expands upon the third: that the controlling narrative often leads to moral and political conclusions that ignore or cavalierly override individual rights and freedoms in a manner incommensurate with the premises of democratic society.

Let me address these points in turn, not now numbered but descriptively subtitled…

~

Thus began my missive to Pacifica. Although its contents quickly grew beyond the limits of anything I could reasonably send, its drafting ended up serving another notable purpose: initiating the writing of this, my *Covid Chronicle.*

Chapter 2

SETTING THE SCENE FOR COVID-19: EARLY (NON-)TREATMENT

In reviewing those features of the mainstream narrative open to serious question, one stands out above all others. It does so both on account of its preeminent practical importance and the particularly dubious character of the official stance on the matter. Indeed, I believe it fair to regard at least one major element of the controlling Covid narrative as not only questionable but—according to the most highly credentialed scientific authority—demonstrably false.

From the first, a puzzling anomaly has characterized the approved response to Covid-19. Measures to prevent spread and the race to mass vaccination have been emphasized, but exploration of prophylaxis and early treatment of disease symptoms—treatment administered upon the first appearances of symptoms, and so typically preceding, by up to two weeks, any necessary hospitalization—has not only been downplayed but positively discouraged. We therefore witness the strange phenomenon of health professionals declining to attend to symptomatic persons and so forfeiting the opportunity to fend off a worsening of the disease. Indeed, if ailing persons do show up at their doctor's office or hospital, most are sent away to await, more or less helplessly, the dire consequences that too often follow such inaction.

This situation would be rationally explicable only if there were in fact no safe and effective treatments available. That indeed has been the position promulgated by reigning health experts and counts as a key element of the controlling Covid narrative. That narrative would have us believe not only that Covid is a devastating disease constantly posing a frighteningly high risk to everyone, but as well that, if you *do* contract Covid, nothing can really be done about it until (if you happen to be one of the unfortunate persons whose natural defenses prove insufficient) you end up in a hospital with a tube down your throat on the brink of death.

According to the testimony of extraordinarily qualified physicians in both the United States and Canada, this is simply not true.

Anyone interested in a window into Covid politics should watch the YouTube video of the United States Senate hearing on early outpatient treatment for Covid convened by Senator Ron Johnson on November 19, 2020.[9] At that session, three physicians presented convincing evidence, substantiated by peer-reviewed theoretical analysis, ample high quality empirical research data, and their own extensive firsthand, practical experience treating Covid patients that a mixture of several readily available and inexpensive substances provides a safe and very effective means of treating high-risk Covid patients within the first two weeks of contracting the disease.

As part of a helpful analysis of the larger Covid picture, one of the doctors (Dr. Peter McCullough from Baylor) displayed a chart outlining the four pillars of pandemic response. These are:

1) Contagion Control (Stop the Spread);
2) Early Home Treatment (Minimizing Hospitalization and Death);
3) Late Stage Treatment (In-hospital Safety Net for Survival);
4) Vaccination ("Herd Immunity").[10]

Dr. McCullough emphasized, with great urgency, that while the first and last pillars have commanded tremendous attention and resources, the second—early treatment—has been largely ignored, a gross omission that has too often led to an overwhelming of hospitals and to unnecessary casualties.

Dr. Harvey Risch, from the Yale School of Health and the Yale School of Medicine, elaborated upon this disturbing fact:

> We're now finally coming to address why, over the last six months, our government research institutions have invested billions of dollar in expensive patent medications and vaccination development, but almost nothing in early outpatient treatments, the first line of response to the pandemic. And it is not that we've lacked candidate medications to study; we've had a number of promising agents.[11]

It is not, moreover, that government agencies have merely neglected or overlooked early outpatient treatment options. Rather, the relevant agencies have taken extraordinary steps to discourage and indeed block research, development, and use of agents suitable for early outpatient care. The case of hydroxychloroquine (HCQ) is the most notorious instance. Although HCQ is and has been used prolifically throughout the world for decades, and is available over the counter in many countries, it has recently been mysteriously branded as unsafe by the FDA. At the same time, that agency has granted EUA to unproven and expensive drugs such as remdesivir, prompting Dr. Risch to accuse the agency of applying an "egregious double standard" in its regulatory work. As Dr. Risch notes:

> So now we've spent the last six months with formal government policies and warnings against outpatient treatment. The government has invested very large amounts in vaccines and expensive new treatments that have yet to be proven, while there has been almost no support for evaluating inexpensive but useful medications.[12]

Dr. Risch continues, "Every outpatient study of HCQ has shown benefit; there are no studies...that do not show benefits."

Dr. McCullough, for his part, laments what he deems the fundamentally *anti-scientific* attitude governing present policy on early outpatient treatment. He emphasizes that, with respect to *all* critical viral infections (including, for instance, HIV and shingles):

> The principle is always early (treatment). I can't think of a single viral infection when the best advice is to wait two weeks before we start treatment in the hospital. *That's the current NIH recommendation.* Americans are appalled by this.[13]

If Americans are so appalled, they are not moved enough to make much political noise about it. That noise, and all those government resources, seem reserved for promoting not the second but the fourth pillar of pandemic response.

I should interject here that the three doctor-advocates (McCullough, Risch, and a third I've not mentioned, Dr. George Fareed, who contributed his own eloquent testimony to the Senate) were not unopposed. Dr. Ashish Jha, the minority (Democratic) invitee, represented the party line, and his testimony included "evidence" of the inefficacy and dangerous character of HCQ as well as (ironically) his own complaints about political interference with science.

I invite everyone who imagines that most critical questioning of the mainstream narrative involves the sowing of "misinformation" to watch the exchanges between Dr. Jha, on the one hand, and Dr. Risch and McCullough, on the other, and to judge for themselves just who is really guilty of that crime. Dr. Risch effectively rebutted Dr. Jha's central allegations by pointing out that the studies to which the latter referred involved use of HCQ in an *inpatient, hospital setting*, a circumstance utterly irrelevant to its prescribed use as an early outpatient method of treatment. As determined by the degree of progression of the disease, the relevant medical conditions are entirely different in the two scenarios.

Speaking in rebuttal on a slightly different though related point (the poison indications that *supposedly* justified the novel FDA warning against use of HCQ, but, upon close expert examination, turned out to be spurious), Dr. McCullough commenced his own repudiation of Dr. Jha's, and the majority party's, disinformation campaign[14] by asserting that he considered Dr. Jha's testimony "reckless and dangerous to the nation."

Yet why, one is naturally inclined to ask, would the government and health authorities effectively block widespread implementation of the kind of "national plan" for early outpatient formulated, for instance, by Dr. Fareed, and which the latter sent to all relevant authorities, including Dr. Anthony Fauci?

After a career that included graduation from Harvard Medical School and research in virology involving a stint at Dr. Fauci's own National Institute for Allergic and Infectious Disease, Dr. George Fareed, wanting to "make a difference" in persons' lives, ultimately became a boots-on-the-ground Family Medical Specialist in California. Of all the physicians present at the hearing, Dr. Fareed could (in dramatic contrast to Dr. Jha) boast of the most extensive practical experience in actually treating Covid patients. According to Dr. Fareed's sworn testimony, appropriate treatment involves no untested formula but instead what he called a "viral cocktail," including several agents (HCQ and zinc among them), each of which performs distinct and complementary antiviral functions. Dr. Fareed administered that formula to thousands of patients in California with excellent results and *no* adverse effects, Dr. Fareed mentioned, too, that additional promising agents (ivermectin, for instance) might also be added to the arsenal of effective treatment substances pending further study.

Doctors Fareed, Risch, and McCullough all agreed, unequivocally, on the fundamental facts of the early outpatient treatment matter, and *all* clearly thought it the *urgent* obligation of the government to make safe and effective outpatient treatment *widely and readily available across the entire country,* an effort that—unlike the development of a vaccine or alternative exotic and unproven treatment methods (remdesivir or plasma replacement, for instance)—could *be easily, rapidly, and inexpensively accomplished* with appropriate support from relevant authorities and agencies.

A logical—albeit deeply objectionable—answer to the question as to why this has not been done is all too easy to formulate. 2020 electoral politics aside (although these undoubtedly played a huge role), powerful interests were and are *heavily* invested in the all-eggs-in-the-vaccine-basket scenario. Moreover, *Emergency Use Authorization of vaccines cannot be legally granted unless no alternative treatments are available.* Consequently, denying the availability of such treatment—then and now—functions as the prerequisite for any Covid-19 vaccination program. Legally, psychologically, and practically speaking, a robust "national plan" promoting safe and effective early outpatient response would likely preempt and preclude development of novel mRNA Covid-19 vaccines. But it was precisely such a program that those powerful interests were banking on. Big-time.

Chapter 3

SOME PRETTY BAD ACTORS: AVENUES OF PHARMACEUTICAL INFLUENCE

It is really no secret that pharmaceutical companies are out to make money—lots of money. Yet just how much money they actually do make may be of some interest. In 2016, for instance, Johnson & Johnson and Pfizer made more than $71 billion and $52 billion US, respectively. For comparative purposes, that is more than the individual gross domestic product of at least 120 *entire countries.* As far as the poorest countries of the world are concerned, those figures amount to more than the *combined* gross domestic product of roughly *forty* of such countries.[15]

Nor is it much a secret that said companies are often ruthlessly unscrupulous in their pursuit of their astronomical financial goals. On the contrary, it is a matter of public record. Most of the major companies, including Pfizer, AstraZeneca, and Johnson & Johnson, are serial offenders, having been accused, repeatedly, of one or another form of fraud, including crimes of *unlawful promotion, kickbacks,* and *concealment of data.* As a consequence, such companies have paid millions of dollars in settlements. Collectively, the ten worst offenders (including Pfizer, Johnson & Johnson, and AstraZeneca) paid over $35 billion in fines between 1991 and 2015. Pfizer and Johnson were second and third on that list, settling thirty-one and nineteen cases for close to four and three *billion* dollars respectively.[16]

Nor have matters improved over the last five years or so; on the contrary.

The opioid crisis represents the most notorious recent case of nefarious pharmaceutical malfeasance. As recently as June 26, 2021, it settled an opioid related suit with New York State for over $230 million.[17] The suit also sought to bar Johnson & Johnson from dealing in opioids. Still more recently (July 22, 2021), a longstanding suit brought by attorneys general from fifteen states targeting leading pharmaceutical companies—including Johnson & Johnson—and major distributors was settled for $26 billion,[18] the second largest cash settlement in history (trailing only the $246 billion 1998 tobacco settlement).[19]

Many such settlements entail a denial of any wrongdoing on the part of the company. According to the company's own account of the matter, Johnson & Johnson is a model citizen, for whom public welfare is always the chief concern. Yet anyone at all familiar with the broad outlines of the opioid crisis knows that such professions of innocence are disingenuous. I will resist the temptation to use less delicate language in describing the industry's complicity in precipitating a crisis that has exacted a toll which, according to official account, is roughly comparable to the official count of Covid death (on the order of half-a-million persons)—and still going strong.

It is a rather dark mystery to me how, as soon as it comes to the matter of vaccines, such weighty moral and practical facts are so readily forgotten or swept under the rug. Perhaps that is a testimony to the public relations acumen of the pharmaceutical companies. It certainly bears witness to the enormous political power linked to their gigantic financial stature.

That power, I believe, accounts for a good measure of the stupendous force driving the controlling Covid narrative and orchestrating the indefensible (and ongoing) blockage of early treatment initiatives. As previously noted, the active obstruction of that option qualifies as an indispensable element of the mainstream narrative and the salvation-by-vaccine formula central to it. Yet how, in the face of expert testimony and proactive initiatives on the part of exceptionally qualified scientists and physicians such as doctors McCullough, Risch, and Fareed, has this policy of obstruction and concealment—so manifestly contrary to public health and welfare—been effectively implemented?

The following passage from Cernic's *Ideological Constructs of Vaccination* (2018) provides a general answer to this and diverse related questions:

> To better understand the problem of vaccination from the point of view of the almost fanatic and uncompromising promotion of vaccines as lifesaving, safe and efficient, despite heaps of data and studies which cast doubt over this generally accepted image, it is necessary to touch upon the issue of the pharmaceutical industry. Its influence on science and medicine is huge, omnipresent and all-embracing. Of course, it is not the only actor and it would be wrong to blame the pharmaceutical industry for everything that goes on in medicine, overlooking numerous other (historical, ideological, cultural, political and economic) factors which co-create the medical reality of today.
>
> However, it is a fact that, particularly in the recent decades, the chemo-pharmaceutical industry has become one of the most important and powerful actors in all areas of health. This is how Gajski describes it: "What

> has created the belief among doctors and patients that statin prolongs life, insulin saves eyes and kidneys, hypertension medications postpone heart attack and alendronate reduces the number of fractures and deaths, while the truth is very far from it? The answer is that *the pharmaceutical network, supported by science and education which it instrumentalized and subordinated to its own interest, has been deliberately building up a system of creating a perception of efficacy, safety and cost-effectiveness of its own products. In parallel, it has been creating an artificial need for medications and, within the political sphere, favorable conditions for their placement* (emphasis Cernic's).[20]

Let me here note two correlative or supporting but—given what has been said so far—distinctly unsurprising facts. First, pharmaceutical companies spend a prodigious amount of money on marketing. Cernic notes that in 2001 the pharmaceutical industry spent, by its own admission, more than $19 billion on marketing. Today, this should hardly startle anyone whose eyes and ears are open. More and more billboard-size ads for drugs accost one in the airport, and more and more advertisements for pharmaceutical products peddle the company's wares on NPR and other mainstream media outlets. Let us again return to Cernic's words:

> The pharmaceutical industry has by far the largest lobby in Washington—and that's saying something. In 2002, it employed 675 lobbyists (more than one for each member of Congress). The job of these lobbyists is to prowl the corridors of power in Washington to promote drug company interests. According to the advocacy group Public Citizen, from 1997 through 2002, the industry spent nearly $478 million on lobbying. Drug company lobbyists are extremely well connected. In 2002, they included 26 former members of Congress, and another 342 who had been on congressional staffs or otherwise connected with the government. The industry also gives copiously to political campaigns.[21]

One additional ingredient to this rather unsavory stew: as is the case in all too many departments, there exists a revolving door between the pharmaceutical industry and government agencies—such as the FDA and NIH—charged with its oversight and regulation. The potential for corruption that bends public health policy decision away from objective considerations of public health and toward outcomes that benefits powerful vested interests is not anomalous but built into the way things work.

Today, in leftward leaning circles, "institutional racism" is all the rage. This perspective encourages understanding that racist attitudes operative in the nation are not merely a matter of personal opinion and prejudice but, to a significant degree, are "baked into the system" of governance, law enforcement, education, and other departments of human life. Yet for all the trendy magnetism of the concept, the fact of institutional racism is hardly news to this writer, or anyone who has been paying attention to one or another sector of the public sphere for the last fifty years (or more). My father, a public interest lawyer based in my childhood city of Chicago, has spent over half a century fighting the nefarious forms of discrimination built into public housing policy at the city, state, and federal level. Last year, he published a book titled *A Brief History of the Subordination of African Americans in the U.S.: Of Handcuffs and Bootstraps*[22] that chronicles, in gory detail, the history of discrimination written into our federal government's policy and lawmaking from slavery and reconstruction to the present. My own first creative nonfiction book, *Rue Rilke,*[23] revolves around the institution of capital punishment and engages the racism written into the abominable institution that represents the tragic apex of our criminal justice system.

Being thus acquainted with forms of bias written into the institutional fabric of American life, I confess myself mystified as to why generally liberal-minded persons, now famously "woke" to this sort of entrenched bias, seem so blind to the fact that the purview of the principle applies not only to matters of race (or gender, or class) alone but infects attitudes involving other issues as well. Those would include views respecting good health practices, pharmaceutical drugs and vaccination.

I hasten to add that I do not mean artificially to confuse or conflate the profound psychic wounding associated with institutional racism, which revolves around a personal factor (skin color) that is not a matter of choice or opinion but indelibly inscribed on the body itself, with the less immediately visible matters implicated in health policy. Nonetheless, it is naive to imagine that the "health experts" charged with governance of public-health policy are *not* systematically subject to both the degree of dogmatism inherent in their position in an entrenched medical establishment *and* the sway of special corporate interests regrettably entangled with government. Indeed, it is utterly implausible to believe that health officials are immune to financially motivated forms of bias generated by their association with those special interests or that their decision-making is typically based on nothing but morally impeccable concern for the public welfare and the north star of true science. To recognize that such thinking represents not fact but wishful fantasy is *not* indiscriminately to impugn the integrity of all mainstream doctors and public-health personnel but to recognize that, *in this sphere as in every other,* critical awareness and independent objective review of facts and evidence is requisite. Blind (or, even worse, politically motivated) trust in officially sanctioned "expert" opinion represents a sorely inadequate response to the present crisis, one that falls far short of the conscientious citizenry essential to democratic—as opposed to autocratic—society.

My principal claim here is simply to point out that powerfully entrenched forces, operating at systemic and institutional as well as at personal levels, habitually work to legislate certain outcomes in the public-health and medical policy sector. It follows that the authority of public-health officials should not be held as absolute but must be open to critical question and public review. Why is this perspective, so readily accepted with reference to many other domains of sociopolitical concern, so anathema to liberal-minded individuals? Do such persons imagine we are back in the eighteenth century, championing, with Voltaire and Diderot, the cause of rationally enlightened science in the face of violence perpetrated in the name of God by rabidly superstitious French Catholics? I would urge that as far as both scientific integrity and the virtue of tolerance are concerned, the Covid shoe today does not fit the left foot. Are most so-called progressive persons so hoodwinked by the *veneer* of "science" painted over everything related to the administration of public-health policy—and vaccine policy in particular—that casting any sort of questioning eye upon officially sanctioned medical proceedings earns not respect but automatic dismissal and social castigation? Since when has the political left been so ready to take the side of government authority, in preference to its historic guardianship of individual civil rights and liberties? Why has it been so willing to respond to propagandist dog whistles—"misinformation," "anti-vaxxer," "conspiracy theory"—as if the mere invocation of those words obviates the need for substantive debate of competing views and positions?

What, after all, is supposedly meant by the phrase *conspiracy theory,* used so liberally to damn most any question of the controlling Covid narrative and its central vaccine clause? To speak of a conspiracy implies that multiple persons or forces act together to achieve a certain (often morally questionable) end, the success of which generally involves elements of disguise, dissimulation, and deception. If we were, objectively, to review the government's reception of doctors McCullough, Risch, and Fareed's initiative—their urgent plea that the powers that be institute a national plan of safe and effective early outpatient treatment for Covid-19—I think it would be fair to say that the callous and unscientific stymieing of that initiative qualifies as the kind of low-grade "conspiracy" inherent to a system of medical and health administration beholden to enormously powerful special interests. Indeed, the historical record makes perfectly clear that, within the huge orbit of the pharmaceutical industry influence, conspiracy is nothing special but, rather, business as usual. This, I would claim, is not "theory" but cold, hard fact.

Chapter 4

DEADENING DIALOGUE: SCIENCE, SOCIETY, AND (*WHAT?*) FREEDOM OF SPEECH

From the first, the Covid controversy has been attended by aggressive and widespread suppression of freedom of speech. Individuals and organizations (Stand for Health Freedom, Children's Health Defense, the Informed Consent Action Network, and others) questioning one or another element of the controlling Covid narrative—no matter how well-grounded those questions and concerns may be—were and are typically subjected to merciless condemnation and, all too frequently, outright censorship and even dangerous harassment. Media giants consistently deplatform material on the basis of industry "fact-checkers" whose own independence and objectivity are not open to publicly visible oversight and review. Relevant publications are denied normal means and channels of distribution.

All this is ostensibly done in the name of "the public good." But preemptively precluding robust public dialogue on matters of concern to every citizen *never* truly serves the public interest, least of all when the issues at stake are of such compelling importance. It is, instead, a recipe for authoritarian overreach on the part of entrenched institutions and powerful interests and thus poisons the lifeblood of democratic society.

This egregious sort of abuse applies, ongoingly, in both the private and public sectors and notably, too, in that scientific community, which—by virtue of its defining commitment to impartial objective truth—should be especially zealous in the protection (not prosecution!) of those freedoms. I still clearly remember when, several months after the pandemic had commenced and health professional were first gaining a sense of how deadly—or not—the disease really was, two Kern County, California doctors[24] carefully and respectfully questioned the wisdom of the extreme measures (including wholesale lockdown) that had been instituted. The grounds for their criticism were medical and immunological as well as economic and social. They emphasized that, in the case of infectious disease, it had *never* been accepted policy to quarantine the healthy or to deny the entire population the enormous benefit of outdoor activity. They feared that along with the inestimable economic and psychological fallout from extended isolation, such hiding away of people from nature and from each other would eventually result both in increased susceptibility and in newer, stronger waves of disease upon emergence from the lockdown.

Whether or not their perspective was more or less valid than that of the mainstream (and I believe it was rather more than less)[25], they, as qualified professionals, were entitled to express their views openly, which the doctors themselves saw as hardly heretical but, on the contrary, very much in line with the traditional understanding that might be taught in Immunology 101.[26] Instead of the respectful dialogue which the presentation invited, the two doctors were immediately subjected to an avalanche of insulting criticism, much of which impugned their persons and not even their ideas. Moreover, within no more than a day or two, they were officially sanctioned by the professional organization (I do not recall the specific one) responsible for oversight of their area of practice, *and* the clip of their presentation and interview had mysteriously disappeared from the Web. Consequently, neither I, nor anyone, was afforded the opportunity to be party to any reasoned dialogue that might constructively have ensued but was condemned to suffer the consequences of the hostile atmosphere in silence and disaffected isolation.

This all took place over a year ago but is exemplary of trends and techniques that have continued more or less unchanged to this day, except that the intensity of the censorship—again in both private and professional spheres—has intensified, long ago reaching a fever pitch. While the leadership of the forces armed to patrol this terrain remain more or less in the background, both heavy artillery and cavalry have been effectively deployed to deny fair hearing to any and all who question the controlling Covid-19 narrative, no matter their degree of relevant professional expertise or (just as important) evident personal integrity and compassionate concern for human welfare. This is especially true, of course, if said person or group questions the religious core of the official Covid story: namely, the sanctity and salvific power of the Covid vaccines.

One recent poignant instance of this pattern as it plays out in everyday social circles involves the life of a recent graduate of Earlham College.[27] Cait Corrigan was a model student, so much so that she had been slated to speak at Earlham's 2021 graduation last month. Yet Cait, who is a Quaker, did not wish to comply with the college's order that all who wished to attend the graduation in person were required to undergo vaccination. She accordingly notified the college that their refusal to recognize her religious exemption (one that had been in force since her entrance to the college) was an illegal violation of Indiana state law. Although the college at first refused to change their position (the college president's revealing response to her initial request for recognition of rights consisted of three letters: "*LOL*"), when Cait availed herself of legal aid as well as assistance from her state senator, the college was forced finally to back down and allow her attendance.

This, however, did not represent an unqualified success, because near universal social persecution stepped in to enforce the judgment precluded by law. Not only was Cait summarily and forcibly dropped from the roll of a class for which she was registered, shunned and reviled by erstwhile friends, and denied the privilege of speaking at the graduation (at which she was forced to stand alone, apart, and at a distance), but the professor who had been a mentor and indeed her personal adviser repeatedly and aggressively harassed her about her vaccination status, offered to pay her *not* to attend, and threatened to retract a letter of recommendation he had written to the Boston University graduate program which she hoped to attend. Finally, offended persons sought to slanderously compromise Cait's integrity in the eye of her supervisor at the charitable organization where she had long worked as an intern so that she might be fired from that post.

All of this goes beyond reasonable difference of opinion or concern for personal safety on the part of Cait's compatriots. Because of her principled refusal to surrender her lawful personal freedom, she was singled out for persecution as surely and viciously as if, like Hester Prynne in Hawthorne's famous novel, she'd had a Scarlet Letter—a gaudy mark of a shameful sin, subversive of the very fabric of society—emblazoned on her clothing.

As disheartening as this story is, many further stories stemming from within the precincts of medicine, government, and the halls of research science itself are even more so. To illustrate, let us shift the scene slightly and look into some official proceedings of our Canadian neighbors north of the border. What has recently transpired there could well be considered shocking *if* it were not so much of a piece with all that has been long going on in the United States.

Recognizing that an atmosphere of sociopolitical suppression had settled in a thick fog over his land, Canadian MP Derek Sloan issued a public appeal, encouraging Canadian citizens to share with him confidentially whatever concerns might have arisen for them as a result of their own interaction with health professionals and Canadian public institutions. MP Sloan heard from hundreds of people from all walks of life. In order to air the relevant concerns, MP Sloan arranged a June 17, 2021 public Parliament Hill event (a virtual news conference)[28] at which he shared two of the communications he'd received from Canadian citizens before turning over the stage to three scientists and doctors.

MP Sloan first conveyed the story of a thirty-year-old female nurse (unwilling, like many, to give her name because of her fear of job repercussions) who told him that she was pressured by healthcare workers and the media to take the vaccine, having been repeatedly told that the benefits outweighed the risks. In retrospect, however, the nurse realized that she had not been informed of *any* of the potential risks. Four days after her first (and only) Pfizer dose, she was diagnosed with inflammation of and fluid buildup around her heart. As of the time of MP Sloan's sharing of her story, she had been on anti-inflammatory medication for three months, medication that has the potential to damage the only kidney she was born with. The nurse finished by saying (as shared by MP Sloan):

> The media keeps telling us that these cases are rare, and that they typically happen with young men. But so far I know of three other cases of Winnipeg women who have also developed heart issues post-shot, and we are all young; under thirty-five years old. Well, this is all concerning, but the most concerning part is that we are still being advised by our doctors to get a second dose. At this point, it feels as if they are purposely trying to harm us.[29]

MP Sloan then shared the message of a Canadian Armed Forces (CAF) service member who did not wish to be vaccinated but provided a detailed account of the elaborate protocol in place (including repeated mandatory clinic visits and aggressive persuasion by health officials) designed to pressure CAF members into "blindly accepting the process" and submitting to vaccination. The service member remarked:

> I am concerned for my fellow members, because I have witnessed my coworkers suffering from vaccine injury in the past, and am sure that the military will cover up the true devastation it has caused, as it has done before, with suicides...[30]

The service member then expressed his deep fear that the vaccine will be made mandatory for all CAF members later this year and issued a "solemn plea" to MP Sloan that this somehow be prevented.

MP Sloan concluded this portion of the event by observing:

> As you can see, we should be asking questions about the process, but whenever someone does so, they are either intimidated or censored by whomever it is that they are reporting.[31]

As disturbing as all this is, the most telling revelations were shared by the three physicians. To understand the full context of their testimony, as well as that of the citizens just cited, it is necessary to know the extent of the deliberate suppression of scientific inquiry perpetrated by the professional organization that supervises their work. The College of Physicians and Surgeons of Ontario (CPSO) possesses (among other capacities) the power to grant or deny licensure and so exerts a determinative influence on professional conduct within Ontario medical circles and all associated research institutions.

On April 30, 2021, the CPSO issued a directive that could not but exercise a chilling effect upon scientific investigation and medical practice in Ontario. As cited by Dr. Patrick Phillips, the directive stated: "It is the professional responsibility of all physicians not to communicate anti-vax, anti-masking, anti-distancing, or anti-lockdown statements, and/or promote unsupported unproven treatments for Covid-19."[32]

"They were very explicit," added Dr. Phillips, "and threatened investigation or discipline for any physician who expressed any of the negative aspects of any of these interventions *no matter what the evidence says*."[33]

Commenting upon the directive, MP Derek Sloan declared: "The purpose of governing bodies like the CPSO is to protect the public, not to stifle legitimate scientific inquiry or dissent by professional doctors." That reigning health experts (such as those staffing the CPSO) govern in accordance with that dictate is, naturally, the working assumption of all citizens who invest their trust in the professional opinion of appointed authorities. The CPSO's directive represents a clear instance of an influential official body's blatant and programmatic betrayal of that trust, one that should give every right-minded citizen pause before he or she mounts the war horse named "Science" and charges off on a crusade to vanquish heretic infidels like our model student Cait Corrigan, our Winnipeg nurse, our vaccine-hesitant CAF service member, and our three physicians who—despite the significant risks they knowingly incurred by their actions—refused to be ruled by the CPSO's directive.

Dr. Patrick Phillips is a family physician working primarily in the emergency department of an Ontario hospital. Like doctors McCullough, Risch, and Fareed before him, Dr. Phillips spoke to the ready availability of safe and effective methods of Covid prophylaxis and early treatment. He noted that while the Canadian Health Ministry labeled as "fake news" the idea that vitamin D can aid in the prevention of Covid-19, objective review of the available data supports the contrary view:

> Over 85 studies and 27 treatment trials, many of these peer-reviewed scientific literature, have shown a 56% reduction in mortality in patients who take vitamin D compared to those who don't for Covid-19.[34]

Dr. Phillips also strongly endorsed the inexpensive and widely available medication ivermectin as a means of both prevention (especially for high-risk patients) and treatment:

> 97 studies and over 30 randomized control trials have shown a huge benefit to this medication in reducing the risk of death and hospitalization in patients who have Covid. And not only does this treat patients with Covid, especially when you give it early, but there is also a role—there's 14 randomized trials—for prophylaxis, meaning taking the medication for high-risk patients; it can reduce your chances of catching Covid in the first place.[35]

Dr. Phillips further disclosed how the CPSO continued to try to block exploration and use of these—in his mind, safe and effective—methods of prophylaxis and treatment:

> At this point, the College of Physicians has launched investigations against many physicians, including myself, threatening to take our licenses away for promoting what they call unproven treatments but which the scientific peer reviewed literature shows is very well supported. The Ontario Science Table even recommends against vitamin D, which I think is unthinkable, because the harm is…none. This is a natural substance, and they are telling us not to give this to patients despite mortality benefit.[36]

He closed with his personal response to such pressure:

> I knew there was something going wrong, and I knew I had to speak out, no matter what the College does to my license. Because at this point, there are bigger things going on than my career.[37]

Next we have Dr. Donald Welsh, professor of physiology at the University of Western Ontario, who declared, "Science has not been functioning properly for the last fifteen months, as we address Covid-19."[38] Dr. Welsh offered public support for his beleaguered colleagues, as well as an impassioned plea for the restoration of the integrity of scientific process, a method of truth-seeking which, he emphasized, requires rigor, impartiality, and—equally important—humility. Dr. Welsh opined that his country's officially sanctioned health measures—including wholesale lockdowns—had not proven effective and urged the necessity of objective critical review of the scientific situation and associated health policy. Articulating the professional ethic so contrary to the spirit and letter of the CPSO directive, Dr. Welsh cited Nobel physicist Richard Feynman, who observed of science: "If you don't make mistakes, you are doing it wrong. If you don't correct those mistakes, you are doing it really wrong, and if you can't accept that you are mistaken, you are not doing it at all."[39]

Center stage, though, was reserved for the first scientific witness, Dr. Byram Bridle, an associate professor of viral immunology at Guelph University. Dr. Bridle, whose work revolves centrally (although not exclusively) around the health and welfare of children, began by stating:

> Since the pandemic was declared, I have been trying to serve as a voice of objective scientific opinion, so that the public can make the most informed possible decision for themselves when it comes to issues related to Covid-19.[40]

Dr. Bridle alluded to the fact that he is not accustomed to or temperamentally inclined toward public exposure. Nonetheless, because he is a scientist employed at a publicly funded research university, the Canadian public effectively pays his salary. He therefore feels especially obligated not only to perform behind-the-scenes research but to serve the public responsibly in matters related to his expertise, in whatever capacity he can.

Dr. Bridle continued to describe how, two weeks earlier (thus, in early June of 2021, roughly a month after the CPSO's directive), he gave a five-minute interview as part of a segment of a radio program addressing issues related to Covid-19. That interview consisted of his response to a single question. Dr. Bridle rehearses the question and the point of departure of his own answer:

> [I was asked] if I knew whether there could be a possible link between Covid-19 vaccines and cases of heart inflammation that have been reported around the world in young males. In this case, it was twelve young males in Israel. I've been delving into the literature very deeply because I'm a vaccinologist. My entire research program is based on the development of novel vaccines. My publication record is based on publishing information about vaccines. So I have a lot of expertise in this area. And indeed I have, along with a large number of collaborators, both within Canada and internationally, developed some serious concerns about the current

Covid-19 vaccines, so I felt that I could express concern that there might be a possible link between this heart inflammation that is occurring and the Covid-19 vaccine.[41]

To be sure, Dr. Bridle could indeed publicly express his concerns, but the aftermath of the interview proved his belief that he could do so *freely,* without fearing violent and sustained backlash, tragically naive:

> After I did the interview, it was like a nuclear bomb went off in my world, and my life was thrown upside down. I am sure my life will never be the same again. Within twenty-four hours there was a website that was put up using my domain name, a fake twitter account was set up to slander me, and I've been undergoing daily attacks, either through email or people trying to call me, and definitely through social media.[42]

Dr. Bridle continued to note that, while the University of Guelph had stood by him and supported his right to express his views, he had been seriously harassed by a number of colleagues. At least one of those colleagues, moreover, served in an official government capacity. As Dr. Bridle detailed:

> It has even gone so far as to have one of the members of the Ontario Covid-19 Science Advisory Committee.... They were actually the first one to post the link to the slanderous website, and have fanned the flames of this smear campaign quite strongly since then. They even went so far as to release confidential medical information about my parents. This is an egregious act. This is a practicing physician. A practicing physician should know they should not be releasing confidential medical information about people in the social realm.[43]

Dr. Bridle then described how the concerted assault exacted a terrible personal toll on him, depriving him of sleep and turning him into a "walking zombie," until, after three days, he began to find a footing that enabled him to face the vitriol directed his way. A newly formed organization played a significant role in that capacity. Dr. Bridle continued:

> I'm part of the Canadian Covid Care Alliance. This is a group of individuals. In fact, the reason we exist is sad. We exist because we are like-minded in the sense that we all want to be able to speak openly and freely about the science and medicine underpinning Covid-19. And we don't feel safe to do it anywhere else other than our own private group.[44]

After noting that the rapidly growing group has, by now, roughly one hundred members, Dr. Bridle remarked:

> Only two of us are willing to talk to the media.... The others are too afraid for their jobs. They are physicians afraid that they are going to lose their license to practice. And they are academics and other professionals afraid they are going to lose their jobs.[45]

Dr. Bridle further noted that he had developed a comprehensive guide for parents so that they could make an informed decision regarding Covid-19 vaccination for their children. He then went on, briefly but cogently, to detail the solid *scientific* basis of the concerns relevant to the Covid-19 vaccines employing the novel, previously untested RNA technology.

The gist of the concerns focus on the fact that one of the key assumptions involved in the experimental development and use of the vaccines has proven dramatically wrong. As Dr. Bridle explains, in traditional vaccines the active agent remains in the area of inoculation (generally, the shoulder) until critical elements of the immunological response are picked up by the lymph nodes and conveyed to the immune system. The crucial vaccine material itself is thus only selectively diffused and activated. In the mRNA technology, however, the vaccine material is not selectively, but generally, distributed throughout the entire body and thus has the capacity to affect vital organ (including heart) function directly. In fact, experience shows that only twenty-five percent of the vaccine remains in the shoulder; the other three-quarters migrates into the rest of the body where it can have undesirable effects, including inflammation of the heart.

Dr. Bridle additionally expressed concerns regarding inadequate and entirely substandard testing of the vaccines. The Covid vaccines, he emphasized, were tested only on rats—not even humans. While he recognized that this is appropriate and unavoidable at a certain stage of study, it is by no means an adequate basis for evaluating the overall safety of a novel vaccine technology, because, in many regards, rodent physiology differs from that of human beings. Representing "an inappropriate animal model," rat testing cannot really serve as a reliable predictor of possible effects on human physiology. In addition to the issues that prompted the interview—concerns that, figuratively as well as literally—go straight to the *heart* of the matter, Dr. Bridle emphasized that—given that preliminary testing has been restricted not only to rats but in fact to only female rats—one can hardly be entirely confident about the long-range effect of the vaccine on reproductive capacity, a function that might be especially prone to adverse effects precipitated by the novel mRNA technology.

For his part, Dr. Bridle emphasized that when it comes to healthy children, we must be very sure of what exactly we are doing: "Mass vaccination of millions of healthy children demands that the level of safety associated with this, the assessed safety value of this, has to be exceptionally high."[46] Given that children are not generally vulnerable to Covid, and that the reproductive systems of this population represents a uniquely relevant concern, this hardly seems an unreasonable or irresponsible position. Indeed, to many, it would seem the only sane and humanly defensible conclusion. Yet Dr. Bridle had a few words to say about the sociopolitical situation of science and its public reception in Canada, words that must resonate, too, with untold Americans:

> We're polarized right now, we're polarized in Canada. There are people on both sides. You have to understand, we're just as passionate. We feel we are trying to look after people's best interests. We are doing our own cost-benefit analysis; for example, in my own case, with children. And I honestly feel that by proceeding with vaccination right now, without conducting the proper safety tests, we may do harm than good. I'm passionate about that. But I'm respectful of those who hold the opposite opinion, and I ask the same for myself and my colleagues. We can't suppress open discussion of science and medicine in Canada. It's the hallmark of a democratic society.[47]

That may well be, and yet, for speaking out on these matters, Dr. Bridle has been crucified. Dr. Bridle continued:

> By expressing this, my career may very well have been destroyed, and I don't understand that. It's incomprehensible to me that this has happened. As Canadians, we have to ask ourselves, do you want your physicians and scientists... their views suppressed? Right now, I don't recognize the country that I was born into, and I would simply ask all Canadians, please, I simply want us to learn to respect one another again.[48]

What can anyone—Canadian, American, or whatever nationality you call your own—say to that except Amen?

Chapter 5

"SAFE AND EFFECTIVE"— THE WHOLE TRUTH, AND NOTHING BUT?

My reader may by now recognize that the scientific facts of the Covid case and, consequently, any moral and practical deductions that might be reasonably drawn from those can hardly be considered cut and dried. Dr. Bridle's remarks lay bare the theoretical bases for some of the real concerns regarding Covid vaccine safety, but a reasonable understanding of the full range and force of those concerns requires further elaboration.

First, it should be acknowledged that the so-called Covid-19 vaccines are not vaccines at all in the traditional sense of the term. To call them "vaccines" (and Merriam-Webster altered the meanings of the word so that the Covid-19 shots would be specifically included in the dictionary definition) encourages a familiarity and, for many, a sense of security that the public would be unlikely to attach to more controversial terms, such as "gene therapy injection," that make direct reference to the actual, novel mode of intervention employed by mRNA technology. Traditional vaccines work by injecting an inactivated version of a virus or viral cells into the body to elicit an immunological response, thus educating the body and preparing it to combat any live viral assault. The new technology, on the other hand, utilizes lipid-packaged mRNA strands. These instruct the body to *manufacture* the spike protein that the Covid virus employs to gain access to cells, thus stimulating the body to produce antigens capable of fighting the virus.

The two techniques clearly aim for an analogous result: education and stimulation of the body's immunological response. One critical—and unanticipated—difference, however, as Dr. Bridle and others have pointed out, involves migration of the active agent in the novel Covid vaccines. The mRNA travels throughout the body so that the potentially dangerous (*actively* pathogenic) spike protein spreads uncontrollably and can adversely effect vital organs, including the heart, adrenals, reproductive organs, and even bone marrow. This contrasts sharply with the delimited and controlled distribution of the immunogen (the agent that elicits protective response) in traditional vaccines as well as the *inactive* character of that immunogen (which is typically deadened—effectively killed—by intense heating or some comparable process). Concerns associated with traditional vaccines stem as much or more from the adjuvants required for the preparation and production of the vaccine as from the *inactive* viral material itself. The mRNA technology avoids some of the issues associated with these adjuvants, but at the cost of the novel threats (including life-threatening organ impairment and sterility) posed by the distribution of the actively pathogenic spike protein throughout the body.

So much for the theoretical background of the safety concerns pertaining to the Covid-19 vaccines. What light does actual experience shed on the matter? Despite the repeated assurances from government agencies and mainstream media channels—the "safe and effective" mantra constantly drummed into the public ear—an objective review of relevant statistics actually reveals disconcerting, not to say positively alarming, results.

Every week, the CDC publishes data collected by the U.S. government-run Vaccine Adverse Event Reporting System (VAERS). According to the latest (July 16, 2021) report, between December 14, 2020 and July 9, 2021, VAERS registered 463,457 total adverse events related to Covid vaccines, including 10,991 deaths and 48,385 serious injuries.[49] This includes 1,943 deaths and 7,370 serious injuries for the week of July 2 to 9, 2021, alone, which adds up to an average of *roughly 275 deaths and more than a thousand serious injuries per day* over the latest week for which numbers are available at the time of this writing. This, remember, is in the United States alone.

While it may well remain true that the majority of persons do not experience anything more than *relatively* minor side effects in the *immediate aftermath* of Covid vaccination—a fact which may theoretically justify the claim that the vaccines are "safe and effective"—the administration of the vaccine to millions of persons nonetheless clearly results in a *substantial* number of deaths and serious injuries. If, just last week, you were one of the almost ten thousand Americans who suffered debilitating injury or death—or were a family member of one who did—the fact that *most* persons did not do so would probably prove cold comfort. People take vaccines to secure protection from death and disease, not to be martyred for the cause.

It should be noted that VAERS accepts reports of adverse events before medical confirmation of any causal relationship between the vaccine and any reported event. In many cases, though, there is a strong presumption of causal connection, either because such connection has been established between a given disease (e.g., heart inflammation) and vaccination and/or simply because death or injury occurred soon after vaccination. In almost sixty percent of the reported deaths, for instance, death (twenty-two percent) or seriousness illness (thirty-seven percent) commenced within forty-eight hours of vaccination; fifteen percent of reported deaths occurred within twenty-four hours of inoculation.[50]

It is, in fact, by no means safe to assume that the number of adverse events caused by the vaccines is *lower* than the reported numbers. As there is good reason to believe that only a small fraction of vaccine-related adverse events are actually reported to and duly registered by VAERS (Dr. Peter McCullough estimated the figure to be in the ten percent range); *it is likely that the true numbers are significantly higher than those reported above.*

But for now, however, let's work with the official, government-approved numbers. In addition to cardiac disorders (which were responsible for almost one-quarter of the reported deaths), additional afflictions included 127,421 reported cases of anaphylaxis, 9,471 cases of blood-clotting, 5,049 cases of Bell's Palsy, 445 cases of Guillain-Barré syndrome, and almost 3,000 pregnancy-related adverse events, including over 1,000 miscarriages or premature births.[51]

In case you are wondering what such numbers imply with respect to the safety of the Covid-19 vaccines relative to the more traditional vaccines widely used over the past thirty years, here are some benchmarks pertaining, primarily, to incidence of death:

- Historically, the seasonal flu vaccine has been the most hazardous of all those commonly employed. The Covid shots are *500 times more deadly.*
- The reported death rate of the Covid-19 vaccines *exceeds the combined death rate of more than 70 traditional vaccines* in wide use over the past thirty years.
- The number of reported deaths due to the Covid-19 shots over the last six and a half months is roughly twice that of the total number of deaths reported to VAERS for *all other vaccines combined over the last twenty-two years.*[52]

Such statistics, reflecting arithmetic based on officially approved numbers, should be sufficiently unsettling to give anyone pause before undergoing vaccination, let alone before insisting that it is their neighbor's moral and civic duty to do so.

To their credit, the FDA and CDC have recently added warnings to the Pfizer vaccine, noting the increased risk of heart inflammation, and to the

Johnson & Johnson vaccine, noting the (rare) incidence of Guillain-Barré syndrome associated with it. Nonetheless, on the CDC's own Covid website, the tab providing vaccine information includes (right at the top), a section titled: "What You Need to Know." The first of seven bullet points reads: "Covid-19 vaccines are *safe and effective*" (emphasis CDC). Only lower down, in a shaded box, do we read: "Serious adverse events after Covid-19 vaccination are rare but may occur."[53]

This last is a statement of fact, while that all-too-familiar first statement is a matter of judgment. Why, then, do the government and mainstream media *pretend the opposite?* Is the (debatable) judgment trumpeted so loudly in order to drown out the drum roll of fact?

The statistics cited generally apply to the American population as a whole, yet select populations, including persons who have recovered from Covid, children, youth, and women of childbearing age, merit special consideration when it comes to any rational cost-benefit analysis of the value of vaccination. Before, however, exploring that terrain, I would like to turn briefly to that other quality celebrated by the flag-like wand waved over those endless rows of Covid vaccine vials: their effectiveness.

This, like so much concerning Covid, is a numbers game, and it's necessary to keep a sharp eye out as to who may playing fast and loose with these numbers. We are all familiar with the apparently impressive figures associated with Pfizer and Moderna's initial trials; the heralded announcements that the vaccines have proven eighty-five to ninety-five percent effective.[54] Yet limited clinical trials are one thing, the inoculation of millions of persons in the general population amid ever-changing immunological conditions (including the emergence of variants) quite another. As Dr. Risch and fellow doctor, Joseph Lapado, of UCLA, wrote in a June 22, 2021, *Wall Street Journal* opinion piece ("Are Covid Vaccines Riskier Than Advertised"):

> Historically, the safety of medications—including vaccines—is often not fully understood until they are deployed in large populations. Examples include rofecoxib (Vioxx), a pain reliever that increased the risk of heart attack and stroke, antidepressants that appeared to increase suicide attempts among young adults, and an influenza vaccine used in the 2009–10 swine flu epidemic that was suspected of causing febrile convulsions and narcolepsy in children. Evidence from the real world is valuable, as clinical trials often enroll patients who aren't representative of the general population.[55]

Given this truth, genuinely *objective* assessment of the safety and efficacy of vaccines necessitates conscientious and meticulous data collection *after* introduction of the vaccine into the general population. Government agencies intent upon making such an objective assessment (as opposed to angling for results that might justify one or another predetermined position) would naturally take measures aiming to optimize the scope and accuracy of data collected. Unfortunately, U.S. government agencies have arguably done just the opposite, proceeding in a manner that *degrades* both the quantity and quality of information available, thus making the goal of obtaining a clear, big-picture view of vaccine safety and efficacy significantly more difficult to achieve.

Part of the story involves the notorious unreliability of the PCR test employed to register Covid-19 positive cases. Originally, the CDC advised laboratories to employ a cycle threshold of forty when testing for SARS-CoV-2, despite the fact that cycle thresholds above thirty-five were widely regarded as producing an extraordinarily high level of false positives. (One might consider PCR tests analogous to washing machines in a sense, in that both can run more cycles for their own purposes.[56] With washing machines, running more cycles leaves clothes cleaner but perhaps wears them out sooner. When PCR tests run more cycles, that is, employ higher cycle thresholds, forty being exceptionally high, they miss fewer Covid positives but also record higher numbers of *false* positives.[57]) In mid-May of 2021, roughly five months after the first release of the vaccine to the general public, the CDC issued new guidelines endorsing the use of a significantly lower (twenty-eight) cycle threshold *for vaccinated individuals only(!)* and, correlatively, stipulated that it would no longer track breakthrough cases, that is, vaccinated individuals who test positive, *except* when such cases resulted in serious injury or death, thus effectively excluding the lion's share of breakthrough cases from any and all real consideration.[58]

Many knowledgeable persons had long advised employing a lower cycle threshold in order to reduce the high number of false positives, the associated (possibly grossly) inflated case numbers, and the many destructive consequences of this, including overly restrictive measures applied to the "positive" individual as well as the population at large. The timing of the joint directives, however, as well as the wholly irrational practice of lowering the recommended rate only for vaccinated persons, rendered the CDC susceptible to the charge that its policy deliberately favored the appearance of a timely reduction of case numbers so as to artificially bolster the case for vaccine efficacy. Moreover, the CDC's accompanying decision to stop recording all less-serious breakthrough cases strengthened the perception of bias since—if followed—the policy would make it much more difficult to clearly evaluate the effectiveness of the vaccines in actually preventing incidence and spread of Covid-19.

Not surprisingly, diverse physicians, researchers, and concerned professionals (most of whom were clearly in support of the general vaccination effort) swiftly condemned the new guidelines as *antithetical* to the cause of both science and public health. While the CDC claimed that the new policy would "maximize the quality of data collected in cases of greatest clinical and public health interest," a whole chorus of concerned professionals begged—emphatically—to differ.

Rick Bright, a former federal health official currently with the Rockefeller Foundation (a major funder of the vaccination effort), declared:

> Just looking at hospitalizations or cases from people who die is really keeping... blindfolds on your eyes and not fully understanding what is happening with this virus. It puts us at a disadvantage in better understanding this virus and how to end the pandemic. These variants are spreading, and if you're just looking at the small percentage [of hospitalizations and deaths], then you're really missing the big picture.[59]

Ryan McNamara, a virologist at the University of North Carolina at Chapel Hill involved in sequencing samples from breakthrough cases of all grades of severity, asserted:

> Asymptomatic, mild symptoms, hospitalized, passed away—all that information is important. If you're asking what variant is driving worse clinical outcomes, you need both ends of the data.[60]

Ali Mokdad, an epidemiologist at the University of Washington and former senior scientist at the CDC, put his disagreement with his former agency's policy decision in pointed terms: "We are driving blind, and we will miss a lot of signals."[61]

If the professional consensus is so clear that the CDC policy decision positively hamstrings vital vaccine-related research, why would they have made it in the first place? Medical researcher Joel Hirschhorn outlines the regrettable but more or less obvious answer:

> Experts aside, most Americans would probably vote to gather all possible data on breakthrough infections. But getting the most possible data would hurt the government's efforts to compel all people to get vaccinated. Vaccine hesitancy and rejection would surely be reinforced by data in local media

> showing that experimental COVID vaccines are not fully protective. This is inevitable if more people get better informed about natural immunity and a number of cheap, proven, and safe treatments that work as prophylactics to prevent infection, mainly hydroxychloroquine and ivermectin.[62]

Very well, you may say, but as we are addressing the question of vaccine efficacy, what of all those reports that the prohibitive majority (up to ninety-five percent) of persons now hospitalized with Covid are *un*vaccinated? Is that in and of itself proof more than good enough for government work? For all practical purposes, what more need we know?

The question is fair enough. Let me venture a preliminary answer.

First, one needs to recognize that the prohibitive majority of *those* persons would probably not be in the hospital at all if the government had invested in preventative and early treatment options instead of promoting vaccination as the only solution to Covid-19. (Of course, the opportunity of so doing is still very much open.) *Second,* one must frankly and transparently acknowledge the very real, serious, and as yet incompletely known risks associated with the novel "gene therapy" injections known as vaccines. *Third,* one should recognize that, so far as the relative efficacy of the vaccines, select statistics do not tell the whole story and that additional, potentially distressing, information pertaining to the potential downside of full vaccination need to be reckoned with, especially when it involves the newly dominant (as of the time of this writing) Delta version of the virus.

Some doctors, including Dr. Harvey Risch, are purportedly reporting that (contrary to the popular view) a majority of their Covid case load is now comprised of fully vaccinated individuals.[63] Given unknown physiological factors (including the potential for ADE, a biochemical dynamic wherein vaccination *decreases* the body's immunological resistance to viral assault) as well as ever-shifting immunological circumstances (including the emergence of new strains), it may be premature to venture any definitive verdict as to the degree of protection afforded by the vaccines with respect to either incidence or severity of the disease.

To wit: a letter recently sent to tens of thousands of doctors in Europe by Doctors for Covid Ethics details four scientific findings emerging from recent laboratory study. The results emphasize: a) the general resilience and strength of *natural* immune response to SARS-CoV-2; and, disturbingly, b) the very real medical risk of antibody-dependent enhancement compromising that response and heightening susceptibility to serious disease and death. The summary of the letter, which precedes technically detailed elaboration of each of the four findings, reads:

> Rapid and efficient memory-type immune response occur reliably in virtually all unvaccinated individuals who are exposed to SARS-CoV-2. The effectiveness of further boosting the immune response through vaccination is therefore highly doubtful. Vaccination may instead aggravate disease through antibody-dependent enhancement.[64]

This letter, by the way, caught the notice of Dr. Robert Malone, inventor of the mRNA technology, who, judging it to be an "interesting summary," included a link to it in a July 18, 2021 tweet. We will hear more of Dr. Malone shortly.

Along analogous lines of concern, some recently collated data from Europe[65] significantly heightens the degree of uncertainty pertaining to vaccine safety and efficacy. If, for instance, one looks at a recent graph plotting the number of Covid cases in Europe over the last two months (that is, summer of 2021)—the period of time during which the Delta variant assumed dominance—one will see graphic display of a disturbing phenomena. The incidence of cases for the three most-vaccinated countries (the UK, The Netherlands, and Malta) shows a dramatic and steep climb, most especially over the last two or three weeks. Taking a rolling seven-day average of cases as the relevant number, both Malta and the Netherlands were well under 100 at the beginning of July, but have surged to over 300 and 500 respectively since then; the UK was below 100 in May and early June, but, over the last month has (like the Netherlands) surged to a figure well over 500. Meanwhile, the fifteen least-vaccinated European countries (Slovenia, Serbia, Slovakia, Croatia, Latvia, Montenegro, Romania, Albania, North Macedonia, Bulgaria, Moldova, Kosovo, Bosnia and Herzegovina, Belarus, and Ukraine) remain essentially flat or show a gradual downward trend. All but one (which comes in at right around 100) register, in mid-July, a figure of somewhere up to fifty cases per day on average. The vaccination rate of these countries is fairly evenly spread out between the low of five percent (Ukraine) and the high of forty-one percent (Slovenia), while that of both the UK and Netherlands is just about sixty-seven percent (almost the same as that of the United States). Meanwhile, Malta—the most vaccinated country in the Western world—registers a vaccination rate of close to eighty-five percent. The visual contrast between the "flat plain" graphs of the least-vaccinated countries and the "alpine ascent" of the most-vaccinated is both striking and disturbing.

If you are inclined to regard such data as a kind of statistical mirage not worthy of real concern, you would find yourself in disagreement with no less of an authority than Dr. Robert Malone, the inventor of the mRNA technology, who himself just recently shared the viral thread displaying the relevant graphs, tweeting: "This is worrying me quite a bit."[66] In response to questions on the topic, Dr. Malone posted a more in-depth series of tweets[67] that clarified his overall position on the Covid vaccination program, one I believe worth reproducing in full. Dr. Malone on July 19, 2021:

> OK, time for another one of these. My positions—
>
> 1. Bioethics requires full risk disclosure and free choice. Neither of these is being met.
> 2. For high risk populations, the risk benefit ratio for the USA vaccines seem to make sense
> 3. We do not know all the risks yet
> 4. For pediatric and young adult populations, the data do not currently support adequate risk/benefit for USA vaccines. So stop.
> 5. Mandating vaccines is wrong
> 6. Censorship is wrong
> 7. Attacking other's credibility as a way to win arguments is the refuge of the stupid
> 8. Dr. GV Bossche is completely correct as a virologist and vaccinologist in everything that I have read of his. Time will prove him right.... But IMO as a physician, the death and disability in the high risk populations still merits vaccination.
> 9. There is a concerted effort to suppress information and dissent in support of the noble lie
> 10. The noble lie is—
>   a. We have to reach herd immunity for economic recovery and to minimize death and disability
>   b. These genetic vaccines are the only path to herd immunity
>   c. These genetic vaccines are perfectly safe.
>
> Each of these statements are demonstrably false.

~

Dr. Malone here makes his own position amply clear. Taking a cue from him, let me conclude this section by turning to the topic of the advisability of vaccination for populations that either are at peculiarly low-risk from Covid (persons who have recovered from the illness and children and youth) and/or may be at especially high-risk for vaccine-related adverse events (pregnant women).

Addressing the overall question of vaccine safety and efficacy, doctors Lapado and Risch offer a cogent overview of both the medical and sociopolitical situation, before focusing on critical subpopulations:

> Some scientists have raised concerns that the safety risks of Covid-19 vaccines have been underestimated. But the politics of vaccination has relegated their concerns to the outskirts of scientific thinking—for now.... *The large clustering of certain adverse events immediately after vaccination is concerning, and the silence around these potential signals of harm reflects the politics surrounding Covid-19 vaccines. Stigmatizing such concerns is bad for scientific integrity and could harm patients*.... The implication is that the risks of a Covid-19 vaccine may outweigh the benefits for certain low-risk populations, such as children, young adults and people who have recovered from Covid-19.... And while you would never know it from listening to public health officials, not a single published study has demonstrated that patients with a prior infection benefit from Covid-19 vaccination.... That this isn't readily acknowledged by the CDC or Anthony Fauci is an indication of how deeply entangled pandemic politics is in science.[68]

The doctors' assertions regarding natural immunity conferred by infection can be readily substantiated by reference to multiple studies, including one from the Cleveland Clinic showing that *not one* of 1,359 employees who had recovered from Covid suffered reinfection (even as significant numbers of non-vaccinated *and* some vaccinated employees did). Also, a recent British study following 2,800 previously infected persons for several months likewise registered *zero* reinfections.[69] On the theoretical level, Shane Crotty, virologist at the La Jolla Institute for Immunology, studied immune cells and antibodies for almost 200 persons recovered from Covid. His conclusion: "The amount of (immune) memory (gained from natural infection) would likely prevent the vast majority of people from getting... severe disease for many years."[70]

That the government does *not* publicly recognize these well-established facts (like its sanctioning of PCR tests with high-cycle thresholds, inevitably bloating Covid case counts, and its protocols resulting in conflation of deaths *by* Covid with deaths *with* Covid, likewise artificially inflating death counts) provides a clear window into why so many persons distrust the official line on most every aspect of Covid policy. Because of the government's enormous power, its scientifically faulty and ethically irresponsible policy (comprehensible only in conjunction with a careless disregard of the risks associated with vaccination) inevitably radiates out into society, resulting in tragic harm and unnecessary social division.

Fabio Berlingieri's seventeen-year-old son was required to undergo vaccination in order to play soccer, despite having previously recovered from Covid. A week after his first Pfizer dose (in 2021), the teen complained of severe pain in the heart region. He was soon forced to exchange a much anticipated prom date for an urgent trip to the ER, where he was treated for acute heart injury that precluded *any* strenuous activity (including soccer, of course) for an indefinite period of time.[71]

How would you feel if it happened to be your, or your son's, health that was so pointlessly sacrificed? My own twenty-one-year-old son suffers the other side of the same coin. He, too, has recovered from Covid, but because he chooses not to be vaccinated, he has been excluded from all group interaction at the company for which he works—this, despite the fact that science shows that he poses *less* of a risk to others than all the vaccinated employees. So does the government's own de facto disinformation campaign help rend the social fabric.

In general, healthy youth or young adults are at low risk of suffering serious illness or death from Covid and, if anything, at higher risk for vaccine-adverse events such as heart inflammation. As doctors Risch, Malone, and others suggest, rational, scientifically based analysis (rather than any calculus driven by fear, politics, and social pressure) would indicate that the costs of vaccination for this subgroup may well outweigh the potential benefits.

As far as children are concerned, the situation is still more clear. Children are at no significant risk of contracting Covid, and consequently (despite fabricated and scientifically unfounded fears of asymptomatic transmission) pose little real risk to others. This truth has been borne out by widespread school reopenings that have—as the absence of negative news on this front verifies—not resulted in worrisome incidence or spread of Covid-19. On the other hand, when considering vaccination of children, the safety concerns that have already been positively identified (including possible long-term compromise of reproductive organs) should naturally weigh hugely on the public conscience. Indeed, the idea of using a largely untested, experimental mRNA technology, one that *experience as well as theory* flag as potentially hazardous, to vaccinate millions of children against a disease *that poses no threat to them* appears tragically misguided to many informed persons. It is hard to imagine this as anything other than a brand of immoral recklessness conceivable only in a world held in the thrall of ignorance and hypnotized by fear.

Any number of persons have said as much, and said it, in fact, directly to the highest government authorities. Dr. Ros Jones, representing a group of

British doctors and academics under the umbrella of the Health Advocacy and Recovery Team, spoke at an FDA Public Hearing Session before the Vaccine and Related Biological Products Advisory Committee on June 10, 2021. Dr. Jones, in brief:

> We all know that the risk of harm from Covid-19 infection reduces the younger the age group under consideration, but it appears that for side effects, the opposite is true with both thrombocytopenia complications [blood clotting] and myocarditis [heart inflammations] having higher prevalence in younger age groups, and there clearly would have to be a tipping point.... We have no evidence that children need this and we have plenty of evidence accruing that the risk of harm will outweigh any potential benefit....
>
> We're rushing headlong into vaccinating children without adequate safety data, neither short-term nor long-term, and the ethics of that is, quite, I think, horrific. And particularly if we start talking about herd immunity, the ethics of expecting children to take a risk of harm for the sake of older adults is totally unacceptable.... Like the last two speakers, I would plead with the FDA not to rush ahead with any further approval.[72]

Diverse knowledgeable and articulate voices are speaking to these most urgent issues; of this, there is no doubt. As to whether the powers that be are really *interested in listening and making relevant information and perspectives available to the public*—well, to quote a character well acquainted with mind-forged manacles: "*That* is the question."

The possibility of the Covid vaccines adversely affecting fertility is yet another matter of import. The matter is highly controversial, with some highly qualified and experienced individuals (e.g., Dr. Janci Chunn Lindsay, who holds a doctorate in biochemistry and molecular biology and can point to thirty years of scientific work in toxicology and mechanistic biology) detailing grounds for urgent concern,[73] and others dismissing these as unfounded. I will not wade into these troubled waters except to observe that in this connection, too, it would seem that common sense would indicate that extreme caution is in order, especially in light of VAERS recording significant numbers of pregnancy-related adverse events.

Such deliberate circumspection, however, does not comport with the swift implementation of the vaccine program promoted by the pharmaceutical industry as well as the government. Indeed, Moderna is set to kick off a pregnancy-related study of its Covid vaccine on July 22, 2021. Over a thousand women over eighteen years of age will be enrolled. According to the brief summary of the trial, the object of the study is "to evaluate the outcomes of pregnancy in females exposed to the Moderna Covid-19 vaccine (mRNA-1273) during pregnancy."[74] Commenting on the forthcoming Moderna trial, one highly qualified (RS, MSN) nurse declared the obvious in rather blunt terms: "It's bass-ackward to release the vaccine to pregnant women before doing a clinical trial or proper animal studies."[75]

To conclude, I believe it fair to say that the "safe and effective" mantra drastically oversimplifies a complex, incompletely known, and, in many respects, deeply troubling picture. Meanwhile, the United States government, with the majority of the still panic-stricken populace in tow, shows little or no reluctance about barreling full speed ahead with what it continues to regard as the final solution to the pandemic problem. Yet numerous highly qualified professionals (a great many of whom are respected establishment figures and anything but "anti-vaxxers") do *not* see an overzealous vaccine campaign as the light at the end of the long Covid tunnel. Instead, such persons regard the no-holds barred vaccine push as a rash, risky, and fundamentally unethical gambit that could conceivably result in an indefinite extension of darkness.

Chapter 6

NEWSBREAK: A FEDERAL LAWSUIT AND DATA ANALYST JANE DOE

Naturally, news continues to break even as I work on this book. While it is impossible to stay on top of all relevant developments, a lawsuit filed in Alabama District Court just a few days ago (July 19, 2021) bears special mention, both because it summarizes many of the key arguments against vaccine mandates and because it reveals dramatic new evidence underscoring the potentially lethal risk run by those who submit to vaccination.

America's Frontline Doctors (AFLDS) filed a motion in Alabama Federal District Court seeking to halt the Emergency Use Authorization (EUA) of the Pfizer, Moderna, and Johnson & Johnson vaccines for three groups: persons under the age of 18; persons who have recovered from Covid; and all other Americans who have been denied the right to *informed consent* as required by federal law. The Children's Health Defense *Defender* summarized the 67-page suit's chief arguments in a number of bullet points.[76] I reproduce these here, reordered and slightly edited:

- There are adequate, approved, and available alternatives to vaccines.
- Vaccines do not diagnose, treat, or prevent SARS-CoV-2 or Covid.
- Known and potential risks of the vaccine outweigh their known and potential benefits.
- There is no bona fide emergency, which is a prerequisite to issuing EUA [Emergency Use Authorization] and EUA renewals for Covid vaccines.
- Healthcare professional and vaccine candidates are not adequately informed.

I have discussed the first and third points at some length; the second is more or less self-evident so long as it is recognized that the incidence of mild breakthrough cases is likely quite high. Let me briefly amplify the final two.

I have already highlighted the truth (the paramount importance of which can hardly be stressed enough) that granting of the EUA, and its repeated renewal, depends upon the tangibly false supposition that alternative treatment methods are not available and so should be regarded as largely politically motivated. The AFLDS suit elaborates additional facts that put the validity of the government's original emergency declaration, and its repeated renewals, in grave doubt.

Drawing upon Human Health Services (HHS) death data, the suit alleges that SARS-CoV-2 has an overall survivability rate of 99.8 percent. When adjusted for those under seventy years of age, that rate increases to 99.97 percent, a rate comparable to seasonal flu.[77]

The motion furthermore alleges that on March 24, 2020, HHS altered the rules applicable to all those responsible for producing death certificates (coroners and certain health professionals) so as to falsely attribute sole or primary causation to Covid-19. The new rule states: "COVID-19 should be reported on the death certificate for all decedents where the disease caused *or is assumed to have caused or contributed to* death" (emphasis mine). The latter clause is clearly dangerously ambiguous and open-ended. Indeed, according to the suit, HHS statistics showed that ninety-four percent of deaths attributed to Covid-19 involved no less than an average of four additional comorbidities.[78] What proportion of those cases should truly properly be attributed to Covid is anybody's guess.

Correlatively, the suit alleged that the use of highly unreliable PCR tests for diagnostic purposes artificially inflated *both* case and death counts. In this connection, it may be noted that both Alameda and Santa Clara Counties in California recently recognized the patent illegitimacy of the practice of attributing a death to Covid simply because the decedent may have tested positive for Covid-19, thus conflating death *by* Covid with death (possibly) <u>*with*</u> Covid. The counties accordingly reduced their official Covid death count by almost one-quarter. The *San José Spotlight* noted the following:

> Santa Clara County used to count COVID-19 deaths by including anyone who died while infected with the disease, even if it was not the cause or a contributing cause. For example, an individual who died in a car collision but had COVID at the time would count as a "COVID-19 death."[79]

So much for the (in)validity of the EUA. The most dramatic revelation associated with the AFLDS suit emerges in connection with the last point listed above: the quality of the information available to both health professionals and the public at large bears on the legal right to *informed* consent.

The filers of the suit attached the sworn statement of a whistleblower alleging that the number of deaths transpiring within 72 hours of receiving a COVID vaccine is actually dramatically highly than that officially published and acknowledged by VAERS. A computer programmer with professional expertise in healthcare data analytics, the (anonymous) whistleblower works for the government in the area of health fraud and enjoys privileged access to Medicare and Medical data available to the Centers for Medicare & Medicaid Services (CMS). Her declaration states:

> I am fully competent to make this declaration and I have personal knowledge of the facts stated in this declaration.
>
> This declaration is submitted in support of legal actions to revoke the emergency use authorization for COVID-19 injections and in support of a preliminary injunction to immediately block the emergency use authorization for COVID-19 injections.[80]

The conclusion, and gist, of the declaration reads:

> It is my professional estimate that VAERS (the Vaccine Adverse Event Reporting System) database, while extremely useful, is *under-reported by a conservative factor of at least 5.* On July 9, 2021, there were 9,048 deaths reported in VAERS. I verified these numbers by collating all of the data from VAERS myself, not relying on a third party to report them. In tandem, I queried data from CMS medical claims with regard to vaccines and patient deaths, and have assessed that *the deaths occurring within 3 days of vaccination are higher than those reported in VAERS by a factor of at least 5. This would indicate the true number of vaccine-related deaths* was at least *45,000.* Put in perspective, the swine flu vaccine, which was taken off the market, only resulted in *53* deaths.
>
> I declare under penalty of perjury under the laws of the United States of America that the forgoing is true and correct.[81]

In its suit, the AFLDS called attention to the rather shocking character of the disclosure and maintained that informed consent *cannot* truly be operative when pertinent safety data is either suppressed or patently misleading. The motion opines:

> It is unlawful and unconstitutional to administer experimental agents to individuals who cannot make an informed decision as to the true benefits and risks to the vaccine on an independent basis. They must be of an age or a capacity to make informed decisions and have been provided with all of the risk/benefit information necessary to make an informed decision.[82]

After you read this and other sections of this letter, and you avail yourself of whatever additional information you deem relevant, I encourage you to make your own objective and reasoned judgment as to whether the government's actions in the case of Covid-19 meet relevant legal criteria, ensuring *informed* consent to all Americans considering whether or not to undergo vaccination. I encourage you, as well, to consider, whatever one's own personal decision may be, the morality as well as legality of seeking to *compel* others to act against their own best judgment in what is, after all, a matter of life and death.

CHAPTER 7
DISSING DEMOCRACY: POWER AND MISINFORMATION

Most proponents of the controlling Covid narrative (in government, in industry and science, and in the populace at large) have one sure-fire way of dealing with all the questions and concerns raised in this letter, namely: Stick to your guns, and shoot down (with a loud *bang!*) any and everything coming your way as "mis-" or "disinformation." No matter how factually reliable the relevant material; no matter how authoritatively expert its source; no matter how well-grounded and reasoned the argument; no matter how civil the delivery or humane the motives of the messenger; *no matter what*, wheel the heavy artillery into place, aim, and shoot (vitamin D, HCQ, and effective early treatment options—***bang!***—unreliable PCR tests and inflated case and Covid-death counts—***bang!***—a dangerous spike protein, its distribution throughout the body, 10,000 to 45,000 or more dead from Covid-19 vaccines—***bang! bang! bang!***).

Yet shooting down offending messages only goes so far; it is more efficient to shoot the offending *messengers*. And in doing so, it seems they do not aim to kill but to incapacitate or, still better, by show of superior force, to preemptively keep them from serious engagement altogether. (Remember the CPSO: "*It is the professional responsibility of all physicians not to communicate anti-vax…*" and MP Sloan, "*They were very explicit…and threatened investigation or discipline.*) Of course, the more potential critics one can neutralize or marginalize with any given salvo or strategy, the better. Thus, our politically polarized society proves a convenient backdrop for demagoguery targeting the whole class of those questioning the mainstream story as right-wing extremists and worse. A March 21, 2021, Bloomberg piece titled "Are mRNA Covid Vaccines Risky? Here's What the Experts Say" includes a short section titled "Who's spreading disinformation about the vaccines?" It reads:

> Traditional anti-vaccine activists have increasingly joined forces with figures on the alt-right, a primarily online political movement based in the U.S. whose members espouse extremist beliefs typically centered on ideas of white nationalism. High-profile conservatives including Fox

News personality Tucker Carlson have raised doubts about Covid vaccines generally. According to the U.S. State Department, several online platforms linked to Russian Intelligence have spread disinformation about mRNA vaccines; Moderna and Pfizer are U.S.-based companies.[83]

So, we are given to believe that the likes of doctors McCullough, Risch, and Malone are probably really alt-right white supremacists *masquerading* as concerned physicians and compassionate human beings. And, of course, by this reasoning they may well be Russian tools, too, while the likes of doctors Byram Bridle and Ros Jones are undoubtedly subversive foreign agents. And, remember, this comes in a section purporting to inform us about *who* is spreading disinformation!

To its credit, the Bloomberg article does follow up with "rebuttals" of some of the disinformation spread by evil actors. These, however, rely, for their eminently questionable conclusions, upon the very government agencies whose facts and judgment are called into question by scientists and citizens less beholden to the system. Here, for instance, is the Bloomberg article's answer to the questions raised by reports of adverse vaccine effects:

> [Critics allege] that we don't know the long-term effects of the vaccines. That's always the case with new vaccines. But vaccine side effects usually show up within the first couple of months of vaccination, which is why the FDA insisted upon two months of safety data before authorizing them. Adverse event reports since then have not detected patterns of death that would indicate a problem with the vaccines, the CDC says.[84]

"*The CDC says…*"! But this blatantly contradicts the VAERS numbers which, at this juncture, indicate that the Covid vaccines are responsible for an *unprecedented* number of deaths. This would be at least *five times more true* if the whistleblower Jane Doe's sworn testimony has merit and it is, in fact, the CDC itself, that is deliberately producing and disseminating deadly disinformation.

Rhetorical combat of this sort, however, hardly exhausts the means employed to control the narrative and prevent the spread of purported misinformation and disinformation. Blatant censorship—that is, simply denying those who question the mainstream narrative access to public platforms—functions as a still more powerful weapon. That it is patently undemocratic, not to mention potentially unconstitutional, does not seem to faze the zeal of relevant authorities, including, lamentably, the United States President, who, in view of sagging vaccination numbers (at the time of this writing), has recently blessed a new initiative to crackdown on the supposed enemies of the regime.

On July 15, 2021, Dr. Vivek Murthy, the U.S. surgeon general, issued an alarming advisory, asserting that spreaders of health misinformation and disinformation have "threatened the U.S. response to Covid-19 and continue to prevent Americans from getting vaccinated, prolonging the pandemic and putting lives at risk." The advisory calls upon Big Tech and social media outlets to take more aggressive steps to prevent the dissemination of views that contradict the "best available evidence" as to the safety and efficacy of vaccines. Evidently aware that science does not speak with one voice on the matter, Murthy takes pains to cover his tracks, declaring that "claims can be highly misleading and harmful even if the science on an issue isn't yet settled.... We can meaningfully *improve the health information environment even without a consensus definition of misinformation* (emphasis mine)."[85]

Let's be clear about what this boils down to. Translated into plain English, it means *government and industry's policing of science* and suppressing what should, as a rule, be considered constitutionally protected freedom of speech. While it may be true that some related information spread on the web is inaccurate and misleading, this is evidently true on *both* sides of the Covid coin, and the winnowing of fact from fiction needs be left to the free market of mind, *impartial* science, and public opinion. *Censorship* based upon the *presumed* "truth" of any given position (such as the safety and efficacy of vaccines and the danger and inefficacy of other treatment methods) is manifestly subject to ideological and political bias and cannot be in the interest of objective inquiry, public health and welfare, or democratic society. Yet the surgeon general, acting at the behest of the U.S. President, seems to be advocating—indeed commanding—exactly that. The only reason the advisory may not necessarily qualify as a dictatorial and unlawful control of intellectual discourse is that the government here more or less orders tech companies and platforms to do its democracy-defying dirty work for it.

And none of this is theoretical, as it has been and is in force. Take the recent case of Bret Weinstein and his wife Heather Heying, two biologists who host the podcast *DarkHorse*, which commentator Matt Taibbi assures us "by any measure is among the more successful independent media operations in the country," broadcasting via two YouTube channels, a main channel and excerpted clips from those shows. According to Taibbi's article ("If Private Platforms Use Government Guidelines to Police Content, Is That State Censorship?"[86]), YouTube flagged the Weinstein's shows eleven times over the last month, targeting material addressing two medical health subjects: (1) The efficacy of ivermectin as a Covid-19 treatment, and (2) What Taibbi calls "the third rail of third rails: the possible shortcomings of the mRNA vaccines produced by companies like Moderna and Pfizer."[87]

It behooves us here to pause for a moment to look upon the spectacle unfolding before our eyes. Here we have a "democratic" government, the administrative leadership of the more "liberal" wing of American politics, the party that imagines itself the jealous guardian of the equality of *all* citizens, openly endorsing (and indeed practically enforcing) a dictatorial suppression of the right of freedom of speech—that very right which serves as the foundation stone of any republic and the careless compromise of which threatens the temple of democracy with imminent ruin. It is doing so, moreover, with the full-throated approval of much of its so-called liberal constituency, which somehow suddenly seems to have forgotten that the First Amendment is designed to preserve and protect the public domain as a forum of free and unprejudiced exchange of ideas and opinions.

This dangerous abuse of governmental power is naturally justified in the name of the greater public good, as, historically speaking, such abuses always are. Material ends, however, almost never justify undemocratic means, and the abrogation of the rights and prerogatives of individual citizens serves as fertile ground for social and political decay. As the high republican ideals fueling the French Revolution devolved into a bloody reign of terror, any person who showed the slightest disinclination to march in lockstep with the party line risked losing his or her head. Here in America, those who hold alternative views about the wisdom of universal vaccination do not have to fear literal decapitation; no, they only risk their professional and social position and the freedom to participate as full citizens in modern society.

Yes, you may say, but that incendiary comparison is not in the least bit apt. The Jacobins who blithely guillotined the Girondists, or the *sans-culottes* who thought nothing of reporting any countryman who displayed the least lack of revolutionary zeal: these parties were serving grotesquely distorted visions of truth and of right—unholy forms of unholy power—whereas we vaccine advocates are hardly caught in the thrall of any tainted ideology but merely championing rational, scientifically proven measures meant to ensure the life and greater liberty of *all* members of society.

Such protest rings peculiarly hollow. Why? Because it is just this premise that remains open to question—*and urgently needs to be kept open to question*—open to free, fair, *uncensored* public debate. After all, if truth and right are on that side, do you not trust that that side will win out *without* violating the foundations of science and democratic society by the forcible silencing of critics? Is not the necessity of censorship and suppression itself an admission of the uncertainty of the supposedly self-evident truths espoused?

Earlier this month, YouTube decided to demonetize Weinstein and Heying for their "offenses." According to Bret Weinstein, that drastic measure *halves* their income. As if that wasn't bad enough, Taibbi writes:

> YouTube's decision with regard to Weinstein and Heying seems part of an overall butterfly effect, as numerous other figures either connected to the topic or to *DarkHorse* have been censured by various platforms. Weinstein guest Dr. Malone, a former Salk Institute researcher often credited with helping develop mRNA vaccine technology, has been suspended from LinkedIn, and Weinstein guest Dr. Pierre Kory of the Front Line COVID-19 Critical Care Alliance (FLCCC) [Dr. McCullough's organization] has had his appearances removed by YouTube. Even Satoshi Omura, who won the Nobel Prize in 2015 for his work on ivermectin, reportedly had a video removed by YouTube this week.[88]

Taibbi points out that, whereas other deplatforming decisions involved electoral politics or suspicions of foreign intervention or incitement, the Weinstein and Heying case did not but *does* raise fundamental constitutional concerns hinging upon "the possible blurring of lines between public and private censorship."

Taibbi advances the cogent argument that if YouTube is consulting with federal agencies such as the CDC, FDA, and NIH as it develops its moderation guidelines with respect to health-related misinformation and disinformation, then persons such as Weinstein and Heying are in fact suffering from what is not only de facto but indeed de jure state censorship, in direct violation of the First Amendment. Such practice creates a situation in which government agencies are not only making public health policy but also controlling the parameters for private and public debate of the relevant issues. (As Weinstein himself observed of YouTube's moderation guidelines: "If it is in consultation with the government, it's an entirely different issue."[89]) Yet this, as Taibbi confirmed by way of conversation with YouTube representatives, is precisely what is going on. As Taibbi quoted the YouTube representatives: "When we develop our policies we consult outside experts.... In the case of our COVID-19 misinformation policies, it would be guidance from local and global health authorities."[90]

Taibbi goes on to document two specific exchanges in which Weinstein and Heying's podcast ran afoul of YouTube's misinformation guidelines: first, Dr. Robert Malone affirming, emphatically, that the mRNA spike protein is cytotoxic and dangerous and saying that he warned the FDA about that risk "months and months and months ago"; and second, where:

> entrepreneur and funder of fluvoxamine studies Steve Kirsch mentioned that his carpet cleaner had a heart attack minutes after taking the Pfizer vaccines and cited Canadian viral immunologist Byram Bridle is saying that the COVID-19 vaccine doesn't stay localized at the point of injection but "goes throughout your entire body, it goes to your brain and your heart."[91]

According to Taibbi:

> *Politifact* [YouTube's fact-checker] rated the claim that the spike protein is cytotoxic as "false," citing the CDC to describe the spike protein as "harmless." As to the idea that the protein does damage to other parts of the body, including the heart, they quoted the FDA spokesperson who said there's no evidence that the spike protein "lingers at any toxic level in the body."[92]

If I were betting on the truth of the matter, I'd put my money on Dr. Byram Bridle (who has risked his reputation to speak out in the interests of truth and children's health and safety) and Dr. Malone (who, as the putative inventor of mRNA technology, probably knows a thing or two about it) over faceless federal "fact-checkers." What about you? Think about it, pretending, for a moment, that—as in a game of Russian roulette—your life depends on it.

In any event, perhaps you are beginning to understand why, if you've generally relied upon readily available mainstream sources for your own Covid information, much of what I have shared so far may well be news to you. This is because the authorities are working tirelessly to make sure that, as a general rule, whatever prose or podcast or video clip *might make you think twice*...is simply not there.

Earlier in this book, I made an imperfect analogy between institutional racism and bias in public health policy. Taibbi offers a more accurate nomenclature for the mechanism at work: "regulatory capture." Taibbi writes:

> As with financial services, military contracting, environmental protection, and other fields, the phenomenon of regulatory capture is demonstrably real in the pharmaceutical world. This makes basing any moderation policy on official guidelines problematic.... If platforms like YouTube are

> basing speech regulation policies on government guidelines, and government agencies demonstrably can be captured by industry, the potential exists for a new kind of capture—intellectual capture, where corporate money can theoretically buy not just regulatory relief but the broader preemption of public criticism. It's vaccines today, and that issue is important enough, but what if in the future the questions involve...[93]

Taibbi finishes that sentence with his own examples, but I'd encourage you to use your imagination to fill in other options. The field of—not dreams, but—nightmares is nigh endless.

Matt Taibbi has hardly been the only one to recognize that *if* acts of Web censorship can tangibly be traced to government influence and interference, then such acts represent (as stated earlier) an unconstitutional violation of the First Amendment. Both government officials guilty of thus corruptly wielding power and the companies bowing to such illicit influence should be held accountable for such misdeeds. Accordingly, in December 2020, Informed Consent Action Network (ICAN) filed suit in the San Jose Division of the United States District Court alleging that, in response to government pressure, YouTube and Facebook illegally deplatformed content—most important, Del Bigtree's popular internet talk show *The HighWire*—in order to forestall any legislative action that would adversely affect their business. The complaint begins:

> One of the fundamental tenants of our democracy is that the First Amendment prohibits government officials from censoring speech they dislike or disagree with. For this principal to have meaning, a government official cannot use a private actor as a cat's paw to censor speech they dislike or disagree with. Nevertheless, this matter presents just such a situation, where government actors used threats to Defendant's businesses to force them to censor speech that the government actors knew they were prohibited from censoring directly.[94]

The circumstances surrounding the alleged violation revolve around Section 230 of the 1996 Communications Decency Act. That act, passed in the early days of the Internet, aimed in part to ensure the free flow of information and discussion on the Web. Section 230 plays a pivotal role in this respect. Protecting internet providers from liability for speech acts posted on their platforms, it frees companies from concerns about costly defamation suits. As the Internet evolved, the act, while indeed promoting free speech, simultaneously came to function as an integral part of the business model of companies such as YouTube and Facebook. As the complaint states:

> Typically, social media companies like the Defendants [e.g., YouTube and Facebook] thrive on user traffic. The more people who come to the sites, the more advertising the companies can sell. This business model, coupled with protection from section 230, meant that before 2016 there was little incentive for Defendants to censor their users' free speech. Even if the Defendants disliked or disagreed with postings—like efforts to influence an election—the Defendants still could make money selling ads on those disfavored postings.[95]

The year 2016 stands out as the time that the threat of foreign (especially Russian) interference emerged as a clear and present danger in the context of that year's presidential election. In response to this threat, Congress not only undertook numerous investigations but additionally instituted measures requiring social media companies to share information that might aid in the government's effort to prevent illegal foreign interference. According to the ICAN complaint, in order to finally secure the cooperation of the Internet companies, Congress "openly questioned whether to eliminate section 230 in order to make companies like Defendants [YouTube and Facebook] more 'accountable' for what users put on their sites."[96]

The ICAN complaint recognized the legitimacy of government actions taken in order to curb illegal interference in the American political process. At the same time, the complaint describes how such action effectively set the stage for future governmental abuse of power. The mere threat of revising or revoking Section 230—the legal clause which provided protection indispensable to YouTube and Facebook's business operations—could conceivably be employed to coerce Internet companies to cooperate in an effort to restrict legitimate and legally protected speech by American citizens, if such speech were viewed as undermining the official position on one or another matter of public policy.

In the case brought by ICAN, the relevant government official happened to be Congressman Adam Schiff, and the relevant matter at hand, Covid-19 vaccines. Alluding, first, to the (justifiable) governmental action taken to preclude foreign interference in American elections, the complaint asserts:

> However, having found a tool in Defendants [such as YouTube and Facebook] to limit speech for a justifiable purpose, Chairman Schiff decided to use this same tool to limit other speech that, while not illegal, he did not like. Chairman Schiff considered so-called "vaccine misinformation" to be dangerous. Therefore, he wrote letters to Defendants probing into

the steps taken by Defendants to combat what he defined as "vaccine misinformation."[97]

These letters, the complaint alleges, produced the desire effect: the censoring of *The HighWire* and other ICAN content that contested the officially sanctioned Covid narrative and its relentless championing of vaccines as *the* answer to the problem.

The verdict in the case is still pending. Whatever the court ultimately decides, however, it seems evident that we have here all the ingredients of what Taibbi calls "intellectual capture."

It is not Congressman Schiff's, or the CDC's, or any government official or agency's role to monitor or control legal speech on this or any issue of public import, and the exercise of such control cannot be justified by the debatable presumption of the "danger" represented by one or another position. The violation of First Amendment rights and "broader preemption of public criticism" affected in this and similar instances need be seen for what it is: government overreach that amounts to dangerous authoritarianism.

In other contexts, Congressman Adam Schiff has shown himself to be a passionate and articulate defender of the public weal. That in this case it is he who is alleged to have abused the power of his position sets in stark relief the moral darkness shrouding all things concerning Covid, and, in particular, *the insidious capture of the liberal conscience by unprincipled, illiberal, and finally antidemocratic forces.* This destructive development finds expression, too, in another Covid-related legal circumstance.

When I was growing up in the suburbs north of Chicago, my father—at the time, a lawyer for a prestigious Chicago firm—satisfied his higher moral obligations by engaging in intensive pro bono work for the American Civil Liberties Union (ACLU). In our house, above all, the ACLU stood for defense of the hallowed principle of freedom of speech. Its most notorious case revolved around the organization's controversial defense of a Nazi group's right to public demonstration in nearby Skokie, a heavily Jewish suburb where my uncle happened to reside.

Much more recently, my father almost severed his lifelong connection with the ACLU because of its position on *Citizen's United.* Evidently, the ACLU's reverence for freedom of speech is so expansive as to include corporate expenditures under that sacred aegis. Judging, however, from its complete quiet on the Covid front, a Nazi group's right to demonstrate not so very far from a Jewish cemetery and the right of giant corporations (such as Pfizer) to spend money in their own political interest represents constitutionally protected speech, but the considered opinions of knowledgeable physicians and conscientious and informed citizens on urgent matters of public health and welfare does not. Squarely confronted with what may well be considered the preeminent freedom of speech issue of the twenty-first century, the ACLU, that vaunted champion of the liberal cause, does not roar like a lion, nor even squeak like a mouse, but maintains an ominous, deathly silence.

Chapter 8

NEWSBREAK: HOLDING THE LINE: JOURNALISTS AGAINST COVID CENSORSHIP

It is not only social media platforms such as YouTube and Facebook that have effectively suppressed free speech and fair discussion of all things Covid-19. *The New York Times, Washington Post, San Francisco Chronicle,* and the like mainstream news sources home and abroad have done and continue to do likewise, even though, given the intrinsic differences in these forms of media, the mechanisms for suppression inevitably differ. Even if journalists do write stories offering perspectives that contest the controlling narrative, publishers and editors typically decline to run those stories. Such practice contravenes basic journalistic principles and operates as a mechanism of de facto violation of freedom of the press internal to the industry itself. It goes without saying that the consequent (mis)shaping of news inevitably (mis)shapes public opinion as well. If revelation of truth, rather than ideological conquest, be the objective, there is never just one side of any story worth telling.

Recently, almost thirty UK journalists formed Holding the Line: Journalists Against Covid Censorship, a group dedicated to calling attention to and redressing this destructive dynamic.[98] One of the group's members, investigative journalist Sonia Elijah, described the group's motive and aims:

> It's been unprecedented the way Covid-19 has been reported in the UK but not just in the UK, worldwide. There's only been one official narrative played out in the mainstream media.... There's only been one 'scientific truth' allowed to be discussed: the one endorsed by worldwide governmental regulatory bodies, even that has been very selective. This has given the public a distorted view of the truth which has been highly damaging.[99]

Elijah cites lack of relevant context for statistics, inadequate coverage of alternative treatments methods, insufficient scrutiny of PCR testing, relative inattention to adverse vaccine reactions, and the costs of lockdowns as marked deficiencies in media coverage of Covid to date. She stresses, too, her deep concern regarding online censorship channeled through the Trusted News Initiative (TNI), a fact-checking organ that polices so-called misinformation and disinformation by way of politically compromised methods analogous to those employed in the United States.

Former BBC journalist Tony Gosling, another member of the group, added this perspective:

> Our main concern is that there's a very powerful lobby behind many of these Covid measures, including treatment, lack of treatment and vaccines, obviously, but there isn't much of a lobby in the other direction. And I think that most of us feel that our employers of various sorts have not been representing both sides. My own aim is to provide balance.... And also to point out to the public that journalists don't always get to choose what gets published. It's the owners and the editors that have final say. So there's always an editor somewhere just saying no, I don't want this, and particularly through this pandemic that's the way it's been, people have found it difficult to get stories in, and it's been frustrating.[100]

The group's secretary, who, like most of the group members, chose to remain unnamed, highlighted the oppressive atmosphere that prevents the news industry from fulfilling its appointed mission:

> It's a difficult time for journalists to go against the grain and we have heard examples of freelancers being blacklisted and of those, with legacy media contracts, being criticised by their managers for wanting to cover stories on vaccine harm and the fallibility of the PCR test. But we are not holding a stance one way or the other on any issue, we just want newspapers and the broadcast media to host balanced debate and for that debate to take place without fear of reprisals in newsrooms.[101]

The last comments go to the heart of the civil liberty concerns bound up with Covid-19. Liberalism prides itself on its supposedly enlightened views on matters of liberty, equality, and human community, yet those holding the mainstream "liberal" line on Covid would do well to recollect the sentiment famously (but probably incorrectly) ascribed to Voltaire: "I disagree with what you say, but I will defend to the death your right to say it."[102] The most important subtext associated with Covid-19 does not revolve around one or another view of the relevant science but whether or not the true spirit of the Enlightenment—which also happens to be the foundation stone of democracy—will be respected and sociopolitically preserved or, on the contrary, deliberately "dissed" and seriously, if not fatally, compromised.

Chapter 9

LINES OF FORCE: UNDERMINING THE COMMONS

Having completed my exposition (supplemented by newsbreaks) of the five points of concern enumerated near the beginning of this volume, I now wish to assess, in still more critical and rather more theoretical terms, the sociopolitical dimension of the Covid debate, recognizing that, as philosopher Paul Feyerabend argued in his classic works *Against Method*[103] and *Science in a Free Society*,[104] this dimension materially affects (what passes for) science in any given day or age.

Indeed, the most important issue at the core of the whole Covid matter is not, ultimately, the safety or efficacy of vaccines or the merit of alternative treatment options but the integrity (or lack thereof) of democratic process in American society today. The solution to one or another pressing scientific or policy question is less important than the often hidden sociopolitical and institutional dynamics determining *how* such questions have been and are being negotiated in the public and private spheres—in the internal workings of, and all-important interfaces between, science, industry, government, media, individual citizens, and the populace at large.

To be sure, the whole complex Covid dilemma ultimately crystallizes around attitudes and policies regarding vaccination. That focus has, as I have sought to show, effectively been written into the script from the first. Even so, to *fixate* at present on the pros and cons of vaccination *as if moral and practical consideration of that question could be lifted out of the context of the whole complex history of Covid to date* represents a dangerously myopic perspective—one, I fear, that intensifies the destructive polarization of society that has marked Covid politics from the first.

As an individual currently opposed to vaccine mandates, I would ask those who believe it right and just to impose the same to take a step back and consider all that has transpired in government, industry, science, Big Tech, and the press to have created—or at least fed into—the situation we find ourselves in at the time of this writing. While one or another contention advanced in the course of this volume may well be debatable, I would propose that the weight of the collective evidence points to a pervasive and systematic pattern of duplicity, coercion, and suppression of dissent on the part of those actors, known and unknown, responsible for generating and sustaining the controlling Covid narrative. PCR tests were known, from the outset, to be notoriously unreliable and indeed, at the high-cycle thresholds positively recommended by government agencies, virtually useless as a diagnostic tool. Nonetheless, numberless individuals who tested positive without showing symptoms were, and indeed continue to this day to be, logged as Covid cases. Hospitals were financially incentivized to chalk up countless deaths to Covid after an inexplicable change in death certificate protocol cleared a path to do just that. The combined effect of these two duplicitous practices alone has played, and continues to play, an enormous role in the public perception of the elevated risk of mortal danger posed by Covid. Concomitantly, the *real* as well as *perceived* threat posed by Covid has been and continues to be immeasurably magnified by the refusal of government agencies to invest virtually any resources in the research, development, and use of non-vaccine preventative and early outpatient treatment measures. While it is certainly fair to debate the efficacy of treatment protocols like those advanced by Dr. Peter McCullough, Dr. Pierre Kory, and the Frontline Covid-19 Critical Care Alliance (FLCCC)—and these *should* be *freely* debated in the scientific and public forums—the charge that responsible government agencies have neglected and indeed sought to block any and all initiatives responsive to the urgent need for prophylaxis and early prevention can scarce be gainsaid.

Such compound errors of omission and commission, justified, in significant part, by the spreading of what may well be regarded as misinformation and disinformation (for instance, suddenly declaring, for spurious and fabricated reasons, long-popular HQC unsafe) produces the impression of a deliberate pattern of distortion profoundly, indeed, tragically, deleterious to public health and welfare. (President Biden heatedly charges dissenting parties with "killing people," but how many lives have been lost, and how much suffering needlessly sustained, on account of the United State government's recalcitrant refusal to promote prophylaxis and early outpatient treatment?) That pattern, moreover, seems logically explicable only in light of the appalling notion that corrupt influences have rendered critical organs of government *more* interested in promoting the severity of the pandemic itself and the vaccine-only solution to it than in exploring and pursuing policy initiatives that prioritize public health and welfare. Correlatively, and just as tragically, the systematic suppression of free speech and demonization of dissent that (taking its cue from on high) has spread throughout the populace cannot but strengthen this odious impression, even while highlighting the huge political costs exacted by the dangerous notion that public health ends tied to the vaccine agenda justify undemocratic and likely unconstitutional means of intellectual and social control.

Knowledge of certain hidden details pertaining to unholy contracts between government and the pharmaceutical industry further enhance the appearance of bad faith and illicit collusion between government and industry. In the earlier chapter "Bad Actors," I alluded, in general terms, to ways and means by which the pharmaceutical industry exercises influence over government agencies, but it is all too easy to supply multiple disturbing particulars. According to one reliably iconoclastic source:

> Conflicts of interests are present at all levels, including our most prestigious public health agencies. While the US Centers of Disease Control and Prevention has long fostered the perception of independence, claiming it does not accept funding from special interests, the agency has in fact made itself beholden to Big Pharma by accepting millions in corporate donations through its government-chartered foundation, the CDC Foundation, which funnels those contributions to the CDC after deducting a fee.
>
> Several watchdog groups—including the US Right to Know (USRTK), Public Citizen, Knowledge Ecology International, Liberty Coalition, and the Project on Government Oversight—filed a petition urging the CDC to cease making these false disclaimers. According to the petition, the CDC accepted $79.6 million from drug companies and commercial manufacturers between 2014 and 2018 alone. This is beyond unacceptable, as the CDC was created to be a public health watchdog.... It has tremendous influence within the medical community, and part of this influence hinges on the concept that it's free of industry bias and conflicts of interest.[105]

The hold exerted by pharmaceutical companies and its potential for not merely influencing but determining public-health policy emerges in the recently leaked contracts[106] setting the terms of government purchase of the Pfizer Covid-19 vaccine. While the documents discovered disclose contracts signed with Albania and Brazil, not the United States, Pfizer typically employs a set template for its contracts so that, while cost may vary significantly from country to country, the basic protective clauses of the contract may be expected to be largely the same. It is consequently revealing that the contracts clearly convey that Pfizer, *not* the governments purchasing from it, effectively holds all the power cards. Not only does the contract protect the company from all legal liability for harm or injury resulting from its product and releases the company from the necessity to meet any particular delivery deadlines, it includes a clause stipulating that no discovery of any other effective drug or treatment method can lawfully release the government customer from the financial obligations incurred in the contract. Such financially binding commitment to the vaccine solution (already over a year prior to this writing, the U.S. committed roughly *$2 billion* to the purchase of the Pfizer vaccine) *clearly discourages robust pursuit of alternative, potentially far less expensive, preventative and treatment options.* In the words of the individual who discovered and disclosed the document:

> If you are wondering why ivermectin was suppressed, well, it is because the agreement with Pfizer does not allow them to escape their contract, which states that even if a drug will be found to treat Covid-19 the contract cannot be voided.[107]

The commitment to a vaccine-only solution has not only conditioned government policy, it has led to official revision of the very *language* employed to think about what constitutes a pandemic and, perhaps still more critically, the chief means of escaping from one—that is, herd immunity. Prior to the 2009 swine flu pandemic, the WHO's definition of "pandemic" included a clause stipulating that a pandemic involved "enormous numbers of deaths and illnesses." In the months leading up to the onset of that flu, however, that clause was excised so that a "pandemic" could be declared in the face of any "worldwide epidemic of disease," *regardless of whether or not such disease caused excess mortality.*[108] This perhaps seemingly minor alteration opens the door to a much looser use of the psychologically loaded term. That change is peculiarly significant to the case of Covid-19, because data from 2020 actually reveals *no* excess of mortality,[109] a fact that could and has been interpreted as reinforcing the supposition that many deaths attributed to Covid were actually caused by a variety of other comorbidities. Instead of one column (heart disease, for instance), the relevant statistic found its way into another *without* significantly altering the overall sum.

One could perhaps contend that this amounts to quibbling—that it is patently obvious that the world is indeed in the throes of what, by any reasonable definition, can rightly be called a pandemic. I will not argue that here (though no few knowledgeable persons would do so) but rather point to the still more significant redefinition of the crucial concept of *herd immunity,* one that critics of the WHO see as a deliberate stratagem intended to frame vaccination as the only viable solution to any and all pandemic disease.

As recently as June 2020, the WHO's website defined "herd immunity" as "the indirect protection from an infectious disease that happens when a population is immune either through vaccination *or immunity developed through previous infection.*"[110] In mid-November of 2020, however, the WHO updated its website, which now describes herd immunity as *"a concept used for vaccination,* in which a population can be protected from a certain virus *if a threshold of vaccination is reached.*"[111] The ideological and political intent of this difference should be obvious. The new phrasing effectively endorses an agenda of mass vaccination and entirely eliminates the key idea, central to immunology for a century or more, that human beings possess immune systems *naturally* designed to adapt to and defend against illness. The new WHO website additionally advances the at best dubious and at worst dead wrong claim that "herd immunity is achieved by protecting people from a virus, not by exposing them to it."[112]

A piece for the American Institute for Economic Research offers the following commentary on these emendations:

> The World Health Organization, for reasons unknown, has suddenly changed its definition of a core conception of immunology: herd immunity. Herd immunity speaks directly, and with explanatory power, to the empirical observation that respiratory viruses are either widespread and mostly mild (common cold) or very severe and short-lived (SARS-CoV-1).
>
> The reason is that when a virus kills its host...the virus does not spread to others. The more this occurs, the less it spreads....When it happens to enough people...the virus loses its pandemic quality and becomes endemic, which is to say predictable and manageable.
>
> This is what one would call Virology/Immunology 101. It's what you read in every textbook. It's been taught in 9th grade cell biology for probably 80 years. And the discovery of this fascinating dynamic in cell biology is a major reason why public health became so smart in the 20th century. We kept calm. We managed viruses with medical professionals: doctor/patient relationships....
>
> Until one day...the World Health Organization suddenly decided to delete everything I just wrote from cell biology basics.... *It has removed with the delete key any mention of natural immunity....* This change at WHO ignores and even wipes out 100 years of medical advances in virology, immunology, and epidemiology. It is thoroughly unscientific.

> What's even stranger is the claim that a vaccine protects people from a virus rather than exposing them to it. What's amazing about this claim is that a vaccine works precisely by firing up the immune system through exposure.... *There is simply no way for medical science completely to replace the human immune system.* It can only game it via what used to be called inoculation.[113]

The writer of this report accuses the WHO of "shilling for the vaccine industry in exactly the way the conspiracy theorists say that WHO has been doing since the beginning of the pandemic."[114] The criticism is a harsh one, but how else is one to interpret the evident bastardization of long-established semantic and scientific norms? Such conduct can readily incline a rational mind toward considering what might instinctively be regarded as "fringe" conspiracy theory as not so very far-fetched after all but, on the contrary, reasonable if not probable. This is all the more so if one takes into account the WHO's widely recognized deep financial ties to persons heavily invested in the pharmaceutical agenda (the Bill and Melinda Gates Foundation).

Very well, you might say, *I see how one may perhaps credibly discern a pattern of systematic deception, but some degree of corruption is more or less endemic to political institution, and these various threads do not necessarily weave together into any coherent design that would fundamentally alter my view of the facts on the ground. Just because there may be some influence peddling inherent in the operation of governmental and international agencies—well, I'm sure that's not the whole or most important part of the story or sufficient reason for me to revise my overall picture of what is really going on. And surely trusted liberal news sources—the* Washington Post, The New York Times*—are not part of any collusion that may be taking place but exercise independent investigative and critical judgment before delivering their versions of the truth or arriving at their editorial positions. Ultimately, when it comes to the most pressing practical concern—in this case, the value of vaccination—the facts upon which I base my own practical and moral judgments more or less speak for themselves.*

Yet I would contest the truth of all these suppositions, not excluding (like the British journalists and newsroom staff who formed *Holding the Line*) this last. In an article for *The Pulse* ("Want to Get to 70% Vaccine Coverage, Mr. President? Here's How You Do It"[115]), Dr. Madhava Setty, an unvaccinated physician who declares himself perfectly open to undergoing vaccination *if* both scientific and sociopolitical considerations convince him that it is the right thing to do, sets out nine conditions, the fulfillment of which could move him in that direction. In the course of expounding his fifth point ("Call off the censorship dogs and unqualified 'fact-checkers'"), Dr. Setty provides an example of how, even as content challenging the prevailing narrative is often summarily and unfairly dismissed as misinformation or disinformation, mainstream media outlets (such as the *Times* and the *Post*) seemingly own a free pass to traffic in what amounts, finally, to patent falsehood. Dr. Setty notes:

> The Washington Post, widely considered an example of balanced and thorough reporting, published an article titled "The Unseen Covid-19 risk for unvaccinated people" in May, 2021. In it they present dozens of graphs that seem to demonstrate the growing difference in disease incidence, hospitalizations and deaths between the vaccinated and unvaccinated population. This is pure speculation based on the *assumption* that the vaccine is, and continues to be, 85% protective with regard to infection alone. This assumption is hidden in their "methodology" section at the end of the article. The diverging plots of the vaccinated and unvaccinated are purely the result of a mathematical artifact that grows as more people get vaccinated. They didn't add up the number of people who were getting sick/hospitalized or dying based on vaccination status. They couldn't. That data is not available (see request #1). Where are the fact checkers and advisory bots with warnings of "missing context" and "partly false information"? Instead, they drew their pretty graphs using terms like "rate adjusted for vaccinated" to imply that the unvaccinated are doing much worse. They further had the audacity to use this assumed efficacy for reducing infection rates and apply it to hospitalizations and deaths as well. This is pure prevarication. The casual reader will easily conclude that vaccines are having a phenomenal impact. We cannot make that conclusion.[116]

The full list of Dr. Setty's conditions of reconsideration is worth noting. It reads:

1. Show me the Data.
2. Put proven prophylaxis and treatment alternatives in the [CDC] guidelines.
3. Release documents requested under the FOIA (Freedom of Information Act) without redaction.
4. Mainstream Media must present both sides of the argument before I will accept what they have to say at face value.
5. Call off the censorship dogs and unqualified "fact-checkers."

6. Vaccine manufacturers need to release interim data from their ongoing trials.
7. MSM [The Morehouse School of Medicine] and their band of "experts" need to admit that they completely blew it with regard to lab origin.
8. The CDC needs to explain why they are using a double standard with regard to cases.
9. Stop decrying natural immunity as an absurd hypothesis while insisting that I should trust "the science."[117]

Many (although not all) of Dr. Setty's points reflect arguments already presented in this volume. The last point, of course, alludes to the critical matter addressed in the American Institute for Economic Research piece—namely, the definition and understanding of herd immunity. Setty writes:

> Is it possible that vaccine-mediated immunity for SARS-COV2 is better than natural immunity? If it were, we wouldn't be seeing what we are seeing now. There are only a handful of documented reinfections with SARS-COV2 in the world yet thousands of "breakthrough" infections in the vaccinated populations of this country alone—so many that this likely compelled the CDC to come up with their double standard for diagnosing infections (see request #8).[118]

Setty's discussion of that double standard in his request #8 engages the crucial matter of the *quality* of data available to anyone wishing to make an informed judgment about the benefits and risks of vaccination. Unsurprisingly, the concern harkens back to the seminal issue of the (un)reliability of PCR testing. I give Dr. Setty's lengthy explanation in full because it so graphically illustrates biases written into the handling of the pandemic from the first:

> Our entire understanding of the severity of the pandemic and the efficacy of our response to it is based on a huge question: how accurate is our means of diagnosing the disease? The RT-PCR test is wonderful technology but it is not designed to diagnose an active infection. That means that the actual number of infections and deaths are uncertain. No test is 100% accurate, however, we have little understanding of how *inaccurate* this test is. The sensitivity of the PCR test...and its specificity...both vary with the cycle threshold (the number of amplification cycles used). The more cycles used, the fewer the cases that will be missed (increased sensitivity) while raising the potential for overdiagnosis (decreasing specificity). Fewer cycles used will result in the opposite effect.

> We do not know what the optimal cycle threshold is; however, we should at least expect that our authorities on the matter would have standardized that number from the very beginning. They have recently done so but only with regard to breakthrough infections, i.e. after vaccinations became available. During the early months of the pandemic there were no limits placed on cycle thresholds. Some labs were using cycle threshold numbers of 30, 35, or even more. Now when considering infections in those that have been vaccinated a case is only a case if a PCR test returns a positive result using a cycle threshold of 28 or below *and* the person is hospitalized or dies. There are still no standards for the unvaccinated. This unquestionably will raise the incidence of the disease in the unvaccinated while lowering the incidence in those who receive the jab.
>
> Let's use an example to demonstrate how egregiously biased this double standard is. If you have been vaccinated and then come down with Covid and get hospitalized, you *do not* count as a breakthrough case if your PCR test was positive using a cycle threshold of 29. On the other hand, if you have not been vaccinated, have no symptoms and get tested in order to return to work or school after going on vacation and your PCR test comes back positive after 40 cycles you *do* count as a case...The end result: the efficacy of the vaccine is being artificially enhanced while simultaneously the presumed risk of remaining unvaccinated gets amplified. Until the CDC explains itself, their edict to vaccinate should be considered disingenuous at best.[119]

I began this chapter by asserting that any fair weighing of the merit of vaccination (and, consequently, any possible justification for *mandating* vaccination) *cannot* be rationally conducted unless it is accompanied by critical review of certain crucial sociopolitical lines of force and their influence upon the relevant scientific information base. What I have shared so far may perhaps persuade you that this is no abstract imperative that a conscientious citizen can casually override by recourse to common-sense evaluation of self-evident empirical realities. To be sure, a certain indeterminate number of persons are suffering from Covid-19. That much can be confidently stated, but the moment we move beyond that relatively firm footing, any attempt to come to an objective view of the whole complex Covid situation rapidly mires in quicksand. Most every aspect of the controlling Covid narrative has been, and continues to be, conditioned if not determined by profound systematic biases in industry, government, and the media. Those biases, in turn, translate into partisan censorship that, as Dr. Donald Welsh and many others have so passionately stated, impugns the integrity of what is called "science" and manipulates public opinion.

I would submit that no one who chooses to blithely ignore all these lines of force can really make an informed decision as to the merits of vaccination for their own selves, let alone claim the intellectual and moral standing to legislate that decision for others. This is all the more the case if such a person stubbornly refuses even to grant a hearing to others who, far from being irrational and antisocial lepers, may in fact entertain deep, and deeply considered, concerns about these Covid-associated matters. Heated condemnation of dissent, regrettably exemplified by none other than President Biden himself, wounds American democracy by supercharging what is already a terribly destructive dynamic: the transformation of the public commons into what is, at best, a condition of hostile standoff and, at worst, a field of war.

Dr. Setty's article begins with a description of how he and his wife encountered another couple at a social gathering who asked if they were vaccinated. Dr. Setty and his wife admitted that they were not and were anxious to engage in a civil and mutually respectful exchange on the topic. The male in the other party, however, was not open to any such dialogue and exhibited such evident hostility that the Settys soon felt compelled to leave the gathering altogether. To that end, Dr. Setty's article, while primarily a vehicle for elaborating his chief concerns respecting the mainstream Covid narrative, also sounds a plea for the kind of civic dialogue defeated by minds closed shut in dismissive disdain. It concludes:

> So, to the couple at the party who couldn't understand our reasoning, I hope you know that we all want the same things: to live long and healthy lives, to enjoy the company of others, to exchange ideas openly without being attacked or dismissed. We aren't completely closed to hearing your side. In fact we have been hearing your side loud and clear for a while now. Have you heard our side? *Or are you only listening to what your side is saying about our side*? Those are two entirely different things.
>
> I cannot speak for every one of us but I certainly would be willing to discuss these matters so that we can understand each other better. If these requests seem flippant or poorly thought out to you I can understand why you would wish to exclude us from your lives or talk about us behind closed doors. You may think we are paranoid, intractable and irresponsible, but please don't call us uninformed or easily seduced by false narratives. Those labels do not apply to us.[120]

For my part, I would be tempted to add, which of the parties here is likely *"too easily seduced by false narratives?"* Yet as Dr. Setty's firm but courteous tone implies, it is necessary, too, to lay our foils aside if we are ever truly to touch each other again. We desperately need to reclaim, in the private as well as public sphere, a space of civil discourse. Dialogue is the life breath of society, and in its absence, democracy chokes and dies.

Chapter 10:

NEWSBREAK: A JOURNALISTIC CONFLICT OF INTEREST? REUTERS, PFIZER, AND THE TNI

Still more news about news: how it is laundered, routinely washed, and dried clean of all matter regarded as detrimental to certain vested interests. The venerable name "Reuters" probably conjures images of journalistic objectivity, of transparent transmission of the latest facts courtesy of an array of dependable sources. Did you, however, know that, after signing contracts with Facebook and, a week before the time of this writing, Twitter, Reuters has recently gone into the ever more popular business of fact-checking social-media posts? This particular service, though, does not stop at comment boxes noting "missing context" or "false or misleading content." Reuters creates a commentary on relevant fact-checked content and publishes these in the form of what appear to be snippets of current news. In accord with the terms of the Facebook and Twitter contracts, this "trusted news" pops up in response to relevant searches on the part of millions of users.[121]

The Thomas Reuters Foundation that sponsors and orchestrates this endeavor presents itself as "the corporate foundation of Thomas Reuters, the global news and information company." As per its website, the foundation professes to help "local media to produce *accurate, impartial, and reliable journalism*." The foundation trains "reporters around the world, promoting *integrity, independence, and freedom from bias* in news reporting."[122] All this sounds very salutary. What is decidedly less so—and indeed stands in flagrant contradiction of these noble aims—are the Foundation's undisclosed ties to other entities that enmesh it in multiple conflicts of interest, namely the TNI, Pfizer, and the World Economic Forum (WEF).

Reuters and its Institute of Journalism are members of TNI, which describes its chief aim to be to "protect audiences and users from disinformation, particularly around moments of jeopardy, such as elections." In December of 2020, TNI announced a new initiative responsive to the world crisis precipitated by the spread of the coronavirus. Presuming, without substantive debate, that mass vaccination represents the chief means of combating the virus, TNI declared that since the success of any vaccination program depended upon public trust, its mission would henceforth include a focus upon preventing the dissemination of vaccine disinformation.

As noted in the earlier introduction of the new British group Holding the Line, the British Broadcasting Corporation acts as an official partner of TNI and is closely associated with it. By the BBC's own report, TNI's other partners include Google/YouTube, Facebook, Microsoft, *The Washington Post* (owned by Jeff Bezos), Twitter, the Associated Press, Agence France-Presse, CBC/Radio-Canada, European Broadcasting Union, the *Financial Times*, First Draft, and *The Hindu*.[123]

In its December 2020 press release, TNI elaborated its reason for its new focus:

> With the introduction of several possible new COVID-19 vaccines, there has been a rise of 'anti-vaccine' disinformation spreading online to millions of people.
>
> Examples include widely shared memes which link falsehoods about vaccines to freedom and individual liberties. Other posts seek to downplay the risks of coronavirus and suggest there is an ulterior motive behind the development of a vaccine.
>
> TNI partners will alert each other to disinformation which poses an immediate threat to life so content can be reviewed promptly by platforms, whilst publishers ensure they don't unwittingly republish dangerous falsehoods.[124]

This is absolutely breathtaking. We are looking here at an official body, one whose stated mission is the protection of objective truth, undertaking to police, both systematically and aggressively, the "free" press and social-media outlets in (chiefly) the United States, Canada, and Europe. What is most disturbing is that TNI *evinces no consciousness whatsoever* that its professed project exhibits a mindset fully worthy of authoritarian and even totalitarian rule, an ideological blindness that one might well expect in Communist China or, yes, a protofascist state such as that of Germany in the run-up to Hitler's rule.

I know that such claims are sensational and usually readily dismissed because of their implausible extremity, but I urge you to read over TNI's language again and ask yourself this: what is the material difference between the behavior of such dictatorial regimes and the TNI's own with regard to the all-important matter of the freedom of expression and free press? We are speaking, remember, of the liberty *to speak out publicly and debate an issue of overriding societal import*—a right essential to democratic society and indeed its central pillar. But the TNI, like some supreme leader or ruling party, exhibits no compunction about simply *assuming* that it knows the truth of the matter and, consequently, knows what is right and good for all, imagining that it is serving the best interests of humanity by eliminating all discourse that dares to disagree.

Indeed, in the indoctrinated mind of the TNI, the very concept that mandating vaccination may infringe upon protected individual freedoms cannot be tolerated or allowed expression in public discourse. Similarly, the mere suggestion that those promoting the vaccine agenda may have "an ulterior motive" proves ground for dismissing content as heretical falsehood. The notion that anything other than virtuous intent may be part of the universal vaccination campaign is, of course, really quite beyond the pale! The TNI's attitude seems to be that Big Pharma executives are not fallible humans prone to the usual temptations of power and greed but guardian angels in disguise. And TNI holds that if you so much as doubt or dispute that, or dispute any other clause of the vaccine catechism, you naturally deserve to have your dangerous thoughts expunged from the public record.

If TNI had its way, I should not be free to express any of the thoughts and concerns contained in this book, nor, indeed, to independently consider and judge for myself what may be true and good. That should be the left to TNI and its unseen and, according to Robert Malone, largely unqualified, "fact-checkers." Isn't it comfortable to have all your critical thinking done for you by the all-knowing, all-mighty, all-beneficent powers that be? Isn't it wonderful to be a citizen of the great United States, the UK, or France, those bastions of liberal democracy, and not—let's say—North Korea, Russia, or the PRC?

Reuters, remember, is a TNI member. Even so, the fact that Jim Smith, former president and current chairman of the Reuters Foundation and CEO and director of Thomas Reuter Corporation, also sits on Pfizer's board[125] cannot be grounds for suspecting any ulterior motives or conflict of interest, can it?

Naturally, Robert Malone disagrees. After calling attention to Jim Smith's position in both organization, Malone tweeted on June 28, 2021:

> Regarding the "Trusted News Initiative" and censorship of information regarding COVID vaccine safety, please be aware of the link between Pfizer and Reuters. I would call that a journalistic conflict of interest. What do you think?[126]

And yes, for having the audacity to raise this question, Malone was, for a while, disappeared. He later observed:

> What we have here is this horizontal integration across pharma, big tech, big media, government and traditional media. It's not just the Trusted News Initiative. It goes beyond. The same thing is true with Merck and all the others. Pfizer is really playing quite aggressively here.[127]

In an interview for *The Defender* (online organ of Children's Health Defense), Malone elaborated on the multiple negative ramifications of the biased, incompetent, and censorious fact-checking typical of TNI and other such organs. *The Defender* reported:

> Malone expressed concern, not only about the conflicts of interest he disclosed, but as well about the "lack of transparency" involved in the process of defining and labeling "misinformation." Furthermore, Malone told *The Defender,* based on his research, most fact-checkers don't have a background in science or health. Yet even without such qualification, and without working off of a transparent definition of "misinformation," fact-checkers are able to shut down online communication between scientists and physicians by flagging or deleting posts.
>
> Worse yet, Malone said, if the fact-checkers label posts by a physician, like himself, as "disinformation," the fact-checker's claim potentially could be used as a justification for revoking a physician's license.
>
> Malone asked: "How is this in the public's best interest?"[128]

How indeed?

Believe it or not, though, with regard to the conflict of interest question, the plot gets still thicker.

I expect you know something about the WEF, a group founded in 1973 by German economist Klaus Schwab. If you do not, it might be a good idea to learn. Schwab's key idea revolves around something called "stakeholder capitalism," a notion that strategically situates private corporations (that would, of course, include Big Pharma) to act as responsible trustees of the public weal. This is desirable, naturally, because democracy doesn't necessarily do a very good or neat job of looking after the best interests of society.

Lest this whole idea seem at all suspect or even perverse to you, rest assured that the WEF, according to its website, "is independent, impartial and not tied to any special interests." Never mind that the same website discloses that WEF's partners include Pfizer, AstraZeneca, Johnson & Johnson, Moderna, Facebook, Google, Amazon, the Bill and Melinda Gates Foundation, and news organizations such as TIME, Bloomberg, and *The New York Times*.

Reuters is not listed as one of the WEF's partners. Yet a significant link nonetheless exists in the person of none other than Jim Smith. Smith is a member of WEF's International Business Council and, too, its *Partnering Against Corruption Initiative.*[129] There is no irony in that, is there? Yet it means that an individual who sits on Pfizer's board and plays an official role in the WEF's initiative to orchestrate international business operations and "fight" corruption happens to be the current chairman and director of Reuters, a global news and information company that willingly subjects itself to the censorious activity of the zealously and unabashedly pro-vaccine TNI.

In case any of this is cause for discomfort, just remember that we know, without a shadow of a doubt, that all parties promoting the vaccine agenda are pure souls with naught but public welfare at heart and need never be suspected of harboring any ulterior motives, financial or otherwise. If your faith in this self-evident truth is so weak that you may be tempted to ask for proof, just look at how much money is given to charity by someone like Bill Gates.

And oh, yes, there's also a connection between Gates (who is strategically positioned to profit greatly by Covid-19 vaccine sales), Microsoft, and (you guessed it!) Reuters.[130] But I'll let you look into that yourself, if you are (dis) interested. At the moment, I've had just about enough of all this so-called conspiracy theorizing. What about you?

CHAPTER 11

THE TALE OF THE UNTOLD: CURRENT (ADVERSE) EVENTS

Vaccine injury may be a *relatively* infrequent occurrence, but it is not one that any person or society can afford to ignore. A world of difference looms between "rare" and "nonexistent," although the controlling Covid narrative—and the media sources promoting it—constantly works to elide that difference. Consequently, a *felt* sense of the frequency and severity of vaccine-induced injury and death qualifies as a chief casualty of the systematic biases written into news today. Media inevitably shapes and even determines our perception of reality. The power of this obvious truth is not exactly taken for granted; most persons are more or less keenly aware of it. Even so, it is a challenge to interiorize and take sufficient account of the potential for bias and distortion inherent in this facet of sociopolitical existence.

Take the case of Covid-19—its incidence and severity. For much of the pandemic (especially in its earlier phases), my own local paper, the *San Francisco Chronicle,* has been running regular stories documenting, in often novelistic detail, the human suffering occasioned by Covid-19. Not infrequently, the stories revolve around healthy persons whom one would not expect to be especially vulnerable to the disease. The cascade of tales, along with the bold, red figures listing case and death counts, effectively produces the impression that Covid could easily strike down anyone at any time, and that death and misery were and are loose abroad, stalking every citizen around every corner.

The *Chronicle* stories are, I am sure, true; they are not "fake news." At the same time, it bears repeating that Covid is not and never has been *that* deadly a disease. It is not Ebola or the bubonic plague. If one happens to be a healthy person under the age of seventy, your chances of dying from Covid-19 were and are quite minuscule. (In a June, 2021 Senate hearing, Senator Rand Paul noted that if you are under twenty-five years old, that chance is one in a million, something one would never know from the aggressive promoting of vaccines for younger and younger populations.[131]) Risk of suffering long-term effects was and is more worrisome, but the chief fact that need to be remembered in this connection is how dramatically that relatively small risk would be further reduced *if* affected persons were routinely to receive appropriate, early outpatient treatment. Yet there has been nary a whisper of this critical perspective in the *Chronicle*. Instead they have only shared a steady stream of horror stories, creating the impression that people were, and may still be, dropping like flies—or at least would and will be if not largely locked down, masked, distanced, and—now, that the jab is available—vaccinated.

The CDC estimates that between 12,000 and 60,000 persons die annually of flu. The number of hospitalizations runs at least ten times that number. In 2017 to 2018, over 60,000 persons died of the flu and over 800,000 suffered hospitalization. (The official count of Covid casualties dramatically exceeds those numbers but, for reasons I have repeatedly stressed, are highly unreliable.) These flu numbers *do* represent a significant toll. In any given year, it would be easy for the *Chronicle* to publish regular stories detailing the human misery and death caused by the flu. But it doesn't. It is not news. Therefore, incidence of flu (except, perhaps, in a very bad year) does not manifest as a phenomenon of dramatic consequence in the consciousness of most persons. I have some vague recollection that 2017 to 2018 was a bad flu season, but that is all. For the most part, that fairly grim reality did not intrude upon my awareness.

My point? What is perceived as consequential, what registers as *reality itself*, is, to an extraordinary extent, selectively determined by the slant and focus of the news sources we consume. If those sources are ideologically invested in a particular perspective, this bias inevitably translates into a very partial and potentially distorted view of the reality of the entire situation. If, for instance, you read umpteen stories about Covid casualties and *none* about those persons who suffered death or serious injury from Covid vaccines, the fact of the latter will appear nebulous, an inconsequential theoretical possibility that can, *if* acknowledged at all, be easily brushed aside as insignificant, a grain of sand that bears little or no weight on the cost-benefit scale of society and the world at large.

So it may be until, one day, reality hits you—you, or someone you know: a neighbor, a colleague, friend, or family member.

These, however, are the stories—and there are tens of thousands of them—that do not get told. Or, if they are told, those who tell them, or enable their telling, are, too often, accused of heretical betrayal of the larger cause and effectively silenced. Senator Ron Johnson held a June 28, 2021, press conference to provide a platform for six severely vaccine-injured persons (including a twelve-year-old girl, whose mother spoke for her) to be seen, heard, and believed, so that the realities they represent might, in some way, be recognized and reckoned with. Senator Johnson was widely vilified for this sacrilege. Evidently, the world wishes to continue pretending that those aggrieved persons (and many others like them) whose lives have been irrevocably altered and even largely destroyed, *no longer really exist.*

It is also revealing that, although we are speaking of previously healthy persons who suffered adverse effects more or less immediately after vaccination, the doctors caring for them typically declined to confirm any causal connection. If, after all, I look out the window of my house and see my child climbing the old oak tree in the backyard and, a few minutes later, find him on the ground writhing in pain because of a broken limb, I cannot *know* that he was injured by falling out of the tree.

This refusal to "confirm" cause is, unfortunately, only par for the course in a surreal world in which the only immutable truth is that *the vaccines have been proven to be "safe and effective."* If your personal experience belies that claim, it is not that mantra itself that comes under suspicion but, in one or another twisted manner, *you.* Fallen from grace for some unidentified sin laid unjustly at your door—perhaps the sin of honesty, or perhaps openness—you become, overnight, an *ideological untouchable.*

However, this does not only happen sociopsychologically but practically and financially as well. Although you are a victim of vaccine injury, neither the (inconceivably rich) pharmaceutical companies that manufactured the product nor the government that first urged and then demanded that you vaccinate will take responsibility for your physical, financial, and social ruination. If you are fortunate, your individual insurance may take care of some of the astronomical costs you may incur, but many in your position will probably not qualify.

This, as the exiled injured will tell you, is another one of the morally repugnant features of the overzealous vaccine campaign, one that—morally, humanly, psychologically—hurts almost as much as the physical agony. It represents the archetypal instance of *adding insult to injury.* You chose to vaccinate not only in hopes of protecting yourself but also out of a sense of social and civic responsibility. Yet, as soon as your own catastrophic misfortune bears witness against the storyline all wish so fervently to believe, you are deserted, not comforted and cared for by the society for which you, in part, sacrificed your most precious treasure—your health and wellbeing, or that of your child. You are cast out and cast aside, the truth your very body represents willfully denied. Only then do you discover, contrary to the terms of what you thought was a fair social contract, that you as a person, as an individual body and soul, count for next to nothing.

And so I ask this question to all who so fervently believe it is the moral and social responsibility of everyone to vaccinate: if that is so, and that categorical imperative truly flows not merely from craven fear and calculated self-interest but from a sound ethical source—and so, too, from a fount of compassion—would not the companies, the government, and society at large gladly attempt to take good care of those who suffered from the social or legal code it urged and enforced? Are we speaking here, of enlightened human community or mobbish members of what remains a primitive and savage tribe? Should we not, by all rights, add the following as another, tenth clause of Dr. Setty's list of conditions to be met before considering vaccination a *reasonable* option: that government and society acknowledge and take care of those who suffer, catastrophically, from fulfilling what has been presented as civic duty, from doing what was loudly called "right"? Otherwise, who can blame a moral philosopher for suspecting that your whole theory of good citizenship or social responsibility is rotten to the core?

So let us turn, now, to those stories: to the stories you will not, as a rule, read in the press. I myself, unvaccinated, remain, in my own estimation, at least, sound in body and mind, but I have friends who have suffered serious adverse consequences, ranging from severe fatigue and dizziness lasting several months to muscular, neurological, and cognitive dysfunction that persists after months of a single dose. These instances (which I cannot describe in great detail on account of privacy concerns) are traumatic enough yet nonetheless involve affliction less severe than those suffered by many, as those testifying at Senator Johnson's hearing can attest. In a 2021 opinion piece for *Newsweek* titled "No, the Unvaccinated Aren't Selfish or Ignorant. Here's Why I'm Not Vaxxed" (plaudits to *Newsweek* for publishing!), Suri Kinzbrunner writes:

> A colleague of my parents reportedly died from complications of the Moderna vaccine, a friend suffered from deep vein thrombosis, and a teenage nephew of another friend now has chronic cardiac issues. These are three examples from my immediate network of family and friends, and I know many others with their own stories. And while it's true that these are anecdotes and do not represent the majority, they are powerful nonetheless.[132]

We do not hear much, if anything, from relatives of the dead. They do exist, in significant number, as VAERS and the CDC whistleblower's data analyses attest. After all that has been said in this volume, do you really wonder why not?

Yet let us move on to a more fully told personal story. Here, courtesy of Emily Jo, is another case of a young person, fourteen-year-old Aiden, who suffered myocarditis after receiving the vaccine.[133]

Emily Jo, Aiden's mother, was bullish on vaccines. She took her son for his first dose of the Pfizer Covid vaccine on May 21, 2021, which she recalls may have been the very day the CDC cleared it for adolescents. Aside from asthma, Aiden had been a healthy youngster.

On June 10, 2021, a few days after his second dose, Aiden awakened his mother in the middle of the night because he was experiencing chest pain and extreme difficulty breathing. Emily acknowledged that she had been aware that heart inflammation had emerged as a concern in connection with the Pfizer vaccine but had been led to believe that the condition, if it did occur, was a mild one, and that, in any event, the risk of experiencing any side effect was "one in a million."

Emily took her son to the emergency room. When tests indicated significant abnormalities, Aiden was transferred to the acute cardiac unit. The cardiologist did report the incident to VAERS and, by way of communication with the CDC, established that Aiden was indeed suffering from post-vaccine myocarditis. Emily Jo said, "The biggest problem is that they [CDC] are not explaining what mild myocarditis means. Aiden's cardiologist told us no case of myocarditis is 'mild.' That's like saying a heart attack is mild."

Two months after his release from the hospital, Aiden still cannot risk any physical exertion: no gym class, no recess, no chasing around with schoolmates, friends, siblings. He can *never* run, only walk, and—until his condition improves—he needs extra time to get from one class to the next to ensure that his heart is not subjected to any additional stress. On August 6, 2021, Emily noted:

> My kids are playing outside with friends. They are running and my son has to walk. At the same time, I'm terrified that he will come in again with shortness of breath or chest pain. It feels like this should be called long myocarditis.[134]

Emily said she'd experienced unpleasantness from those opposed to vaccines after vaccinating Aiden, and now many proponents have been criticizing her for sharing Aiden's story.

> I was one of those jerks who was like, 'Oh, it's your fault. You're the reason everybody needs to get vaccinated,' so this has flipped everything for me upside down.... They [the CDC and APA, American Academy of Pediatrics] have lost me and they're going to lose a lot of people. When you lose trust in public health, we have a big problem.[135]

Emily Jo also volunteered that, knowing what she knows now, she would not have vaccinated her children. Indeed, she feels authorities who advocate doing so are overzealous and misguided because, in reality, the vaccines are not truly effective, and children are very low risk.

> I know the Delta variant is serious. I take this all seriously. I have never been someone to downplay the virus. We masked, we distanced. We did online learning. I just don't see enough...and the way that they're pushing—the APA—pushing this through. This is just disgusting to me.... I've known many, many children who've gotten COVID. This is anecdotal. I know there are serious cases but anecdotally, I have seen 15-20 kids who have had COVID. They had *sniffles* and my kid is the one who ended up in the hospital because of the vaccine.[136]

Emily Jo further acknowledged that before she found herself dealing with her son's adverse reaction, she did not realize that the manufacturers of the vaccine bear no liability. She feels parents should be conscious of the fact that, if something does go awry, they are left largely alone to deal with the consequences. The injustice of that circumstance deeply disturbs her:

> I think another thing parents need to understand is that myocarditis is not covered under the National Vaccine Injury Compensation Program, and the Countermeasures Injury Compensation Program only covers if you're incapacitated, wheel-chair (*sic*) bound or dead. We have incurred thousands and thousands of dollars in medical bills. We have insurance but they don't pay all.... I don't feel I should have to pay for doing what I was told to do by the government. Hey, we are all in this together and then you get a vaccine injury and you're just completely ignored—and not just ignored but beat up from both sides.[137]

In fact, not only are pharmaceutical companies not answerable for any damage caused by their products, as Emily Jo, to her chagrin, discovered, but the relevant government agency (the Department of Health and Human Services) also "bears zero responsibility." She cannot comprehend how the government can mandate an action but refuse any responsibility whatsoever for adverse consequences that might result from following the official order. "Why,"

Emily lamented, "are these boys just shoved into a corner as collateral damage as if it doesn't matter?"

Meanwhile, the Advisory Committee on Immunization Practices (ACIP), a committee within the CDC, held a meeting on June 23, 2021, to review data and form recommendations. Incidence of heart inflammation in youth was on the docket, with the CDC acknowledging 1,200 cases of heart inflammation in sixteen- to twenty-four-year-olds. Pediatric doctor Elizabeth Mumper audited the entire meeting. Mumper later observed:

> I was surprised that a working document was presented in which the ACIP was leaning toward recommending a second COVID vaccine in patients who experienced heart inflammation after the first dose, as long as the patient had improved. I was also surprised that some ACIP committee members seemed to be making the assumption that the cases of myocarditis and pericarditis would not cause long-term harm. We simply do not have the evidence to make COVID vaccine decisions on that assumption.[138]

How do you think Emily Jo would rate ACIP on quality of logic, caution, and compassion? As for Dr. Mumper's concluding remark, how many other Covid vaccine decisions have been made on equally shaky grounds? How intelligent is it to plan to *build* our shining city *back better* on the San Andreas fault?

CHAPTER 12

ACTION ALERT: A LETTER WITHIN A LETTER

As I expect my reader may well imagine, composing this book, initially intended as a letter, has required far more time than initially anticipated. It has, as well, naturally been challenging to respond to the new developments transpiring almost daily. It is thus hardly surprising that, while still in the process of writing, I received, on July 29, 2021, an update from the president of Pacifica, one that by no means excluded the possibility that vaccine mandates might be instituted as a condition of the reopening of the campus in 2022. Recognizing the urgency of the situation and, too, that the length of this—as yet unfinished!—letter to him rendered it entirely unsuitable for its original purpose, I interrupted the writing of this longer piece in order to compose a much shorter version, one that I could in good conscience—and quickly!—send. The beginning and end of that more concise effort frame the question at hand in a fashion that crystallizes my own moral logic. I thus continue this longer exposition by inserting material from near the beginning and end of that one.

July 30, 2021

Dear President Cambray:

> ...The controlling narrative tells us that Covid is a deadly disease for which no safe and effective treatment is readily available, so that universal vaccination represents the chief means of combatting Covid and restoring a modicum of normality to human life. With the spread of the Delta variant, the temperature is rising again, and one hears a chorus of voices asserting that unvaccinated persons are driving a new surge and persevering in reckless behavior that endangers the life and liberty of all.
>
> This narrative is built upon four critical assumptions: (1) That Covid poses a serious mortal threat to the entire human population. (2) That no safe and effective means of prevention or early treatment are readily available. (3) That the vaccines themselves are safe and effective. (4) That contrary views on all these matters represent misinformation or disinformation stemming, primarily, from irrational, irresponsible, often right-wing

sources. I believe, however, that each of these assumptions is open to serious question...

After a brief exposition which serves as a kind of abstract or synopsis of the main points of *this* much longer epistle, my short letter concludes:

What I have been able to share here barely scratches the surface of all that could be said on the Covid issue. Let me draw to a close by bringing these thoughts to bear on the practical matter at hand with reference to the distinctive character of Pacifica and its unique mission.

The body is the locus of personal identity and individual autonomy. Any significant decision impinging upon a person's freedom of choice with respect to their body cannot help but be of inestimable psychological as well as sociopolitical importance. I would think there would need be *an extraordinarily high bar of truth and consequence* before even *beginning* to consider abrogating the right of individual freedom of bodily choice by making vaccination a prerequisite for participation in academic life. While advocates of the mainstream Covid narrative may imagine that high bar vaulted by Covid-19, I see a very different story.

If Covid-19 truly posed a severe mortal danger to the whole of the population *and* the government had assiduously explored and promoted safe and effective means of prevention and early treatment; *and* the Covid vaccines had been rigorously and extensively tested and shown to be at least as safe as traditional vaccines; *and* free, fair, and open debate on relevant issues had been protected in the community of science, the public forum and the Web; *and* (despite all countermeasures) Covid remained a serious menace; *then* an argument could be made that every person should certainly vaccinate. *If* all these conditions had been fulfilled, however, mandating vaccination would likely be redundant, because most everyone would voluntarily choose that course. In fact, however, these conditions have *not* been fulfilled.

I do not believe that our current health challenges can be blamed on those who question the flawed premises of the controlling Covid narrative and the coercion to which it is leading. Down that path, I fear, lies not greater "normality," but more intense division and polarization. Genuine freedom of speech is always, in its moment of consequence, freedom to *dissent from* and *actively contest* prevailing opinion and—most especially—government authority. Censorship of and discrimination against conscientious and informed citizens who question the controlling Covid narrative and so make different personal health choices simply cannot be squared with the premises of a democratic society.

As an institution of higher learning dedicated to the education of the mind and sovereignty of the soul, I respectfully urge that Pacifica *not* institute vaccine mandates. Doing so would, in my mind, not only contravene essential civil rights, but also belie the depth psychological imperative to respect the autonomy of the individual soul.

Emerson:

> A political victory...raises your spirits, and you think good days are preparing for you. Do not believe it.... Nothing can bring you peace but the triumph of principles.

Respectfully Yours,
Daniel Joseph Polikoff, Ph.D.

CHAPTER 13

TWO ROADS

I am not sure I have yet adequately articulated why I feel that mandating vaccination is so profoundly wrong. The popular opinion these days, of course, is just the opposite: that it is evidently the right thing to do, and all rational persons who possess a modicum of human conscience and compassion should hold that stance. I, however, have taken some pains to show that the supposed rectitude of that position rests upon a rotten foundation, the integrity of which has been eroded by duplicity, corruption, and bad faith; a whole maze of power single-mindedly directed toward the end of mass (and that means, finally, compulsory) vaccination. So I would ask: can the logical culmination of a program of dishonest, self-interested, censorious thoughts and deeds, the *coronation* of an agenda not distinguished by virtue but rather infected with vice, conceivably serve *the Good?*

I do not doubt that most conscientious persons who endorse vaccine mandates believe, sincerely, in the ethical propriety of that edict. Yet goodness, which Kant associates with practical judgment, always depends upon truth. *If* the ground of your judgment of what is true *now* rests upon a whole history of falsehood, and *if* your present practical judgment depends upon and (by eschewing critique) tacitly *sanctions* a string of prior immoral acts, and *if* your judgment of what is right effectively extends the life of a corrupt and antidemocratic system of power indefinitely into the future (Pfizer is already lobbying for boosters and assuring its stockholders that the revenue stream of its vaccines will likely achieve permanence, as if its pharmaceutical solutions were the fixed stars in some financial sky), can, under such conditions, your judgment possibly be *Good?*

What then are we to do, as a human community, about Covid-19? What measures can we take so that we can, without fear, once more mingle in the school and the office, the market and the theater, the gym, the café, the club, the museum, the mall, and the music hall and so lead a recognizable American life once more? Is not universal vaccination our best passport to the restoration of so much of what we know and love of human life and the surest means of keeping the spike of death from the door of our heart?

With all due respect, *I think not.* I believe this a mirage, a chimera, a charade. Look at much-vaccinated Israel; look at my own beloved Bay Area, with its high vaccination rate—and, according to officialdom, climbing case counts, and new and more repressive measures every day, measures that give some what I believe to be a false sense of security, while making countless others sick with frustration and rage.

Many doctors, including some endorsing the vaccine, affirm: coronavirus will not go away. No vaccine will stamp it out any more than flu shots will wipe out influenza. It is not smallpox, nor polio, but a respiratory virus, and as such the natural course of affairs is for the virulent strain to take a toll and, eventually, as resistance builds up in the population, become more transmissible but less deadly, endemic instead of pandemic, and so manageable, like the flu. The flu does kill tens of thousands of persons every year. Death is, after all, part of life. But we do not turn the world upside-down and cease to be and live and begin to hate our neighbors because of the flu.

If, moreover, prophylactic measures and early treatment protocols were widely disseminated, the public as well as medical community accordingly educated, and appropriate care readily and routinely available—*as doctors McCullough, Risch, and Fareed desperately urged in the United States Senate long, long ago*—very few people would have to fear for their lives, or fear for serious consequences for their health. This agenda, empowering personal responsibility and the human capacities of care and healing, could yield to a sense not of desperation in an ill-fated battle against ever-shifting pandemonium but to a real, calm, and measured sense of competence and managed control. Such a program would also, of course, go hand in glove with the aim of truly boosting the whole population's naturally engendered and thus *genuine* herd immunity—not one based on an artificial vaccine threshold.

This, I believe, is the crux of the matter: that spurious change of definition—that WHO-sponsored deletion of natural immunity. Let me quote the American Institute for Economic Research: "There is simply no way for medical science completely to replace the human immune system. It can only game it via what used to be called inoculation."[139]

Read that again: *there is simply no way.*

Are these words, perhaps, a sign of the times?

At this critical juncture, Americans—no matter our class, creed, or color—are all New Englanders standing in a yellow wood at the divergence of two roads. One is the road posted with the WHO's redefinition of "herd immunity"—and we are, at present, all being prodded to stampede down this road so that we may be duly branded and identified as property belonging to Big Pharma's O.K. Corral. Down this road lies, I suspect, a fearful, uncertain future—a future without a human face. This way lies no real security from disease and illness but instead an ever-shifting battle against new mutant strains, and (count on it!) ever more boosters or new shots—even a vaccine treadmill run by ever-changing stories of efficacy and risk and, too, ever more vaccine damage covered up and over. It is the road leading to more authoritarian restriction of individual freedom, and more and more violent jostling in the holding pen. It is the stony road, at last, toward ever more division and conflict in a society stuck together not by the cohesion of love but by the force of coercion.

The other road, the road less traveled by, may initially look more frightening to those who have absorbed the mainstream narrative most deeply. It is the path not of ever-ballooning corporate profits, repressive official edicts, technocratic control, and popular mobbishness but of what is both a more natural and more cultured humanity. It is a way that depends upon our capacity to take personal responsibility for our bodies and minds and to treat our fellow beings humanely, a way that encourages us to drink in the vitamin sun and partake of the dark bread of the earth and so to fortify and build natural immunity to diverse strains of disease. It is a path that trusts not in one-size-fits-all injections but in individual choice and in doctors empowered with knowledge and resources to treat their patients, and treat them right. It is the road of reason and imagination, of trust and love and faith and hope instead of deceit, fear, control, and coercion. It is the road, finally, of freedom: the long, winding road down which the soul walks with God, looks death in the eye, and speaks with Emerson, Sojourner Truth, and the spirit of the living Christ: *I am.*

> I shall be telling this with a sigh
> Somewhere ages and ages hence:
> Two roads diverged in a wood, and I—
> I took the one less traveled by,
> And that has made all the difference.[140]

PART II

INCREASING F(R)ICTION

We have been relentless—relentless—in our efforts to get people vaccinated. Our whole-of-government response will continue its relentless efforts to end this pandemic.[141]

—Jeff Zients, White House Coronavirus Response Coordinator

The bottom line for me, and perhaps others who are seriously ambivalent about the COVID-19 vaccine, is that trustworthy information guidance is key. And those of us opting out of the vaccine are not doing so out of ignorance or selfishness. We have simply been paying attention to the mixed messages, the hypocrisy, the changing standards, and the censoring of counterevidence. And we have not been convinced that this is something we need to do, for our own good or that of our communities or country.

The COVID-19 vaccine remains one effective tool among many in the fight against COVID-19. Clear, transparent information about what the vaccine does, what its risks and limitations are, and what other options exist, especially for prevention and early treatment, are what is needed to restore trust.

The mandates, bribes, social pressure, censorship, and ever-changing policies that don't present clear scientific rationale need to stop. But at least the doctor/patient relationship should be prioritized in the meantime, so that we as individuals can make informed decisions for ourselves, enabling us all to emerge sooner rather than later from this seemingly never-ending health crisis.[142]

—Suri Kinzbrunner, *Newsweek* op-ed

Chapter 14

A PANDEMIC OF THE UNVACCINATED?

News certainly breaks fast these days: no sooner has one penned a conclusion and put down the figurative pen, than novel developments call for again taking it up, and adding on.

Donning the Covid-colored lenses that are *de rigueur* today, I find that the world on this morning of the 20th of August 2021 looks different, and yet darker, than it did when I began this extended epistle at the end of June seven weeks or so ago.

As alluded to in my short letter within a letter, the rise of the Delta variant has once more precipitated a widespread sense of a crisis out of control, and restrictions and vaccine mandates have begun raining thick and fast: healthcare workers, teachers, college students, therapists, law enforcement personnel, and firefighters—the list, like a Whitmanian inventory of the rich and diverse walks of life of Americans, goes on and on. Recently, San Francisco became the first city to require proof of vaccination for indoor spaces, including restaurants and gyms; theaters and concert venues are doing likewise for those who wish to partake of the cultural fare that is the food of love. I hear laws or regulations are under consideration which would preclude unvaccinated individuals from boarding an aircraft (no negative test option offered), condemning creatures such as myself to the sorry plight of birds with clipped wings.

This is all, of course, based on the presumed superior truth of what I have called the controlling narrative, which is not only a matter of *controlling the story* but also employing *story as a vehicle of control.* That narrative has recently acquired a new twist, one essential to sustaining its coherence and persuasive power in the face of ever-changing circumstance. As the story has, from the first, revolved around the vaccine-only solution to the pandemic problem, *if* that problem persists or even worsens after rollout, it follows that there can be only be one logical explanation: that those recalcitrants who remain unvaccinated are the chief cause of the new phase of the plague. Thus, what we are now experiencing has been officially christened "a pandemic of the unvaccinated."

The only issue with that new twist is that it is, indeed, like so much of the story, *twisted;* at best, it is a very partial truth, and, at worst, it is a distortion that *principled scientific reasoning* reveals to be contrary to the truth of the matter.

First, as always, the facts: the evidentiary base of judgment. In mid-July of 2021, with Delta ascendant and case counts on the rise, CDC director Rochelle Walensky declared, "There is a clear message coming through. This is a pandemic of the unvaccinated."[143] That declaration, resonantly echoed by others (including Dr. Anthony Fauci and President Biden), was backed up by repeated reference to statistics supposedly revealing that virtually all Americans (ninety-five to ninety-nine percent) currently suffering hospitalization or death are unvaccinated individuals. The implication to be drawn from such figures is clear: if you do vaccinate, you are close to 100 times less likely to suffer serious consequences than those of your benighted brethren who do not.

On August 5, 2021, the White House Covid Response Team, consisting of Anthony Fauci (Chief Medical Adviser to the President and Director of the Institute of Allergic and Infectious Disease), CDC Director Rochelle Walensky, Surgeon General Vivek Murthy, and Coronavirus Response Coordinator Jeff Zients held a press briefing, as per their weekly custom. After short presentations acknowledging the climbing case counts and sounding a very loud call to arms (literal arms, I mean—more and more of them, not to give but to receive shots), CNN correspondent Caitlin Collins asked a pointed question:

> Several of you and the President have repeatedly cited figures saying that 99% of those who die from Covid-19 are unvaccinated, and 95% who are hospitalized are unvaccinated. With the Delta variant, do you still stand by those numbers, and do you have government data to back them up?[144]

CDC Director Dr. Walensky replied:

> Those data were data from analyses in several states from January through June [of 2021], and didn't reflect the data that we have now for the Delta variant. We are actively working to update those in the context of the Delta variant.[145]

Wait a moment: *January* through *June*? The vaccination program did not even really begin until January (of 2021). On New Year's Day 2021, less than one percent (in fact, half that) of the U.S. population was vaccinated. By mid-April of 2021, only a little less than a third of the population had received at least one shot, and my mid-June of 2021, less than fifty percent (48.7 percent) were "fully" (and so, for statistical purposes, tallied as) "vaccinated."[146] (Remember that, for the Pfizer and Moderna two-dose protocol, one is not considered fully vaccinated until *two weeks* after the *second* shot. As that second shot may be given up to six weeks after the first, many if not most persons would not qualify as "vaccinated" until almost two months after receiving their first shot.) This means that the data employed to establish that *virtually all persons dying or hospitalized on account of Covid-19 are unvaccinated* registers data from a time period during which *the vast majority of all Americans were—unvaccinated!*

Contrary to the manner in which it was presented by government officials, the data does not prove that full vaccination eliminates almost all risk of hospitalization or death from Covid-19, nor can it be legitimately used to compare the vulnerability (or resistance) of a vaccinated individual vis-à-vis that of an unvaccinated individual. Moreover, and this is critical, when it comes to the newly dominant Delta variant, the much-touted data say *nothing at all.* After all, on August 5, 2021, Dr. Walensky openly acknowledged that the relevant data had not yet been updated. As of that date, and during the time that officials were trumpeting news of "a pandemic of the unvaccinated" (the catchy title of the new, most recent chapter of the official Covid story), we did not have official numbers addressing overall incidence of hospitalization and death in the recent, most relevant Delta era.

This reference to Delta is not ancillary but absolutely central, theoretically as well as practically. Why? As Sherlock Holmes was wont to say, "It's elementary, Watson." Viruses naturally evolve new strains in order to circumvent the defenses mounted by vaccine-induced immunity. In point of fact, since August 5, 2021, it has become more and more evident that the Covid vaccines are demonstrating less and less efficacy in the relatively new Delta era. In particular, the power of the Pfizer vaccine to protect against infection appears to be effectively halved. Consequently, and not unpredictably, health officials are already recommending boosters as a way "to keep ahead" of the virus.

But this is a potentially counterproductive, and even a dangerous, game, as our Canadian friend and neighbor Dr. Byram Bridle explains. Explicitly asked whether it might justly be claimed that we are in the midst of "a pandemic of the unvaccinated," Dr. Bridle did not mince words:

> Absolutely, it's untrue to be calling this a pandemic of the unvaccinated. And it's certainly untrue…that the unvaccinated are somehow driving the emergence of the novel variants. This goes against every scientific principle

that we understand. The reality is, the nature of the vaccines we are using right now, and the way we're rolling them out, are going to be applying selective pressure to this virus to promote the emergence of new variants. Again, this is based on sound principles.

We have to look no further than... the emergence of antibiotic resistance. The principle is this: If you have a biological entity that is prone to mutation—and the SARS-CoV-2, like all coronaviruses, is prone to mutation—and you apply a narrowly focused selective pressure that is nonlethal, and you do this over a long period of time, this is the recipe for driving the emergence of novel variants.

This is exactly what we're doing. Our vaccines are focused on a single protein of the virus, so the virus only has to alter one protein, and the vaccines don't come close to providing sterilizing immunity. People who are vaccinated still get infected, it only seems particularly good at blunting the disease, and what that tells you therefore is that these vaccines in the vast majority of people are applying a nonlethal pressure, narrowly focused on one protein, and the vaccine rollout is occurring over a long period of time. That's the recipe for driving variants.[147]

Asked, furthermore, if it was fair to blame those who decline vaccination for our current plight and to discriminate against them by denying access to services and the like, Dr. Bridle was no less direct:

It is ridiculous. If anything, the unvaccinated are likely acquiring, probably in pretty substantial numbers, naturally acquired immunity, which I would argue, from an immunological perspective, is going to be much more protective than vaccine-induced immunity against novel variants.[148]

Dr. Bridle here engages the crucial concern I addressed earlier in this letter: namely, the WHO's decidedly unscientific and unprincipled (re)definition of "herd immunity," a conceptual as well as semantic revision that ties it, exclusively, to vaccine-induced immunity while eliding all consideration of naturally acquired immunity. When further asked about the human body's potential to protect itself against infection and thus, in certain circumstances render vaccination unnecessary, Dr. Bridle's forceful concluding remarks expand upon this crucial theme:

It is shocking to me as an immunologist. Yes, essentially, *our immune systems actually work*. They do respond to pathogens, and they do protect from pathogens.[149]

After citing several high-quality peer-reviewed papers that confirm these capabilities in the case of SARS-CoV-2, Dr. Bridle continues:

> [These studies show that] naturally acquired immunity against SARS-CoV-2 is very potent, it's very long-lasting, and, importantly, in the context of novel variants, it's very broad in its scope; it's very balanced. We are going to have lots of antibodies and T-cells, and the thing is, it targets multiple components of the virus, not just the spike protein. Variants will occur that are going to be able to bypass the vaccine-induced immunity but these variants aren't going to change the other components that people who have naturally responded are going to be protected against.[150]

Dr. Bridle is, remember, a career vaccinologist. If we presume the soundness of his principles, what had we best bank on: vaccine-induced "herd-immunity" that hamstrings our own best weapon even while launching upon a long (and even endless) war with an elusive enemy adept at guerrilla tactics? Or should we rather rely upon a strategy that depends and builds upon our own natural capability, fostered over eons of evolution, to mount a balanced, broad-based defense, a strategy that can also effectively work to dilute the opponent's power—by inducing conversion to more transmissible but less deadly strains—and even turn enemies into friends? Is not the one-size-fits-all eggs in the vaccine basket the immunological equivalent of the Maginot Line?

Of course, rational choice of strategy depends on your desired outcome. I am assuming that to be a better future for humankind—our collective health and welfare as well as freedom from fear and undue constraint. If your principal aim happens to be a never-ending revenue from ever more injections, or a human population ever more subject to strictures of technocratic control, your calculus and your conclusion may look quite different from mine.

Chapter 15

A COLOSSAL BLUNDER

Dr. Bridle is hardly alone in his fear that a flawed vaccination campaign could backfire and, because the vaccines are nowhere near capable of delivering any sort of knockout blow, end up strengthening the virulence and adaptability of the virus more than our immunological defenses. Remember Dr. Robert Malone's list of ten points detailing his own stance? All are largely self-explanatory, except number eight, which reads:

> 8) Dr. [Geert Vanden] Bossche is completely correct as a virologist and vaccinologist in everything that I have read of his. Time will prove him right.... But IMO as a physician, the death and disability in the high risk populations still merits vaccination.[151]

Who, then, is Dr. Geert Vanden Bossche, and what has he said and written about Covid-19?

Geert Vanden Bossche is an eminent, internationally recognized virologist. Anything but an "anti-vaxxer," Dr. Vanden Bossche, after holding academic positions in Belgium and Germany, worked on research and development for several vaccine companies (including Novartis), joined the Bill and Melinda Gates Foundation's Global Health Discovery Team as senior program officer, served as senior Ebola program manager at the Global Alliance for Vaccines and Immunization (GAVI) in Geneva, Switzerland, and worked as the head of vaccine development at the German Center for Infection Research in Cologne. In connection with his role reviewing the safety of the Ebola vaccine, Dr. Vanden Bossche has extensive experience evaluating the safety and efficacy of vaccination protocols developed and employed in the context of a global health pandemic.[152]

On March 6, 2021, Dr. Vanden Bossche took the extraordinary step of putting his professional reputation on the line by circulating an urgent personal letter addressed "To all authorities, scientists and experts around the world, whom this may concern; and to the entire world population." The letter called for an immediate, thoroughgoing review of the worldwide response to the

Covid-19 pandemic in general and to the ongoing mass vaccination campaign in particular.[153]

Dr. Vanden Bossche's chief concern echoes that of Dr. Bridle—or rather vice versa. His lengthy discussion of the topic accents one of the features of the complex epidemiological situation referenced by Dr. Bridle. Not only does a program of nonlethal vaccination promote immune escape and the emergence of vaccine resistant viral strains, but this negative outcome proceeds in synergy with active suppression of the body's natural immune response, thus rendering the vaccinated persons more vulnerable to SARS-CoV-2 infection. How so? Once the body has, by way of vaccine-induced immunity, developed antibodies specifically designed to combat the spike protein of the virus, it will depend upon that targeted response—even if it is not fully effective on account of emergent viral variation—and fail to mobilize its broader-based natural immunological capacities to the same extent it would have done so otherwise.

Ill-timed, nonlethal, mass vaccination thus hits the human population with a double whammy: at the same time that it breeds more infectious and immune-resistant variants, it "fools" the body itself into suppression of its own natural broad-based immune response. While it may be true that the vaccine-induced protection sometimes (though not always!) suffices to prevent serious illness and death, if it does not prevent infection, vaccinated individuals may then become both breeding grounds and potentially asymptomatic spreaders of more resistant strains of the virus. When this occurs, it endangers sectors of the population (for instance, younger persons) whose strong natural immunity would otherwise have effectively defended against viral infection. Consequently, an indiscriminate mass vaccination campaign—one that targets young as well as older populations—can readily result, especially over time, in less protection for naturally less-susceptible subgroups of the population, most notably children and the young. As Dr. Vanden Bossche stated in his letter:

> Suppression of innate immunity, especially in the younger age groups, can, therefore, become very problematic.... Basically, we'll soon be confronted with a super-infectious virus that completely resists our most precious defense mechanism: The human immune system.[154]

Yet another lynchpin of the official pandemic response feeds right into this destructive dynamic, especially, though by no means exclusively, because it touches upon the health and wellbeing of young children. As Vanden Bossche explains, the broad-based "generalist" component of our innate immune system does not come with built-in memory; it develops immunological intelligence and reactivity by way of ongoing learning catalyzed by constant interaction with the environment. That is why it is a terrible idea to try to create a super-sanitized, "germ-free" environment for infants and young children. This cripples the body's necessary immunological exercise and education and ultimately renders it acutely and artificially vulnerable to infection and illness. The same principle applies to the population at large, as those Kern County doctors alleged at the onset of the pandemic: lockdown, social isolation, and excessive sanitation to avoid infection can significantly weaken the body's natural immunological defenses.

Combine this with ill-advised mass vaccination, and Dr. Vanden Bossche—as his urgent letter makes amply clear—sees a disaster in the making. In his March 6, 2021 letter, Dr. Vanden Bossche wrote:

> Widespread and stringent infection prevention measures combined with mass vaccination campaigns using inadequate vaccines will undoubtedly lead to a situation where the pandemic is getting increasingly 'out of control.'[155]

Here we are (at the time of this writing), just short of six months later, and who can say, as many did at the time, that Dr. Geert Vanden Bossche (who draws upon a vast reservoir of peculiarly relevant experience, and whose judgment Robert Malone thought would be vindicated in time) was all wrong?

Dr. Vanden Bossche himself, moreover, is quite clear that the core of the problem inheres in the very topic I have repeatedly foregrounded here: a false reconstruction of the idea of herd immunity and its practical application to the management of a pandemic. The title of a later (July 14, 2021) post on his website could hardly state the gist of the matter more clearly. In the piece titled "Not Covid-19 vaccine-mediated but naturally acquired immunity enables herd immunity," Vanden Bossche writes:

> From their very first conceptualization, it should have been very clear that their S-based [spike protein-based] Covid-19 vaccines are completely inadequate for generating herd immunity in a population, *regardless of the magnitude of the Ab (antibody) titers induced or the ratio of vaccine coverage*.... The propensity of viral variants to propagate on a background of S-directed [spike protein-directed] immune pressure prevents

> 'imperfect' vaccines from establishing herd immunity when used in a mass vaccination campaign at the height of a pandemic. As a result, vaccines are prone to breed naturally selected immune escape variants and serve as asymptomatic spreaders. This is exactly the opposite of what herd immunity is defined as![156]

Dr. Vanden Bossche's prognosis, if we keep on railroading everyone down the vaccine track, is dire indeed:

> Moving the program forward would fulfill all the conditions for driving S-directed viral immune escape to eventually result in full resistance of Sars-CoV-2 to the Covid-19 vaccines.[157]

Nor are those booster shots, while perhaps music to Pfizer shareholder ears, likely to remedy the situation:

> Boosting vaccinal antibodies with 2nd generation vaccines is not going to solve the issue of immune escape even if the immunization with 'updated' vaccines would be repeated at 6 month intervals. This is because 2nd generation vaccines will primarily recall S- specific antibodies elicited by the first generation vaccines…and not be effective against recombinations of Sars-CoV-2 variants, which are likely to occur as a result of co-infection, especially in the most vulnerable.[158]

Five days after his original March 6, 2021, letter, Dr. Vanden Bossche delivered a brief oral appeal. Here is the transcript of that cry of distress:

> Dear Colleagues at the WHO: My name is Geert Vanden Bossche…I am a certified expert in microbiology and infectious diseases. I have a PhD in virology and I've a longstanding career in human vaccinology. I'm urging you to immediately open the scientific debate on how human interventions in the Covid-19 pandemic are currently driving viral immune escape. I'm urging you to invite me for a scientific hearing open to the public and to scientists all over the world on this very topic. *Ignoring or denying the impact of stringent infection prevention measures combined with mass vaccination using prophylactic vaccines is a colossal blunder.* Please do listen to my cry of distress, and let's first and foremost deliberate on a scientifically justified strategy to mitigate the tsunami of morbidity and lethality that is now threatening us. And let's meanwhile devise a strategy to eradicate the steadily emerging highly infectious variants. On behalf of humanity, I sincerely thank you for considering my call.[159]

Unfortunately, Geert Vanden Bossche's call seems to have fallen on deaf ears—at least at the agency to which he appeals. The lack of visible public debate and discussion on this world-important, life and death issue is all too characteristic of the sociopolitical history of Covid-19. Judging from the numerous appreciative *public* responses, many persons seem to think that the WHO, rather than impartially and disinterestedly serving the cause of global health, may have another agenda altogether.

Chapter 16

THE IVERMECTIN ANGLE

If we were to draw conclusions from the relatively brief remarks toward the end of his open letter, Dr. Vanden Bossche's own ideas as to what might constitute "a scientifically justified strategy" for combating Covid-19 involve not the leaky, nonlethal mRNA vaccines but an entirely different sort of vaccine that might be developed. It would be one that capitalizes upon, rather than suppresses, other elements of the body's natural immune system. Vanden Bossche, remember, has spent his career championing—even while critically overseeing—mass vaccination efforts. A prior employee of both GAVI and the Gates Foundation—viewed by many opposed to mass vaccination programs as the public health equivalents of Mordor and Darth Vader—Vanden Bossche is hardly a natural spokesperson for the alternatively minded. His keen and withering criticism of Covid-19 policy is all the more telling for that. Nonetheless, other distinguished doctors and researchers have come forward with promising, more immediately practicable ideas as to how best to meet the global health challenge posed by Covid-19.

The tale of ivermectin undoubtedly represents one of the most compelling subplots woven into the still-unfolding saga of Covid-19 story. While I can hardly do justice to the whole complex matter here, let me nonetheless seek to shed what light I can on the ivermectin angle.

When Covid-19 first emerged as a global threat in early 2020, Dr. Paul Marik, the second-most published intensive care unit (ICU) specialist in the world, recruited four of his closest associates to form a team dedicated to the mission of developing treatment protocols for Covid-19. One of those individuals, ICU and lung specialist Dr. Pierre Kory, emerged as the chief spokesperson for the organization that eventually coalesced—the Frontline Covid-19 Critical Care Alliance (FLCCC)—and currently spearheads the effort to promote ivermectin as a treatment for Covid-19. In his joint appearance with Bret Weinstein on *The Joe Rogan Experience,* Dr. Kory recounted how the team first became aware of ivermectin's antiviral potential:

> [When we first began our work,] we learned everything we could about Covid-19. We just read paper after paper after paper. We followed all the therapeutics that were being trialed and tested around the world.... The first paper was last March or April, but it came out of a lab. It was what is called a cell culture model.... It showed that if you applied ivermectin to these monkey kidney-cells, the virus was essentially eradicated within 48 hours. They could find almost no viral material. Some places around the world took that bench study and brought it out into clinical use. I call that from the bench to the bedside.[160]

Dr. Kory acknowledges that very few substances that show promise in a lab ultimately prove to be of real therapeutic value; most fall off the bridge spanning the gulf between lab bench and human bedside. From the outset, however, two critical factors weighed in favor of ivermectin's as yet nascent Covid-19 career.

First, as detailed on the FLCCC website, ivermectin is no exotic unknown but a familiar pharmaceutical friend with an impeccable safety record:

> Ivermectin is a well-known, FDA-approved anti-parasite drug that has been used successfully for more than four decades to treat onchocerciasis ("river blindness") and other parasitic diseases. It is one of the safest drugs known. It is on the WHO's list of essential medicines, has been give 3.7 billion times around the globe, and has won the Nobel Prize for its global and historic impacts in eradicating endemic parasitic infections in many parts of the world.[161]

Second, Covid-19 did, after all, precipitate a global health crisis. Under such pressing circumstances, many physicians (especially those in less affluent nations that possessed limited resources for vaccine or experimental drug development) found themselves desperate for viable treatment options and were often willing to give anything that offered reasonable hope of amelioration a try—especially, of course, a cheap, readily available drug that posed virtually no risk of harm. Consequently, to cite Dr. Kory's plain words, "People used it." Thus an impressive body of evidence accumulated, the great bulk of which bears witness to the remarkable efficacy of ivermectin as a treatment for Covid-19.

Why then isn't the whole world routinely employing ivermectin as a treatment for Covid-19?

Anyone who has read this letter so far should be able to supply the easy if indigestible answer. It is not principally scientific concerns or public health and welfare concerns that stand in the way of more widespread, government-supported adoption of ivermectin-centered treatment protocols in America and other nations but politics—primarily, although not exclusively, the politics of corporate profit. The very features that, from any rational and humanitarian perspective, should qualify as the drug's greatest assets (efficacy, safety, ready availability, and, perhaps most important, affordability) count as strikes against it in a world ruled by powerful forces inflexibly committed to the controlling Covid-19 narrative.

The economics of ivermectin require an additional gloss, one that will reveal that the controlling Covid narrative is not quite as vaccine-centric as I have pretended. It is not exclusively vaccines that are acceptable solutions to the Covid problem but any pharmaceutically engineered product that can potentially turn a handsome profit for Big Pharma (confirmed by the December 8, 2020, U.S. Senate hearing we will soon discuss). Ivermectin, however, is not only very inexpensive to produce and distribute, *it is also off-patent.* Consequently, even Merck, the pharmaceutical that originally created and marketed it, cannot make real money from it. No one can.

Merck, in fact, has more or less disowned ivermectin as a viable Covid treatment and has for some months been pushing forward with plans to promote a different drug of its own—devising one, of course, that it *could* patent if it proves successful. On March 25, 2021, Bloomberg reported on "Merck's little brown pill" rather glowingly: "The antiviral drug molnupiravir, still in clinical trials, would give doctors an important new treatment and a weapon against coronaviruses." A couple of months later the Fierce Pharma website ran a witlessly revealing piece headed as follows: "With $1.2B deal for molnupiravir, U.S. bets on Merck's oral COVID-19 antiviral." It begins:

> Merck has struggled to develop therapeutics and vaccines to fight COVID-19. But the United States is betting that the pharmaceutical giant at last has a winner in its oral antiviral molnupiravir. On Wednesday, Merck revealed a deal to supply 1.7 million courses of the experimental treatment to the U.S. for approximately $1.2 billion. Molnupiravir has yet to be approved, but it's shown promise for newly diagnosed, non-hospitalized COVID-19 patients.[162]

The article appears beneath a captioned photograph of Merck's classy, glassy research headquarters. The caption reads:

> Merck has failed with two COVID-19 vaccines and another coronavirus treatment. But the U.S. believes Merck might have a winner in molnupiravir, for non-hospitalized COVID-19 patients.[163]

What is wrong with this picture? Just about everything. Here we have the U.S. government investing well over a billion dollars in clinical trials of an unproven drug (the therapeutic use of which in any event is limited to non-hospitalized COVID-19 patients), researched and developed by a company that has done nothing but fail in its repeated efforts to produce something of use in the fight against COVID-19. Meanwhile, here on the shelf sits that company's very own ivermectin, one of WHO's essential medicines, an approved, safe, inexpensive, readily available medication that impressive evidence shows to be highly effective, not only for early outpatient treatment, but *also* for *both* prophylaxis *and* in-hospital care.

Is this too good to be true? Too bad, say the responsible U.S. government agencies and those (fierce!) pharmaceutical companies that can all too easily imagine a drug like ivermectin (or HCQ, for that matter) blowing up the financial bonanza offered by COVID-19.

I am, however, getting a bit ahead of myself, so let's return to a somewhat more orderly telling of the ivermectin story.

After ivermectin appeared on their radar in the spring of 2020, Dr. Kory and the FLCCC doctors commenced and subsequently continued not only their intensive worldwide study of ivermectin but, as well, their own development and practical implementation of treatment protocols. In accord with their specialty, the team of ICU doctors first created a protocol for in-hospital treatment, and soon after proceeded to develop distinct but related protocols for both prevention and early outpatient treatment of Covid.

Meanwhile, despite mounting evidence of benefit, the NIH issued an August 27, 2020, advisory *against* use of Ivermectin for Covid-19 treatment, except in the context of clinical trial. By late December of that year, however, Dr. Kory and the FLCCC team had prepared a research paper reviewing, in detail, the "mountain" of scientific evidence supporting the efficacy of ivermectin as a treatment for Covid in each of the three relevant phases: prophylaxis, early outpatient treatment, and in-hospital treatment. The many studies cited included multiple randomized control trials and reflected a database of some 4,000 persons.

On December 20, 2020, Dr. Kory presented his group's finding at a U.S. Senate hearing (convened once more by Senator Ron Johnson) that represented the official sequel (part 2) to the November 19, 2020, hearing on early treatment featuring doctors McCullough, Risch, and Fareed. Dr. Kory's own chief aim was simple: to convince government health authorities to review the data in the hopes that the NIH and other relevant agencies would recognize the enormous benefit conferred by treatment with ivermectin and revise federal guidelines, policy, and resource allocation accordingly. Dr. Kory's passionate plea effectively echoed doctors McCullough, Risch, and Fareed's earlier call for a "national plan" of early treatment involving multiple complementary substances, except that here ivermectin occupied center stage and the prospective "plan" embraced prophylactic as well as in-hospital care, the first and third as well as the second of Dr. McCullough's four pillars of pandemic response.

Before, however, Dr. Kory, or any of the other witnesses, had a chance to open their mouth, the Senate committee's minority leader Michigan Senator Gary Peters had already begun kicking them around as if they were not so much doctors and citizens as political footballs.

I would like here to formally broach a critical topic I have so far mentioned only in passing. One could well argue that if Covid politics has always reflected the politics of profit, it has also been bitterly and unreservedly partisan. This stems, to some degree, from the timing of the 2020 presidential election. Democrats sought to hang President Trump's inept and inconsistent Covid response around his neck like an albatross that might sink his political fortunes. I am certainly not in the business here of defending President Trump, or his handling of the pandemic, but bring this up merely to call attention to the fiercely partisan political forces that have gathered and clung, like iron filings, to one or the other pole of the powerful Covid magnet.

President Trump generally played down the risk represented by Covid and endorsed certain remedies (such as HQC) that could, if genuinely effective, mitigate the threat it represented. Consequently, there emerged, on the Democratic side, the marked tendency to associate *any* questioning of the severity of the pandemic or the suitability of measures taken to combat it (such as lockdowns, masks, and social distancing) with Trump, his signature mendacity, and right-wing politics in general. This trend continued unabated after the election: thus, most criticism of the Biden administration's Covid response (including the vaccine campaign at its center), *no matter its substance or its source,* has too often automatically been viewed as a partisan Republican power play and, consequently, worthy of the dismissive disdain deserved by all those persons so misguided as to believe ex-President Trump's Big Lie.

This shallow and indiscriminate politicking has drastically degraded the quality of public discourse pertaining to Covid-19 and indeed, as shown by the rampant censorship it bred, has proven a disaster for American democracy. *As I hope this volume makes perfectly clear, the intellectual and moral substance of critical and conscientious resistance to official Covid policy has nothing intrinsically to do with any kind of reactionary right-wing agenda or any sort of assault on truth, science, or civic responsibility. Indeed, precisely the opposite is the case.* Liberals delude themselves and betray their own most cherished ideals if they imagine and construct matters otherwise.

It is true, of course, that certain Republican politicians have made a kind of cause célèbre of resisting the restrictive clauses of the Democratic administration of Covid policy.

I cannot judge here whether this or that politician's position represents a reasoned and principled stand (as appears to me to be the case, for instance, with Senator Johnson's championing of early treatment options) or instead just crass and facile opportunism. Both species (and probably everything in between) find representation in the stream of current political affairs. Yet the antics of a select politician or the biases of certain media personalities should not be magnified to overshadow the genuine and principled concerns that traverse, and indeed transcend, the spectrum of political allegiance.

The truth of that assertion is nowhere better embodied than in the words and deeds of many of the doctors and scientists that have addressed Covid concerns. It is true that the likes of doctors Peter McCullough, Byram Bridle, and Harvey Risch tend to appear not on or in CNN, the *Post* or the *Times,* but on Fox News and *The Wall Street Journal*. This, however, does not mean that these physicians and scientists harbor any overt or covert right-wing allegiances but rather reflects the deeply regrettable fact that the more *liberal media outlets systematically deny them any sort of platform for expression.* Dr. McCullough, for instance, has repeatedly (and so far vainly) sought airtime on CNN. He consequently has had little choice but to resort to an outlet such as Fox News if he is to broadcast his voice and views at all. The superficially illiberal cast of these doctors' media appearances thus reflects political allegiance only insofar as it is an *artifact* of the rigidly ideological partisanship of those so-called liberal channels who continue to deny them a forum for expression.

Automatic repudiation of *all* those who critically question official Covid-19 policy on the grounds of alleged right-wing partisanship is a red herring, and indeed one huge enough to constitute its own Big Lie. This destructive dynamic was on full display in the lead-up to the December 8, 2020, Senate hearing as well as in the hearing itself.

Unfortunately, *The New York Times,* that venerable organ of liberal-minded journalism, has assumed a positively McCarthyesque attitude with respect to any person or group that does not uncritically embrace the Democratic party line on Covid. Throwing truth and journalistic responsibility to the winds, the *Times'* coverage of this world-important matter descends at low tide to the level of tabloid smear campaign (as in the case of its misinformed hit piece on Dr. Joseph Mercola). In the December 8 Senate hearing, Dr. Armand Balboni, a distinguished infectious disease expert with an extensive academic background as well as seventeen years of service as a physician and scientist in the U.S. Army, reacted to the *Times'* preemptive marginalization of his testimony:

> I never thought I would have to say this, but I am a lifelong Democrat with a subscription to *The New York Times*.... I have to say I was quite dismayed this morning when I saw in the news that I was participating as a fringe member of an anti-vaxxer group. That couldn't be further from the truth.[164]

Perhaps nothing better illustrates the illusion-ridden, rabidly intolerant, and dictatorial attitude exhibited by the Democratic establishment in its conduct of Covid-19 affairs than minority leader Senator Gary Peters' opening remarks[165] and subsequent (mis)behavior at the December 8, 2020, hearing. After invoking the drastic toll so far exacted by Covid-19, Senator Peters continued:

> Thanks to the tireless work of our public health agencies, the private sector, and our scientific and medical communities, we've made progress in treating this disease. The FDA continues to use scientific standards to authorize innovative and effective early treatments.[166]

Given the almost total lack of any such treatments, one must wonder what Senator Peters is talking about. Is he simply creating castles in the air? Or referring to largely unaffordable treatments such as ineffective remdesivir or monoclonal antibodies? He went on:

> Unfortunately, today's discussion will not meet that standard. Senator [Johnson], I certainly share your goal of ensuring that patients across the country have access to early and effective treatments for coronavirus, but those statements must be based on evidence and not on politics.[167]

As the substance (or lack thereof) of the rest of Senator Peter's remarks confirm, the hypocrisy here is *off the charts*. After alluding to the prior month's hearing, Senator Peters proceeds:

> Unfortunately, that hearing, and the one before that, amplified unverified theories about treatments that are not supported by the scientific community. Instead of hearing from expert witnesses about scientific developments in coronavirus treatment or how we can improve the pandemic response, the committee was used as a platform to attack science and promote discredited treatments.[168]

After lamenting what he considered the abuse suffered by Dr. Jha in the hearing (remember that doctors McCullough and Risch had the audacity to challenge the veracity of Dr. Jha's conclusions, and Senator Johnson elicited from him an admission that he had never, in fact, treated any Covid-19 patients), Senator Peters continued:

> Sadly, it appears that today's hearing is going to follow the same path, playing politics with public health. It will not give us the information we need to take on this crisis.[169]

It can hardly be said that Senator Peters (who has yet to hear a word from any of the witnesses) is approaching the hearing with an open mind. After complaining of the discourteous treatment Dr. Jha received in November, he turns his attention to integrity of the witnesses themselves:

> The minority was not consulted about the scope of the hearing before it was noticed. The panelists have been selected for their political, not their medical views, and for that reason the composition of the panel creates a false and terribly harmful impression of the scientific and medical consensus. The witnesses have made many harmful and inflammatory statements.
>
> These statements include undermining a Covid-19 vaccine, promoting unproven therapeutics, discouraging common sense measures to stop the spread of the virus such as social distancing and masks, and even comparing physicians who support these interventions to supporters of a Nazi regime.[170]

This is demagoguery, and it is not only because the FLCCC's website actually endorses masks and distancing. Senator Peters continues with his own spurious brand of inflammatory rhetoric:

> We have a responsibility to follow science, to follow facts, not conspiracy theories and not disinformation.

...before concluding with the predictable denoument that casts the vaccine as a kind of divine child that the world, like anxious parents-to-be, awaits with breathless expectation. Are the crib, clothes, and perambulator duly prepared? When, after the event, will the notices for the shower go out?

> In the coming weeks, we expect that the first coronavirus vaccine will become available. We should be conducting strong oversight, including hearing testimony from government officials responsible for vaccine development and distribution. The commerce committee will be holding a hearing on how every American can get a vaccine.[171]

Senator Peter's clearly makes belief in the saving power of the vaccine an article of faith. No wonder that he appears simply to have *left* the hearing after delivering his opening salvo. His mind was not merely closed against anything the witnesses might say but locked, barred, and barricaded.

It bears mention, too, that—as Senator Johnson repeatedly pointed out—the hearing did not pertain to the matter of vaccines at all. All parties acknowledge that effective early treatment options are critical, and remain so even in the event of the development of a successful vaccine. In the context of the topic of this, and the prior hearing, talk of the vaccine was entirely beside the point. Or it *should* have been so, except for the inconvenient, elephant-in-the-room truth that recognizing the efficacy of other forms of treatment (such as ivermectin) could legally jeopardize the EUA status critical to accelerated vaccine deployment.

That said, Senator Peters' penultimate sentence rings with irony: "*We owe it to the American people...to get this right.*"

Upon offering his testimony, Dr. Kory was moved to respond to Senator Peters' intemperate assault:

> I want to register my offense at the ranking member's opening statement. I was discredited as a politician. I am a physician and a man of science. I've done nothing but commit myself to scientific truth and the care of patients. To hear that I am here because of a political angle...I am not a politician. I am a physician.
>
> I want to start by saying that I'm not speaking as an individual. I am speaking on behalf of the organization I'm a part of [the FLCCC]. We are a group of some of the most highly published physicians in the world. We have nearly 2,000 peer-reviewed publications between us. Led by Professor Paul Marik, our intellectual leader, we came together early in the pandemic and all we have sought is to review the world literature on every facet of the disease, trying to develop effective protocols.[172]

Dr. Kory proceeded to lay the groundwork for his presentation of the ivermectin angle, bolstering his personal credibility by way of reference to a prior unconventional recommendation that turned out to be critical for in-hospital Covid care:

> You just mentioned that I was here in May. I recommended that it was critical that we used corticosteroids for the disease when all of the national and international healthcare organizations said we cannot use those. That turned out to be a life-saving recommendation.
>
> I am here again today with a new recommendation.
>
> In the last nine months, in our review of the literature—again, we are some of the most highly published physicians in our specialty in the world—we have done nothing but try to figure out how to identify a repurposed and available drug to treat this illness. We have now come to the conclusion, after nine months . . .[173]

At this point, Dr. Kory interrupts himself to call aggrieved attention to a cardinal point I alluded to earlier: namely, the government's total disinterest in, and lack of support for, treatment options (including employing repurposed drugs such as ivermectin) that did *not* involve novel pharmaceutical engineering. He states:

> And I have to point out, I am severely troubled by the fact that the NIH, FDA, and CDC . . . I do not know of *any* task force that was assigned or compiled to review repurposed drugs in an attempt to treat this disease. Everything has been about novel and/or expensive pharmaceutically engineered drugs, things like . . . remdesivir, and monoclonal antibodies, and vaccines. We have over a hundred years of medicine development. We are expert in the all the medicines we use, and I do not know of a task force that has been focused on repurposed drugs.[174]

Dr. Kory continues to detail how the doctors that now comprise the FLCCC stepped in to address this glaring deficiency. In his own opinion at least, that effort achieved relatively swift success:

> I will tell you that my group, and our organization, have filled that void. That is all we have done: focus on those things we know and the things we do. And I'm here to tell you: we have a solution to this crisis. There is a drug that is proving to be of miraculous impact, and when I say miracle I do not use that term lightly. I don't want to be sensationalist when I say that. This is a scientific recommendation based on *mountains* of data that has emerged in the last three months.[175]

Throughout his relatively lengthy testimony, one can hear Dr. Kory pushing back against the confining strictures of a slow-moving if not unresponsive government bureaucracy, one that is enormously influential in determining how, in fact, most physicians treat (or do not treat) Covid-19:

> When I am told, and I just had to hear this in the opening statement, that we are touting things that are not FDA or NIH recommended.... Let me be clear. The NIH: their recommendation on ivermectin, which is not to use it outside of control trials, is from *August 27th*. We are now in December. That is three to four months later. Mountains of data have emerged from many centers and countries around the world showing the miraculous effectiveness of ivermectin. It basically obliterates transmission of the virus.... It has immense and potent antiviral activity. We've known that from the first study...[ivermectin] has made it from the bench to the bedside.[176]

Dr. Kory proceeded to summarize, to the best of his ability, the "mountains" of data testifying to the efficacy of ivermectin in three distinct and equally important applications: prophylaxis, early outpatient treatment, and in-hospital care. I cannot begin to due justice to that data here, nor could Dr. Kory himself, as he freely admitted. The chief purpose of his testimony was thus to exhort the NIH to carefully review the scientific paper that documented, in detail, the results from the many trials comprising that "mountain of evidence." I will, however, briefly mention a few of the salient results Dr. Kory highlighted in his testimony.

Data pertaining to ivermectin's *prophylactic power* included four large, randomized control trials (the gold standard in scientific research) involving a total of over 1,500 patients. Results showed ivermectin to be, in Dr. Kory's words, "immensely effective" as a prophylactic agent. Dr. Kory additionally mentioned results of a trial recently concluded in Argentina that involved eight hundred health workers. Half of them were given ivermectin as a prophylactic measure; half were not. Whereas *none* of those who received ivermectin contracted Covid-19, 237, or fifty-eight percent, of those who did not, did.

With respect to *early outpatient treatment,* Dr. Kory referenced three randomized control trials as well as multiple observational and case studies, all showing that use of ivermectin on an outpatient basis dramatically decreased the risk of hospitalization and death. Similarly, four large, randomized control trials demonstrated its value for *in-hospital treatment*, as its use in that setting significantly reduced the chance of death.

The most impressive and graphically visible evidence Dr. Kory presented, however, involved population-wide use of ivermectin in locales within three South American countries—Peru, Paraguay, and Mexico—each of which represented a quite distinct experimental circumstance. Eight Peruvian states initiated ivermectin distribution campaigns beginning in July 2020. The number of deaths in patients over sixty (by far the most vulnerable demographic) declined precipitously in August in all of those states, whereas no such amelioration transpired in those areas that did not distribute ivermectin. A not entirely dissimilar scenario unfolded in Mexico. Only a single state, Chiapas, incorporated ivermectin into its treatment protocol in July 2020. The death counts fell steeply in Chiapas, declining from roughly twenty-eight deaths per 100,000 persons in the weeks before August 1, 2020, to four deaths per 100,000 persons thereafter. No other Mexican state showed a steep decline; the vast majority of states, on the contrary, experienced a marked increase in deaths, the number of deaths per 100,000 persons, ranging from twenty-four to more than a hundred, with most states registering figures between forty and eighty—that is, ten to twenty times higher than Chiapas.

Perhaps the most humanly interesting ivermectin story played out in Paraguay. The governor of one region in Paraguay and his brother both contracted Covid-19, took ivermectin, and experienced swift amelioration. But since the federal health agencies in Paraguay, like those in the United States, *discouraged* use of ivermectin, the governor distributed ivermectin under the cover of a "deworming campaign." (Ivermectin, as you will recall, is primarily known as an antiparasitic). After six weeks, that state's hospitals were virtually empty of Covid-19 patients. Meanwhile, other regions of the country were recording between 1,000 and 3,000 cases and twenty to fifty deaths weekly.[177]

Quite a lot more relevant data is available through the FLCCC website.

Dr. Kory ended his initial presentation with a passionate and heartfelt plea that the data be reviewed promptly so that ivermectin might be recommended and widely employed as a means of stemming the tide of illness and death precipitated by the coronavirus. His concluding remarks were marked by agony as well as urgency. Dr. Kory emphasized that, as an ICU physician, he had seen more Covid patients die than could readily be imagined, and knowledge that many could have been saved by appropriate prophylaxis and treatment only intensified the traumatic and tragic character of that experience.

Dr. Kory concluded on a decidedly liberal note, hardly commensurate with the typecasting that too often serves the majority party's straw man tactics:

> Senator, the last thing I want to say is... You know who is dying here? It is our African-American, and Latino, and elderly. It is some of the most disadvantaged and impoverished members of our society. They are dying at higher rates than anyone else. It is the most severe discrepancy I've seen in my medical career. And we are responsible to protect those disadvantaged members. We have a special duty to provide countermeasures. The amount of evidence to show that ivermectin is life-saving and protective is so immense, and the drug is so safe.... It must be instituted and implemented. I'm asking the NIH to review our data and come with recommendations for society. Thank you.[178]

It goes without saying that expensive drugs such as remdesivir or monoclonal antibody treatment would hardly serve these populations. On the other hand, if the evidence offered by Dr. Kory is any indication, the potential for cheap, safe, and readily available ivermectin to do so can hardly be overestimated.

The NIH did review the paper submitted by Dr. Kory. While that review did produce a tangible result, it was hardly the outcome Dr. Kory envisioned. In February 2021, roughly two months after the hearing, the FDA upgraded its evaluation of ivermectin from "not recommended" to "neutral." The U.S. Government and its relevant agencies (the NIH, CDC, and FDA), did not move to support or promote ivermectin in any way. No funding for additional research was allocated, no positive recommendation that might lead to its incorporation in standard treatment protocols emerged, and certainly no plan for national education or distribution was formulated.

Not all knowledgeable persons evince the same confidence in ivermectin as Dr. Kory. Even so, given the volume and quality of the evidence (the merit of which *did* find tacit recognition in the FDA upgrade), one could reasonably have expected, at least, that responsible agencies would welcome further evaluation and open discussion of the drug's healing potential—*if* ideological and political consideration did not, as usual, stand in the way.

As we have seen, in his testimony, Dr. Kory expressed dismay at the government's apparent total disinterest in repurposed drugs and the correlative lack of the kind of effective, affordable, and readily available early treatment options that must figure as an integral part of any rational strategy to curb the pandemic. Despite Dr. Kory's plea, the government did next to nothing to make him and the FLCCC feel less alone in their effort to fill those huge black holes that continue, to this day, to suck the lives out of innumerable persons.

Instead of active support or even real neutrality, censorship traceable to government opposition to ivermectin continues to actively suppress further scientific and public exploration of the drug's therapeutic value as well as its practical use by physicians. I have previously discussed YouTube's demonetizing of Bret Weinstein's *DarkHorse* podcast on account of the latter's discussion of ivermectin. Believe it or not, Dr. Kory's own Senate testimony (which received millions of views on YouTube in the weeks following its broadcast) was disappeared from YouTube, a circumstance that prompted an angry February 2, 2021, *Wall Street Journal* piece by Senator Ron Johnson titled "YouTube Cancels the U.S. Senate."

In order to counteract such undemocratic measures, popular podcaster Joe Rogan invited Bret Weinstein and Dr. Kory to make a joint appearance on *The Joe Rogan Experience.*[179] Indeed, Rogan thought the mission of providing fair public discussion of the topic so urgent that he moved up the interview several weeks and christened their episode his first "emergency" podcast. In the lengthy interview, Kory and Weinstein not only reviewed diverse aspects of the ivermectin angle but also openly queried why, even in the midst of the ongoing crisis, the reigning health authorities had actively sought to discourage its use and discredit its proponents. Kory and Weinstein emphasized that in light of the potent combination of the drug's strong record of benefit *and* its proven safety, such recalcitrance *simply made no sense at all.*

To be sure, certain questions had been raised about the quality of this or that aspect of the research, but Dr. Kory stressed that obsessive preoccupation with questionable standards of scientific "proof" should hardly outweigh extensive real-time evidence of benefit. And this should be all the more true, naturally, in the midst of a pandemic when: (1) human lives are constantly at risk; (2) no other good treatment option is easily available; and (3) there exists good record of ivermectin's safety, and there is, in marked contrast to the mass vaccination program, *no significant downside to giving the drug a chance to work its magic.*

The official stance, all three discussants agreed, was indeed inexplicable—*unless* one were to admit of the suggestion, considered repugnant by all, that corporate profit rather than public health and welfare was setting the agenda for the government's Covid response. Given the inconceivable human cost of such immoral conduct, neither Kory nor Weinstein—two manifestly intelligent and compassionate souls—were at all anxious to confirm that conclusion. To any rational mind, however, it appears (alas!) virtually inescapable.

At one point in the interview, Dr. Kory made a related, singularly revealing statement. He confessed that his attitude with respect to the government's administration of public health had undergone a sea change over the course of the last year. He had previously always proceeded on the assumption that he could best serve public health by working *with* the government whenever and however possible. Now, though, Dr. Kory, speaking in a rather resigned tone that was quite unlike the tone of fervor he displayed at the Senate hearing, admitted that he more or less took it for granted that, if one wanted to accomplish one's goals, one had to anticipate working not *with* the government but rather *around* it.

As far as the judging the merits of the case for ivermectin is concerned, Weinstein, Rogan, and Kory offered one more particularly insightful angle. *Look*, the trio suggested, at exactly *who* is on *which* side of the debate, and *how* they are conducting themselves. They pointed to one's side proclivity for uniformity and lack of toleration for dissent, and the other side's diversity, independence, and openness to dialogue. Let me, in closing, take that ball and run with it.

On the *one* hand, you have a single controlling narrative, endorsed by a powerful bureaucracy quarterbacked by an authority (Dr. Fauci) personally invested (both financially and ideologically) in outcomes that benefit pharmaceutical companies, and who himself materially contributed to the risky Wuhan lab research that could conceivably have caused the pandemic; government agencies and officials falling in line behind that single narrative and (entangled in an intricate network of special interest and corporate greed) not only evidently intent on suppressing all dissent but ready and willing to employ coercion to that end; media outlets that do not only habitually decline to tell both sides of a story but are manned by faceless, inexpert fact-checkers who, responding to government pressure, carry out a program of systematic censorship and disinformation even while (often groundlessly) accusing alternative voices of doing the same; doctors who having never treated a single Covid-19 patient offering "expert" testimony aimed at discrediting the arguments of those who have treated thousands; and legions of other duly obedient health professionals following a government protocol that, *for no good reason*, aggressively discourages safe and effective treatment options that could well have prevented untold human misery and perhaps long ago helped put the pandemic in the rearview mirror.

On the *other* hand, the individuals and groups contesting the official narrative comprise a heterogeneous group of strikingly *independent* minds and personalities. This ensemble includes exceptionally brilliant and accomplished researchers (Dr. Robert Malone, Dr. Geert Vanden Bossche, Professor Paul Marik, and others); extraordinarily committed and public-minded physicians who have founded or worked with non-for-profit organizations dedicated to alleviating the toll of Covid suffering (doctors Kory, McCullough, Fareed, and others); academics and doctors who have courageously and visibly risked professional careers and reputations in the interest of public service and scientific integrity (all of the above persons, as well as doctors Byram Bridle, Patrick Phillips, and others); journalists and podcasters (Hold the Line members; Bret Weinstein, Joe Rogan) who make it their public mission to resist censorship and seek to tell both sides of any story; and iconoclastic organizations spanning the political spectrum (Children's Health Defense, The Informed Action Consent Network, and Stand for Health Freedom) dedicated to preserving individual American citizens' essential rights and freedoms.

As Bret Weinstein himself emphasized, the people and groups mentioned in the previous paragraph are by no means of one mind on all things Covid-19. There is no Party Line, no one simple, agreed-upon formulaic solution to the Covid-19 problem but rather a positive interest in ongoing and lively debate pertaining to the prevention and treatment of Covid-19.

To follow and have faith in the one side is a fairly simple matter: Distance, Mask, and, above all, Vax, and you'll have discharged your civic duty. (While you are at it, though, make sure others do likewise!) To listen to the many voices that question the hegemony of the controlling narrative is evidently more of a challenge, intellectually, and, I suspect, emotionally as well. Even so, given the profile of the two lineups, to whom do you think we had best listen? Whom, after all, would you sooner trust with your (and our *American* way of) life?

Chapter 17

NEWSBREAK: "YOU ARE NOT A HORSE"

Despite the strenuous efforts of the powers that be, word gets around. Most people have heard of ivermectin and its efficacy in prevention and treatment of Covid-19. This *should* be good news. The government's failure, however, to support further exploration or responsible use of the (by now notorious) drug has opened the door to its misuse. Ivermectin has long been marketed as an antiparasitic for farm animals as well as humans, and in that form can be obtained—without a doctor's prescription—at feed stores. While the substance remains essentially the same in both applications, dosages naturally differ dramatically for creatures with such different body masses. Recently, news outlets reported a spate of cases of persons taking equine-sized doses of ivermectin, an unsafe practice that landed some in the hospital.

This regrettable development (one that could have been entirely avoided by responsible government stewardship) has naturally provided new ammunition for those who oppose use of the drug for prevention and treatment of Covid-19. A lead article in the September 3, 2021, edition of the *San Francisco Chronicle*[180] ("FDA: Don't use horse drug to fight COVID") exhibits this mainstream paper's opportunistic attempt to utilize this unfortunate circumstance to discredit the drug entirely. In so doing, it all too clearly displays the shoddy yellow journalism characteristic of much mainstream press coverage of Covid matters.

The article begins with an ill-humored put-down of those disinclined to trust Covid-19 vaccines even as it casts ivermectin in a decidedly off-color—not to say disgusting—light:

> People who say the COVID-19 vaccine is too dangerous suddenly can't wait to get injected—with horse de-wormer.[181]

The next paragraph continues in the same bestial vein, insinuating (incorrectly, of course) that ivermectin is not for humans:

> The animal drug ivermectin has gotten so popular as an imagined shield against the coronavirus that some shops selling it, like the Peninsula Feed Store in Redwood City, are posting reminders: "You are not a Horse."[182]

After the rhetorical damage inflicted by these opening salvos, the article does get around to reporting some of the notable history of the drug (including its Nobel Prize-winning treatment of river blindness) before playing up the dangers of wrongful use and insinuating that there is no sound biological basis for imagining that ivermectin may be an appropriate treatment for Covid-19. Covid, of course, is caused by a virus, and the *Chronicle* cites an FDA cautionary warning that ivermectin is *not* an antiviral drug. As an antiparasitic, ivermectin may not technically be classed as such; it may nonetheless—as Dr. Kory claims—function as "an immensely powerful antiviral." By the time the article cites Dr. Kory's own words to that effect, however, the reader has been well-prepared, by the edict of federal authority, to doubt the sobriety of his judgment.

The article does proceed to highlight Dr. Kory's dramatic assertions affirming the efficacy of ivermectin as a Covid treatment. But the paper's first line of response? A reference, once again, to horse medicine, and, too, singularly unimpressive medical authority:

> Dr. Graham Walker, an emergency room physician in San Francisco, debunks Kory and his group on Twitter. "I don't want people to take horse medicine," Walker said. "It feels like I have to do something as an ER doctor." He asked that his hospital not be named because he isn't authorized to speak for it.[183]

Needless to say, no reference to farm animals can "debunk" Dr. Kory and the FLCCC's case for appropriate use of ivermectin—least, of all, a random emergency room doctor's Twitter thread. If one checks the relevant feeds, moreover, one will discover that Dr. Graham Walker, while he does reference studies that may raise legitimate questions about some of the data supporting ivermectin efficacy, does not himself begin to do any authoritative "debunking." In fact, Dr. Walker—though an aggressive and polemical proponent of the official position—openly recognizes that its public advocacy has been deeply flawed:

> The anti-vaxx and misinformation people honestly haven't had to do too much to succeed in this pandemic. We've done it for them by publishing misleading, inaccurate, or incomplete data, jumping to conclusions or widely disseminating preprints. We have met the enemy, and it is us.[184]

The rest of the *Chronicle* article certainly bears out Walker's words. To substantiate the supposed "debunking" of ivermectin, the article cites two studies, one a preprint pending publication, showing little or no benefit from treatment with ivermectin. The *Chronicle* presents this as sufficient ground to render a more or less definitive verdict—indeed, so much so that the continuation of the front-page article on page three sports a big bold-face subtitle reading: *"Trials show ivermectin has no benefit for COVID."*[185]

These, however, represent just two of numerous studies, many of which contribute to the "mountain" of evidence that Dr. Kory, Bret Weinstein, and others believe does confirm ivermectin's agency. It is true that data analysis and interpretation can be much less clear-cut than one might expect in scientific studies, and some scientists have raised serious questions as to the quality of the data supposedly supporting ivermectin. Even so, independent data analysis of relevant high-quality data (twenty-four randomized control trials involving 3,406 participants) by accomplished and experienced medical data analysts does confirm significant efficacy.[186]

Moreover, as Dr. Kory himself alleged, overly academic preoccupation with theoretical standards of proof can sometimes result in failing to see the forest for the trees. As a lay citizen interested in practical results, I find the FLCCC's evaluation of the *brand* of evidence most trustworthy in this connection to be quite reasonable. The FLCCC website[187] contains (or provides reference to) an immense amount of evidence of all sorts and introduces one especially relevant section of the *Summary of the Evidence for Ivermectin in COVID-19* with these words: "The reports *most relevant to public health officials* are from the national and regional ministries that employed either distribution or 'test and treat' programs with ivermectin (emphasis mine)."[188]

Results from such programs, quoted from their *Summary,* include:

- Mexico City: "The IMSSS Health Agency compared over 50,000 patients treated early with ivermectin to over 70,000 not treated and found up to a seventy-five percent reduction in need for hospitalization."

- Peru: "A nationwide mass-distribution program called 'Mega-Operación Tayta' (MOT), initiated at various times across 25 states of Peru in May 2020, led to a seventy-four percent drop in regional excess deaths within a month, with *each drop* beginning eleven days after each MOT region's varied start times."

- La Misiones, Argentina: "Health Ministry just analyzed the first 800 of 4,000 ivermectin treated patients and compared to the rest of the population over the same time period, they found a seventy-five percent reduction in need for hospitalization and an eighty-eight percent reduction in death."[189]

The *Chronicle* piece itself doesn't seem to trust the weight of its own scanty evidence, and the close of their piece veers off into truly surreal scare tactics. After reiterating the danger represented by ivermectin overdose, the article continues:

> Dosage is just one safety issue surrounding people who self-medicate with ivermectin. Another involves the extra stuff contained in drugs, like stabilizers and preservatives, said Desi Kotis, UCSF's chief pharmacy executive. Unless such ingredients are also studied, it's impossible to know if the drug is safe to take, she said, noting that heroin users often died in the 1980s not from an overdose, but from talcum power cut into the drug that clumped and blocked blood flow to the heart.[190]

How did we progress from any rational consideration of ivermectin, a drug on the list of the WHO's essential medicines and so safe it has been used 3.7 billion times (at the time of this writing), to "the extra stuff contained in drugs," *heroin,* talcum powder, and fatal blood clots? The logic here escapes me, unless it is an underhanded attempt to associate ivermectin with an infamously illegal, addictive, and too-often lethal narcotic. The *Chronicle* coverage of the pandemic has been more propaganda than news from the first, but I have to hand it to the writer of this piece: as far as irresponsible journalism is concerned, she really pushes the envelope.

Glenn Greenwald, like Matt Taibbi, represents another class of journallist altogether; the kind of independent journalism unflinchingly dedicated to the truth of the matter at hand.

I close this chapter with a duet of tweets, the first from Greenwald, and—in reply—one from the man who has become the public face of ivermection, Dr. Pierre Kory:

> **Covid19Crusher** @Covid19Crusher ~ Sep 2
>
> It is absolutely amazing.
> 44 peer-reviewed ivermectin studies.
> 39 positive.
> And some journalists still proclaim that none exist.
> twitter.com/ggreenwald

> **Pierre Kory, MD MPA** @Pierre Kory. 18h
>
> Hey, @ggreenwald, there are 44 published, peer-reviewed studies
> of IVM in COVID - 11 Double blind RCT's, 12 open RCT's,
> 1 simple blind RCT, 2 PSM OCT's - nearly all showing MASSIVE
> benefits...+ more than 30 non-RCT's show the exact same.
> NIH could give a weak/cautious rec...but won't. Insane.

Chapter 18

THE EMPEROR'S (NOT-SO-)NEW CLOTHES

Ivermectin has shown itself to be an invaluable ally in the fight against Covid-19, but it is not the only tried and true one. In all professionally recommended protocols, it is employed in conjunction with other critical agents, including zinc and vitamin D. Indeed, Dr. Vladimir Zelenko, who published the first effective protocol, states that it is zinc that is really the silver bullet that kills the virus.[191] Zinc, however, cannot itself enter the relevant cells, so the efficacy of that bullet requires one or another "gun" to force its entry. HCQ (the "gun" in the original Zelenko protocol) and ivermectin are both effective "weapons" suited to that purpose.

At the same time, another not-so-secret agent—one that has been around since the beginning of the pandemic—is gaining prominence in the struggle to combat the Delta variant. At the first sign of illness, patients may receive either an injection or intravenous infusion of monoclonal antibodies. The antibodies, available in medicinal form in a product manufactured by Regeneron, work (like other treatment agents) to neutralize the pathogenic spike protein. The procedure, readily performed on an outpatient basis, lasts a painless thirty minutes, and is very safe. The treatment (which is FDA approved, and may, if desired, be employed in synergistic conjunction with ivermectin and other early treatment protocols) is proving very effective in preventing hospitalization and death, Delta notwithstanding,[192] so much so that Texas has recently initiated a program to establish infusion centers throughout the state.

Dr. Richard Bartlett, a general practitioner and ER physician in Texas, is one of the doctors administering treatment with monoclonal antibodies. In an interview with Del Bigtree,[193] Dr. Bartlett bore witness to its great efficacy, saying that illness-related discomfort (including backaches and a range of other symptoms) often decreased or disappeared in the course of the half-hour treatment itself. More important, although I know of no relevant statistics available at this point, there seems to be near-widespread agreement among physicians that the treatment works to the extent of drastically reducing the need for subsequent hospitalization. In the words cited below, Dr. Bartlett gives voice to truths relevant not only to this particular treatment but to an overall view of the whole Covid picture:

> This is all about early treatment. That's what has been ignored, suppressed, minimized, censored: Early effective outpatient treatment. This [monoclonal antibodies] falls in that category.
>
> All the people that were anti-early treatment agree that this works. I think that means that there *is* early effective outpatient treatment. The bottom line is: That's the winning strategy.
>
> There are other [outpatient treatment] strategies that work. There are doctors on both sides on mask or no mask, vaccine or no vaccine...but everybody agrees on monoclonal antibodies.[194]

As the interview continues, Dr. Bartlett addresses the official word on two of those other effective treatment strategies: ivermectin, and another repurposed pharmaceutical, budesonide, that Oxford University studies have recently shown to be yet another quite effective counter to Covid-19. Predictably enough, Dr. Anthony Fauci disputes the efficacy of both of these measures, declaring, of ivermectin, "There is no clinical evidence that this works."[195] Asked by Bigtree to comment on that unequivocal counterfactual statement, Dr. Bartlett responded:

> I heard the same thing about budesonide...He said it's a placebo, it doesn't really work. Oxford University says the opposite. Oxford is the oldest university in the English-speaking world, since 1096, with 72 Nobel Prize laureates. They say that he's wrong. They say 90% of hospitalization and urgent care visits...What has he said that *is* right?
>
> This is the same pattern of information going out from two sources. One has been proven wrong, over and over. I'd say half of the people I am seeing in the infusion center have been vaccinated.
>
> I love people. I have loved ones who have been vaccinated; others who haven't. The problem is the virus, and the problem is there's a tremendous effort to censor information, and interfere with science, and facts. Fauci doesn't talk about facts, and science. He just says something and has nothing to back it up.[196]

To that end, have you ever heard of the tale of the Emperor who had no clothes? When, in this country, will the great mass of people stop believing in the story everyone's been told?

Of course, not everybody is buying into all the fine-spun features of the story handed down from on high. Take, for instance, the controversial subject of the origins of Covid-19.

The lab leak theory has recently progressed from a hypothesis hatched by so-called fringe conspiracy theorists to a plausible idea that many if not most expert persons now regard as the default option for explaining the origin of the pandemic.

From the first, Dr. Fauci has aggressively denied not the possibility of a lab leak but its probability, despite all the common-sense reasons to regard the lab leak as, in fact, the most likely explanation. Take these factors: 1) the failure so far to discover any naturally occurring animal source; 2) ongoing laboratory research on bat coronavirus in the very area of disease-origin, and in the confines of a lab, no less, regarded as falling well short of adequate safety standards; 3) the illness, by coronavirus infection, of personnel working in the lab shortly before the onset of the pandemic; and finally, 4) genetic evidence that qualified experts believe indicate an engineered rather than naturally occurring, zoonotically transmitted virus. The latter point is particularly sensitive because Fauci himself, in his capacity as director of the NIH-affiliated National Institute of Allergic and Infectious Diseases, helped fund (via discrete organizational channels that screened his financial involvement) what may well be judged illegal research in the Wuhan Lab—research of the kind, in fact, that may have led directly to the escape of the virus that caused the pandemic.

The legal question here revolves around whether the relevant work at Wuhan technically qualifies as illicit "gain-of-function" research. Senator Ron Paul, one of those "childish" onlookers liable to believe the testimony of their own mind and body, believes it most certainly does. In a U.S. Senate hearing, Senator Paul, whom I will quote, challenged Dr. Fauci's honesty on this score:

> Viruses that in nature only infect animals were manipulated in the Wuhan Lab to gain the function of infecting humans. This research fits the definition of the research that the NIH said was subject to the pause in 2014 to 2017, a pause in funding of gain-of-function. But the NIH failed to recognize this, defines it away, and it never came under any scrutiny.
>
> Dr. Richard Ebright, a molecular biologist from Rutgers, describes the research in Wuhan [as follows]: "The Wuhan Lab used NIH funding to construct novel chimeric SARS-related coronaviruses able to infect human cells and laboratory animals. This is high-risk research that creates new potential pandemic pathogens that exist only in the lab, not in nature. This research matches…indeed epitomizes gain-of-function research."
>
> Dr. Fauci, knowing that it is a crime to lie to Congress, do you wish to retract your statement of May 11, when you claimed that the NIH never funded gain-of-function research in Wuhan?[197]

The (by now infamous) exchange continues:

> *Dr. Fauci:* Senator Paul...I do not retract that statement. This paper [holds up document] that you are referring to, was judged by qualified staff up and down the chain, as *not* being gain-of-function.
>
> *Senator Paul:* You take an animal virus, and you increase its transmissibility to humans....You are saying that is *not* gain-of-function?
>
> *Dr. Fauci:* That is correct. Senator Paul: [emphatically] you do not know what you are talking about.[198]

Despite Dr. Fauci's heated insistence, it seems perfectly clear that Senator Paul knows precisely of what he speaks. Don't you think that Dr. Fauci's assertion of royal authority ("Senator Paul: you do not know what you are talking about") might well echo what the Emperor, and his crowd of servile admirers, said to the child who dared exclaim: "Look! The Emperor has no clothes!"?

Postscript: Other persons, too, suspect that Senator Paul might not be the party suffering delusions of grandeur here. In early August, ICAN filed a FOIA (Freedom of Information Act) request for any and all documents (or other forms of relevant evidence) corroborating Dr. Fauci's claim that "qualified staff up and down the chain" judged the NIAID-funded Wuhan research as not gain-of-function.[199] By law, FOIA requests must be honored within twenty days of filing. If the relevant party fails to comply, a subsequent motion to enforce compliance can be filed.

Evidently, that staff "up and down the chain" didn't record their assessment in writing. Or if they did, the NIH is not anxious to come forward with the evidence that could exonerate—or alternatively, contradict—Dr. Fauci. The twenty-day deadline has come and gone without compliance. ICAN has filed the follow-up motion to expedite discovery. As I write these words on Labor Day weekend (September 5, 2021), the denouement of Senator Paul and Dr. Fauci's dramatic exchange remains pending.[200]

CHAPTER 19

THE RIGHT WAY TO FIGHT VIRUSES

Monoclonal antibodies represent a very promising antidote to Covid-19. Repurposed pharmaceuticals—ivermectin, certainly, and most likely HCQ, budesonide, and others, as well—can also be game-changers in the fight against Covid-19. Indeed, Bret Weinstein believes that a full-court press employing ivermectin as a prophylactic could eradicate the virus by decimating the number of available hosts. (As mentioned, the Covid vaccines, even regularly boosted, can never do likewise because the vaccines focus solely on the spike protein and do not exert "lethal pressure.") In his session with Joe Rogan and Dr. Kory, Weinstein related how, after lengthy dialogue with a skeptical Robert Malone, the latter finally came around to share that point of view after pursuing his own rigorous inquiry.[201]

Such an initiative, however, is politically improbable—unless relevant authorities were to perform a 180-degree turn. Even if they were to do so, there are likely persons disinclined to take any pharmaceutical as a purely preventative measure. Such individuals, however, are hardly without alternative resources. Indeed, *any comprehensive COVID-19 strategy should be broad-based, and include common health measures that bolster resistance to all viral disease as well as an informed use of nutraceuticals (vitamins).*

This brings us to one of the most critical—and grossly warped—features of the usual Covid story. Once U.S. health authorities (belatedly) recognized the danger represented by Covid-19, they generally behaved as if it were some kind of deadly alien invasion against which all usual lines of defense were singularly powerless. In fact, the etiology of Covid-19 is kin to that of other viruses and (as might be expected) experience shows that while Covid-19 certainly poses its own distinct and dramatic challenge, measures effective in both the prevention and treatment of other viral infections (such as the flu) remain valuable and even indispensable allies in the fight against Covid-19.

Sadly, anyone informed solely by the official response to the virus would never have the least clue of that. In his August 2021 newsletter, "The Right Way to Fight Viruses," Dr. David Brownstein (echoing the sentiment we have heard from concerned physicians time and again) recalls the lamentable circumstances pertaining to the CDC's initial reaction to Covid:

> As more and more patients became ill with COVID-19, the CDC and other powers that be—who were supposed to be guiding physicians and public institutions on how to respond—claimed that there were no treatments available for patients suffering from COVID-19...They could only come up with a few paltry recommendations such as staying home, social distancing in public, eventually mask wearing, and then just waiting for a vaccine. There were no therapeutic treatments offered for those suffering from COVID.[202]

In a concluding section, Dr. Brownstein writes:

> COVID-19 is a constellation of symptoms caused by the virus SARS-CoV-2. At the beginning of the outbreak, the media and other powers that be sent the message that becoming ill with COVID-19 is a death sentence. Nothing could be further from the truth.
>
> COVID is nothing to be taken lightly. Far too many have died. However, the news is not nearly as bad as what was predicted. Research has shown that this strain of coronavirus can be effectively managed with both pharmaceuticals and nutraceuticals.
>
> I have been treating this illness since it began 18 months ago. My protocol of using nutritional and oxidative therapies has shown its effectiveness time and again. Others have reported positive results with pharmaceuticals such as ivermectin and hydroxychloroquine.
>
> We all need to lower the fear level and look at COVID-19 as a treatable illness, not a death sentence.[203]

In the body of his newsletter, Dr. Brownstein tells the tale of his own Detroit-area clinic's confrontation with Covid. He recounted the panic that struck his office; how, in late February 2020, his office manager told him he needed to meet with this staff, many of whom were scared to interact with patients and threatened to leave if the office remained open. When he did convene a meeting, Dr. Brownstein first confirmed that he fully expected Covid to arrive in Detroit in the very near future. He continued by declaring: "I am not closing this office. We know how to treat patients with viral illnesses. We have been treating patients suffering from viral illnesses for decades."[204]

Dr. Brownstein had long been employing nutritional and oxidative therapies to treat patients with flu and other kindred illnesses. Because various types of coronavirus infections trigger roughly one-third of such illnesses, Dr. Brownstein had good cause to believe that his protocol would prove effective in treating Covid-19. He told his staff: "This strain of coronavirus is different. I can't make any guarantees, but I'm confident our patients will do well."

Dr. Brownstein naturally went through a preliminary period of deep concern, fearing that despite his well-grounded conviction to the contrary, his means and methods would not stave off serious illness or death of patients who contracted Covid. His confidence was soon tested. Not long after that staff meeting, the Detroit area became one of the country's first Covid hotspots.

Here is Dr. Brownstein's own summary exposition of his treatment protocol:

At the first sign of illness—such as sore throat, cough, or fever—we instructed patients to take, for four days, high doses (orally) of:

- *Vitamin A (100,000 IU)*
- *Vitamin C (1,000 mg every waking hour until bowel tolerance)*
- *Vitamin D3 (50,000 IU)*
- *Iodine (25 to 50 mg per day)*

Patients (especially those with breathing difficulties) were also advised to nebulize 3 ccs every waking hour of a dilute solution of hydrogen peroxide (0.03 percent) and iodine (one drop of five percent Lugol's solution).

Finally, if they were very ill we had patients come to the back of our office, in the parking lot, where we administered intravenous nutritional and oxidative therapies to them in their cars.[205]

Dr. Brownstein's belief in his principles and methods was soon justified. The therapies did indeed ameliorate the ill effects of infection and aid recovery. At the time of the publication of his August 2021 newsletter, Dr. Brownstein and his associates had treated more than 520 Covid-19 patients. *None* of those patients died, only nine were hospitalized, and roughly 2.5 per cent (13) suffered symptoms associated with "long Covid."[206]

These are good numbers, and generally compare favorably with other treatment methods.

When Dr. Brownstein saw that his protocol was indeed efficacious, he was moved to offer an antidote to the helpless doom and gloom scenario that pervaded the public in spring 2020. As Dr. Brownstein recalled:

> People were afraid to leave their homes. Most thought that they were going to die if they contracted COVID-19, and therefore they were afraid to be around anybody. Worse yet, many people were scared to go to the hospital because the death rate for COVID-19 was very high for hospitalized patients at the beginning of the crisis. I wanted to show people that COVID-19 was a treatable illness.[207]

In keeping with that aim, Dr. Brownstein recorded a series of video interviews with patients, who shared news of their (sometimes quite serious) illness and their improvement upon treatment. Dr. Brownstein called the series: "There is Still Hope Out There."

A month or so after he began posting the videos, Dr. Brownstein received a warning from the U.S. Federal Trade Commission (FTC) to stop making statements about Covid treatment protocols. To cite Dr. Brownstein's words: "Because there was no proven prevention, treatment, or cure for COVID-19, any mention of the protocol I had used to treat my patients was a violation of federal law." The letter directed Dr. Brownstein to remove all video and blog posts within forty-eight hours. Dr. Brownstein consulted his lawyer, who advised him that he could either fight the government or continue treating his patients. Dr. Brownstein chose the latter, and removed all the content.

He did, however, publish a peer-reviewed paper, titled "A Novel Approach to Treating COVID-19 Using Nutritional and Oxidative Therapies." It appeared in the *Journal of Public Health Policy* in July of 2020.[208] He also published a book (his 16th), titled *A Holistic Approach to Viruses.*[209] His lawyer assured him that these publications represented speech protected by the First Amendment. Should there ever have been any reason for doubt on that score?

At the end of his account of his Covid adventures, Dr. Brownstein both emphasized the success of his own treatment protocol—which included *no* pharmaceutical component—and, also, recognized that ivermectin and HCQ have also proven efficacious. He closed with words that sound yet again a theme that echoes throughout the body of *this* book:

> Simply put, COVID-19 is *a treatable illness.* I believe that if patients were treated early in the outbreak, we would not have hundreds of thousands dead. Dr. Peter McCullough, a cardiologist and vice chief of medicine at Baylor University Medical Center in Dallas, estimates that more than three-quarters of the patients who died from COVID-19 could have been saved with treatment. If he is correct, the pandemic could have looked like nothing worse than a bad flu season.[210]

Effective treatment protocols are clearly crucial; equally so, however, are preventative measures, *the most fundamental of which entail essential health practices that help bolster the body's own immunological power and so defend against incidence and severity of viral infection.* While I have neither the expertise nor the space to go into the topic in depth, Dr. Brownstein's newsletter includes a section titled "Six Strategies for Protecting Against Viral Infections" that provides a brief explanation of relevant measures.[211]

The last three of Dr. Brownstein's suggestions are: (4) *Supplements that support immunity (including vitamin D)*; (5) *Iodine*; and (6) *Nebulize with hydrogen peroxide and iodine*. All these are important tools, and the fourth and sixth have already been referenced.

I will not address them further here; those interested can find other sources of information, including, with respect to iodine, Dr. Brownstein's book: *Iodine: Why You Need it, Why You Can't Live Without It*.[212]

Anyone at all health-conscious will, however, immediately recognize the first three of Dr. Brownstein's suggestions, all of which merit brief mention here on account of their inestimable importance:

1. *Healthy diet*. Dr. Brownstein writes: "I can't stress enough the importance of diet, not just for helping overcome a viral infection, but also to give you the best chance for dealing with any stressful situation your body encounters." The first requisites of healthy diet are negative: refined or processed foods (including refined sugars, salt, and oils) are very deleterious; conversely, consumption of fresh (preferably organic) produce provide indispensable nourishment. These dietary facts are, regrettably, keenly relevant to the high incidence of Covid-19 in many minority communities, within which context poor quality and even junk food are often disproportionately consumed and fresh produce (which is sometimes difficult to procure on account of a lack of suitable grocery outlets) correspondingly underrepresented. This most likely is one of the most significant factors contributing to the grossly disproportionate impact of Covid on disadvantaged, often minority communities.
2. *Optimal hydration*. Dr. Brownstein emphasizes that it is crucial to maintain good hydration during any and all illness, including Covid-19. Dehydration exacerbates inflammatory issues and impedes the body's natural capacity to fend off infection.
3. *Daily exercise*. Dr. Brownstein notes that exercise is known to "stimulate and moderate" the immune system. Accordingly:

   > A study of 48,440 adults with a COVID-19 diagnosis found that those who were consistently inactive had a *126 percent greater increased risk of hospitalization and a 149 percent greater risk of death* compared to patients who exercised daily.[213]

He also observes:

> Since the beginning of COVID-19, obese individuals have been found to be at a high risk for a poor outcome from the infection. The authorities should be promoting exercise as an effective part of the regimen for combating this outbreak.[214]

Lockdowns, anyone?

Chapter 20

ICU INTERLUDE: IN-HOSPITAL MISTREATMENT

In prior sections, I have discussed a variety of effective prophylactic and early outpatient treatment measures for Covid-19. Health authorities' willful neglect or active discouragement of these finds unfortunate reflection in the standard protocol for *inpatient* treatment that determines the fate of countless persons who do land in the hospital. Regrettably, there are grounds to suspect that the CDC- and NIH-approved inpatient protocols are every bit as damaging as their policies pertaining to prevention and early treatment. This is unsurprising, as the former represents the (il)logical extension of the latter.

Ivermectin, in an appropriately adjusted dosage, can be effective for prevention, early treatment, *and* in-hospital care. The same holds for nutraceutical treatment. Government prejudice against these measures extends to inpatient care and so ultimately denies sick persons recourse to a variety of means that impede progress of the disease and bolster patient recovery. As a consequence, far too many patients end up much too quickly on a ventilator, at which point the prognosis (as most everybody should know by now) is dire.

In an August 6, 2021, episode of her radio show,[215] Kate Dalley recounts her experience of accompanying her husband as he went in-hospital for treatment for "Covid-pneumonia." Dalley herself was skeptical of the diagnosis reached on the basis of a PCR test run at a cycle threshold of forty. As she points out, such a test is entirely incapable of distinguishing between Covid, flu, pneumonia, or any kindred illness. If her husband actually had simple pneumonia (which, in her mind, remained a distinct possibility), he would have been placed in a regular hospital room, given high-flow oxygen to aid his impaired breathing, and, in all probability, released in a matter of days. On account of his Covid diagnoses, however, he was immediately transferred to the ICU and tracked for treatment in accordance with hospital's Covid-19 protocol.

Already in the ER, after the Covid diagnosis, Dalley and her husband were told that "the next step" would be ventilation. Knowing that the fatality rate of those put on ventilation is extraordinarily high, Kate Dalley demurred, insisting that hers was "a no-ventilator family." The hospital personnel took affront at this and insisted that, in cases such as her husband's, it was standard procedure. When she still resisted, they turned to her husband, saying that it was his life, not hers, and that he might very well suffer brain damage if he did not agree to ventilation.

Unfazed, he did not.

Once her husband was in the ICU, Kate Dalley was informed that he must count on being there for a minimum of seven days—and the confrontation continued. Following recommendations from America's Frontline Doctors, Dalley and her husband requested intravenous injection of high-dose vitamins C and D, as well as zinc. The hospital initially refused:

(Hospital): "It isn't protocol."

(Dalley): "That doesn't matter."

(H): "Well, it's not protocol. We don't do that."

(D): "You don't give vitamins and nutrition to your ICU patients? Why?

(H): "We don't do that. It's not protocol."[216]

"Protocol," according to Dalley, refers to a 341-page document put out by the CDC detailing officially approved guidelines for treatment of Covid-19. If Dalley's experience is representative (and I expect it is), most hospital physicians adhere inflexibly to these. Like most every other aspect of official Covid-19 policy, those guidelines fail to recommend relevant measures that help strengthen the body's natural ability to resist the disease. On account of such omissions, the protocol tends to move the patient more or less inexorably toward ventilation. That may be good for hospital finances (the more Covid patients, the more funds the hospital receives), but it is not good (in fact, it is disastrous) for most patients. Dalley offers her opinion of the situation in no uncertain terms:

> It's not COVID that's killing people. It's the protocol. It's over-treatment. I wanted to "under-treat" my husband with nutrients and vitamins to help fight what he had so he could breathe again instead of overtreating him, overmedicating him, and shoving him on a ventilator too early. Because the death rate on the ventilator is up to 75 to 80%. That's really scary. Yet they were talking ventilator from the minute I got in there.[217]

As Dalley emphasizes, patients can and should insist on the treatment measures they prefer, protocol notwithstanding.

The hospital finally did reluctantly consent to administer intravenous vitamin C. At first, however, they did so at a ludicrously low-dosage level—a level suitable to helping a child get over a cold. Finally, at Dalley's insistence, her husband received appropriate intravenous injection of high-dose Vitamins C and D. (It's not clear from the clip whether or not she succeeded in procuring zinc treatment as well.)

Dalley further bucked protocol by insisting upon use of budesonide, a corticosteroid that fights lung inflammation. While recent studies show that budesonide can be very helpful in treating Covid-19, the official guidelines deem there to be "insufficient evidence" to recommend it.

The same formula applies to all the relevant nutraceutical treatments. The NIH conveniently offers its critical evaluation of vitamins C and D and zinc in one short, boxed section titled "Supplements: Summary Recommendations." Last updated February 11, 2021, it reads:

> **Vitamin C:** *There is insufficient evidence for the COVID-19 Treatment Guidance Panel to recommend either for or against the use of vitamin C for the treatment of COVID-19.*
>
> **Vitamin D:** *There is insufficient evidence for the Panel to recommend either for or against the use of vitamin D for the treatment of COVID-19.*
>
> **Zinc:** *There is insufficient evidence for the Panel to recommend either for or against the use of zinc for the treatment of COVID-19.*
>
> *The panel recommends against using zinc supplementation above the recommended dietary allowance for the prevention of COVID-19, except in clinical trial.*[218]

I don't think Dr. Brownstein—none of whose 520 Covid patients died and only nine of whom landed in the hospital—would concur with the conclusion that there is "insufficient evidence" for relevant nutraceutical treatment of Covid-19. Nor would Kate Dalley or her husband buy that familiar line. Within thirty-six hours of his treatment with high dosage nutraceuticals and budesonide, Dalley's husband's condition improved markedly. He was, by her report, talking, laughing, walking to the bathroom, and watching movies. The surprised doctor remarked, "Wow, he's better off than anyone else in here!"

Kate Dalley's husband was released after a scant three-plus days—half the duration of the minimum time he had been told he would be in the ICU, and a record release time for Covid patients at that unit.

Dalley commented:

> I was told by someone with a medical degree that vitamins didn't work, and budesonide probably didn't do much.... Well, why are you standing

> there, wringing your hands, waiting for the patient to decline and oxygen to get worse? You're not exactly helping the patient to progress. You are just watching them slide down, and then telling everybody...this is the best care we can offer. And then you are slamming them on a ventilator, even young ages...and saying "We did everything we could...but they died because of that killer COVID."
>
> It's the protocol. It's the protocol. I can't say that enough. After having gone through this, and getting to peer behind the curtain: It's the protocol. The protocol coming down from the CDC.[219]

Dalley makes clear that she certainly does not imagine that doctors and nurses are deliberately mistreating patients. For the most part, they do the best they can while *following orders*—edicts from on high. Most doctors, she alleges, do not stay independently abreast of the most recent developments or avail themselves of all relevant information. Dalley concludes:

> Doctors don't read studies. They don't read studies. They are not up on the latest, because they think they've been given the latest by the hospital administration. And that's a problem.[220]

It should, perhaps, be acknowledged that, unlike almost all of the sources cited in this letter, Dalley wears her own political allegiance on her sleeve, and her show packs a patently Republican punch. That certainly warrants critical examination of her slant, as would any like offering from a distinctly left-leaning source. It does not, however, automatically discredit her account, especially since the essential features of her narrative dovetail with so much else I have elaborated on in this volume. I consider Dalley's story all too consistent with the overall picture of the official Covid-19 response that has gradually crystallized in my mind's eye in the course of its writing.

The more I look at it, the more ugly—even grotesque—that picture looks.

Chapter 21

NEWSBREAK: A WINDOW ON PANDEMIC POLITICS

Speaking of politics, a recent episode involving Del Bigtree of ICAN and Tom Porter, a journalist writing for Business Insider, provides yet another illustration of the usual (and usually deplorable) style of public discourse characterizing Covid-19 politics. Bigtree and ICAN are generally regarded, and dismissed, as rabid, right-wing "anti-vaxxers"—a label that tends to be as freely, and damningly, thrown around these days as was the charge of "communist" in the red-baiting 1950s.

Bigtree ranks high on the list of the so-called disinformation dozen compiled by a UK-based "charity" called The Center for Countering Digital Hate and consulted by none other than President Biden. The name of the organization itself represents a glaring instance of the patent doublespeak tainting much mainstream Covid rhetoric. The center's blacklist brands diverse individuals and organizations as subversives with black hearts deliberately plotting to undermine the humane and rational governance reliably provided by reigning authorities.

In reality, ICAN's stated mission is the laudable one of ensuring honest and transparent disclosure of all relevant information that bears upon an individual citizen's legal right to *informed* consent as it pertains to vaccination and other personal health choices. In pursuit of that charter, Bigtree seeks to make available such information while performing, as a rule, due diligence to verify that the positions he ultimately advocates are evidence-based: substantiated by officially approved data (such as VAERS), peer-reviewed scientific publications, and the like. Correlatively, he gives voice to the opinions of top scientists (such as Robert Malone and Geert Vanden Bossche) whose dissenting views are often suppressed or censored.

One does not necessarily have to agree with Bigtree and the positions he advocates to recognize that his efforts are not motivated by any evil or antisocial intent—on the contrary. He is passionate, to be sure; but (as Dr. Bridle expressed in that early Parliament Hill press briefing) he is passionate in defense of positions and principles that he believes to be in the best interests of public health and welfare *and* the preservations of rights essential to a democratic society. Both science and democracy depend, absolutely, on dialogue, which in turn depends, absolutely, on difference and dissent. Blacklisting and censoring Bigtree and others hardly counter hate, digital or otherwise; on the contrary, it inflames and spreads the plague of intolerance that sickens contemporary society.

In the all-too-typical case of Porter and his reporting on Bigtree, the name-calling and social castigation carried out in the name of truth and social rectitude ("virtue signaling") actually traffic in anything but. Porter, angling for an interview, notified Bigtree that he was preparing a piece on him for *Business Insider.* That communication evidently conveyed that Porter intended to characterize Bigtree, as per his high digital hate standing, as a purveyor of vaccine disinformation. In response, Bigtree asked Porter to forward to him any concrete instances of alleged misinformation or disinformation, so that he (Bigtree) could check his sources and evaluate, objectively, whether the claim had merit or not.

Porter interviewed Bigtree privately shortly before his piece, "How a New York Billionaire-funded Anti-vax Group Is Contributing to the Vaccine Hesitancy That's Crippling the U.S. Recovery," appeared in *Business Insider* on August 24, 2021.[221] Toward the close of that interview, Bigtree noted Porter's failure to share, as per his request, any specifics substantiating the charge of his disseminating misinformation or disinformation and reiterated his invitation to do so. Porter never honored that request. Not surprisingly, his published piece eschews informed debate, or indeed *any substantive mention of particular points of contention,* in the favor of two typical tactics: first, sweeping allegations backed up by nothing but the official word of those very agencies whose judgment Bigtree and other critics call into question and, second, guilt by association.

Porter's article is certainly heavy on the latter, aggressively seeking to try to tie Bigtree directly to Trump supporters and the kind of unruly lawlessness exhibited during the January 6, 2020, Capitol riot. It is true, of course, that criticism of the current administration's Covid policy today finds—regrettably—broader welcome in Republican than Democratic circles. It is also true, regrettably, that too many Republicans have themselves shown a singular disregard for truth and due political process in the run-up to and aftermath of the November 2020 election. These political facts in and of themselves should not, however, stand in the way of evaluating principled arguments pertaining to Covid-19 on their own objective merit. As I have sought to show throughout this book, arguments contesting the controlling Covid narrative cannot, as a general rule, rightly be regarded as originally or essentially partisan in nature. Like Dr. Kory and the FLCCC's initiative, they emerge largely from nonpartisan scientific and humanitarian impulses, as well as from the desire—equally dear, one would hope, to true liberals and conservatives alike—to preserve rights and liberties fundamental to democratic society. When partisans of the mainstream "democratic" view ignore this backdrop and summarily dismiss informed dissent without engaging in open, conscientious, and principled dialogue, they merely emulate the kind of truth-free ideologically driven politicking they rightfully condemn in others.

Porter cites any number of sources supposedly confirming Bigtree's Trumpian ties, for instance:

> Ana Santos Rutschman, Assistant Professor of Law at St. Louis University, said ICAN and Bigtree were "taking advantage of the way anti-vaccine messages resonate with many Trump supporters and deliberately propagating vaccine disinformation with those supporters in mind."[222]

Notice that—all too characteristically—Bigtree here stands accused of "propagating vaccine disinformation," without *any concrete instantiation* of that damning allegation. The closest Porter's piece comes to such particulars appears after Porter cites Bigtree's defense of his, and ICAN's, position:

> "We simply are a consumer-advocacy group that seeks to make sure that people are getting the safest products they can. There is a protocol to how we approve pharmaceutical drugs, and we believe that vaccines should adhere to those same protocols and principles," [Bigtree] said.[223]

Porter's article continues:

> He [Bigtree] said public health officials and the Centers for Disease Control and Prevention were wrong to advocate Americans to get the shot: "I believe it's reckless. I believe it's dangerous and I think it is unnecessarily putting people in unknown risk situations."[224]

The quoted statements derive from Porter's interview with Bigtree, which Bigtree made available in full on ICAN's website.[225] Porter, however, *makes no mention of Bigtree's reasoned and evidence-based substantiation of his position,* including his citation of VAERS data and rehearsal of the details of normal testing protocol, which typically includes extensive double-blind trials and lasts years so as to take longer-term risks into account.

Porter delivers his own "decisive" rebuttal of Bigtree's concerns, the solid ground that supposedly justifies branding Bigtree as a purveyor of disinformation, in the following terms:

> Claims that the vaccines have not been properly tested for safety have been squarely rejected by most public-health professionals and infectious-disease experts. The shots have been found in clinical and real-world trials to be safe and effective.
>
> The CDC says on its website that the US COVID-19 vaccines "have undergone and will continue to undergo the most intensive safety monitoring in US history." The Food and Drug Administration fully approved Pfizer's vaccine on Monday, saying "the public can be very confident that this vaccine meets the high standards for safety, effective, and manufacturing quality."[226]

It should go without saying that this parroting of the official position constitutes no reasoned or evidence-based counterargument at all. If dissent is dismissed and discarded not because it is carefully demonstrated to be wrong on the merits *but because it is dissent*—that is, because it contradicts the authorities—then we are no longer functioning in anything resembling a democratic society. We are manifestly sliding dangerously toward tyrannical authoritarianism, because just such automatic repudiation of dissent as such *is* what constitutes authoritarianism per se.

I did not, however, take up the Porter–Bigtree episode with the intention of addressing yet again the distinctly undemocratic profile of Covid politics. The Porter–Bigtree interview caught my special attention because of Del Bigtree's own comments on the topic of in-hospital treatment, which in fact echoed much of what Kate Dalley had recounted. Here, for the record, is the relevant passage, elicited by Porter's question on whether Del Bigtree did not feel guilty when he read of unvaccinated persons dying in ICUs:

> The number one question I ask myself when I hear about someone struggling or potentially dying from this illness is: were they given the opportunity to use ivermectin, hydroxychloroquine, or budesonide, all products that in studies around the world have been shown to be effective? Or were they, as per the reports we hear...sent home [from the hospital]...and told: "Well, your oxygen level is still okay. Come back when you are struggling."
>
> And when they are struggling, they are put on a ventilator—really given no medicine whatsoever, except perhaps, remdesivir, which is just

> a waste of money, and has been proven to be totally ineffective. And then they die.
>
> So I think those deaths, for the most part, should be investigated as medical malpractice…I think the way our hospitals are handling this is deplorable. And I believe we should…investigate how the care for these people was so misguided.
>
> We know that early treatment is the secret to all illness and yet hospitals are sending people home and saying, "Wait until you get more sick." That's why people are dying. And the doctors at hospitals that are following through on that protocol should be held accountable.[227]

The whole interview is well worth listening to. I invite you to do so and decide for yourself which of the two personalities appears the more knowledgeable and conscientiously concerned citizen and whether—judging from the content of both the interview and Porter's *Business Insider* piece—the likes of Del Bigtree deserve to be number two on a blacklist of persons supposedly spewing "hate" and deadly "disinformation."

Chapter 22

CLOSING ARGUMENT: MCCULLOUGH ET AL. VERSUS THE ACLU

Speaking of blacklists and censorship, on September 2, 2021, David Cole, national legal director of the ACLU, and Daniel Mach, director of its program on freedom and religious belief, published an opinion piece in *The New York Times* titled "We Work at the ACLU. Here's What We Think about Vaccine Mandates."[228] Evidently, I can no longer accuse the organization of keeping silent on what I called "the premier freedom of speech issue of the twenty-first century."

Or can I?

The article begins:

> Do vaccine mandates violate civil liberties? Some who have refused vaccination claim as much.
>
> We disagree.
>
> At the ACLU, we are not shy about defending civil liberties, even when they are very unpopular. But we see no civil liberties problem with requiring Covid-19 vaccines in most circumstances.
>
> While the permissibility of requiring vaccines for particular diseases depends on several factors, when it comes to Covid-19, all considerations point in the same direction. The disease is highly transmissible, serious, and often lethal; the vaccines are safe and effective; and crucially there is no equally effective alternative available to protect public health.

The next sentence states the gist of the ACLU's position:

> In fact, far from compromising civil liberties, vaccine mandates actually further civil liberties.[229]

The ACLU, as I know from my father's historic involvement with the organization, can often rightfully boast that its advocates demonstrate incisive legal acumen. It does not, however, take a high-powered lawyer to know that the soundness of your conclusion depends absolutely upon that of the assumptions upon which it is predicated. Here, each of the stated premises upon which Cole and Mach base their stance is, as this book demonstrates, open to serious question, if not demonstrably false.

Perhaps the most pivotal premise—the last stated, deemed "crucial" by Cole and Mach themselves—is the one I have spent the most time debunking. There is not one "equally effective alternative" but many, virtually all of which can be employed synergistically: nutraceutical treatment, pharmaceutical treatment (hydroxychloroquine, ivermectin, budesonide), monoclonal antibodies. Physicians interested in availing themselves of remedy have a formidable arsenal at their disposal. It is, moreover, only the politically motivated repression of these treatments that opened the door for the Emergency Use Authorization of vaccines and the Pandora's box of sociopolitical as well as medical ills that has followed in its wake.

With reference to the article's first stated premise—the seriousness and lethality—of the disease, this too is questionable. Of course, press coverage produces the graphic impression that Covid-19 represents a lethal pandemic, one out of control or ever on the verge of being so. But media-generated appearance and fact-based reality are often dramatically different stories.

What matters most is the mortality risk posed by Covid-19. This, above all, has stirred global panic; it has motivated lockdowns, business closures, and vaccine mandates and generally turned the world upside down. Yet the preprint of a paper[230] likely to be published soon by Cathrine Axfors and John P. A. Ioannidis (a world-renowned, if now controversial, epidemiologist out of Stanford) in the Yale Biomedical Journal sheds light on the *reality* of the risk of death (not the hallucinatory *fantasy*) for different age groups of persons who do become infected by Covid-19. The results of the paper, "Infection Fatality Rate of COVID-19 in Community-dwelling Populations with Emphasis on the Elderly: An Overview," are striking, to say the least.

The paper is based upon seroprevalence (mortality risk) studies covering fourteen countries. Here are the salient results, listed in the form of the percentage of persons in distinct age groups who survive Covid-19 infection:

AGE (YEARS)	SURVIVAL RATIO (%)
0–19	99. 9973
20–29	99.986
30–39	99.969
40–49	99.918
50–59	99.73
60–69	99.41
70+	97.6 (non-institutionalized)
70+	94.5 (all)

These figures indicate that the risk of dying from Covid should rightfully be of compelling (potentially life-changing) concern only for those over seventy. (While not registered here, the risk of death climbs significantly the higher the percentage of persons over eighty-five is included in the seventy-plus age group.) This data confirms the essential soundness of the general approach endorsed, shortly after the onset of the pandemic, by the signatories of the Great Barrington Declaration, which proposed that rigorous preventive measures target high-risk populations more or less exclusively while allowing the rest of society to function normally.

Thus, despite the ACLU's popular assumption to the contrary, for the vast majority of persons, contracting Covid-19 is *not* "often lethal." That description could be justified only for those over seventy, and even for these persons it is by no means (to employ Dr. Brownstein's term) "a death sentence." These numbers, moreover, reflect (cf. ACLU premise #3) a period of time (unfortunately, as yet ongoing) during which effective treatment (both inpatient and outpatient) is not the rule. The figures would undoubtedly be much lower still when (or if) such treatment becomes routine.

Meanwhile, given the genuine safety risks that, as Ros Jones testified, are magnified for younger populations, these numbers indicate that we really have no business vaccinating children, youth, and even young adults, for all of whom Covid represents a statistically negligible risk of mortality. And for older persons?

I myself am sixty-four. In response to the presented question, allow me to share an analogy. I do know that car accidents kill many persons; accordingly, I try to make sure the vehicle I drive is in good working order, and I strive to drive safely, resisting the temptation to pass farm vehicles on curvy back roads. I am not, however, going to stop driving because of the risk of fatality, nor do I think society would condone unduly restricting everyone's right to drive, even if so doing would undoubtedly reduce mortality. Reasonable cost-benefit analysis, conscious and unconscious, is a standard part of society's decision-making mechanism—*except,* it appears, when it comes to Covid-19.

Now, let's look at the other side of the coin: the supposed safety and efficacy of the Covid vaccines. I have shared a good deal on this topic already, but let me add some more recent information pertaining to just how safe or effective the vaccines really are, or are not.

At the time of this writing, the prevalence of Covid in the Delta era, even and indeed especially among highly vaccinated populations, casts a dark shadow of doubt upon the vaccines and their purported efficacy. Israel is one of the most-vaccinated countries in the world. If the Pfizer vaccine (the only one used in Israel) were as effective as advertised, one might have expected that Covid-19 would have been largely subdued in the country. In fact, the opposite is true: cases are currently surging to record levels.

Earlier in this volume, I cited Dr. Peter McCullough's incisive November 2020 U.S. Senate testimony. Since that time, Dr. McCullough (who naturally continues his medical practice, which includes treatment of Covid patients) has stayed as up-to-date as possible on all things Covid, and remains one of the most credentialed and knowledgeable persons speaking on the subject today. In a recent interview with Robert F. Kennedy Jr. (which I will draw upon extensively in the concluding sections of this volume), Dr. McCullough queried:

> As we are really in the midst of this Delta outbreak, which is occurring worldwide, particularly in countries that have higher proportions of the population vaccinated, we are asking the question: how in the world can we have so many vaccinated individuals, but have such a prominent outbreak of the Delta variant among vaccinated and unvaccinated?[231]

In the course of that interview, Dr. McCullough provides a number of relevant perspectives on that crucial question.

First, one may look at certain critical facts that have been clinically, as well as experientially demonstrated. Even if vaccination may reduce incidence of infection (we will soon discuss further to what degree), it does *not* prevent it. Breakthrough cases occur with regularity in the Delta era and, crucially, vaccinated individuals who contract Covid can very well transmit it to vaccinated or unvaccinated others.

Indeed, a just-released (August 10, 2021) preprint in *The Lancet* by Nguyen Van Vinh Chau indicates that healthcare worker vaccinees infected with Delta in a Ho Chi Minh city hospital in Vietnam bore a very high viral load: 251 times higher than persons who had contracted earlier forms of the SARS-CoV-2 virus as measured in March and April 2021 at the same hospital. Moreover, the controlled conditions of the study environment (the hospital went into lockdown) made it clear that the infected vaccinees were freely transmitting the infection to one another. These sentences from the paper's abstract suggest why that was likely the case:

> Neutralizing antibody levels after vaccination and at diagnosis of the cases were *lower* than those in the matched uninfected controls. There was no

correlation between vaccine-induced neutralizing antibody levels and viral loads or development of symptoms.[232]

I understand this to mean that the vaccines (here, the AstraZeneca type) did *not* efficiently stimulate the antibodies, or immunological defenses, necessary for effective protection against the Delta variant. The authors' own interpretation confirms that conclusion:

> Breakthrough Delta variant infections are associated with high viral loads, prolonged PCR positivity, and low levels of vaccine-induced neutralizing antibodies, explaining the transmission between the vaccinated people. Physical distancing measures remains critical to reduce SARS-CoV-2 Delta variant transmission.[233]

The inability of the vaccine to protect against infection and spread of the Delta variant here indicated in all probability derives from the phenomena of immune (or antigenic) escape highlighted by Geert Vanden Bossche, Byram Bridle, and others. Delta may be living proof of the validity of their concerns, as Dr. McCullough notes:

> We knew originally that the vaccines were non-sterilizing, that is, the vaccines could not get the immune system to completely eradicate the virus in the early studies. So the fear was that we were going to create superspreaders.[234]

Does Delta qualify as a "first-generation superspreader"? Perhaps. If so, it must lead one to wonder: If the present vaccination program continues on its appointed course, what will future generation superspreaders look and act like, and is there truly any realistic hope that vaccine technology can match the pace of nature's swiftly evolving mutations?

More on that subject shortly. For now, let us return to facts and perspective on the present efficacy of the vaccine as judged not by clinical trial but by large-scale real-world experience. Dr. McCullough segues from commentary on the Chau study to the latter:

> The message here is that the vaccinated clearly are susceptible to Covid-19 and the Delta variant. The vaccine in this case was...AstraZeneca...but we know separately from Israel, that exclusively uses the Pfizer vaccine, that the Israeli health minister now has the Pfizer vaccine down to 17% efficacy. The Mayo Clinic...using Rochester, Minnesota inhabitants vaccinated with Pfizer; they have Pfizer down to 42% efficacy. *These levels are far below the 50% efficacy regulatory standard to even have a vaccine on*

the market. So it is clear that, whether it is Delta, whether it is AstraZeneca or Pfizer, in these working examples, *the vaccines are failing*.[235]

The failure of the vaccines to perform as expected has been born out not only by the rise of case counts and the reimposition of unwelcome restrictions but, as well, by the call for boosters. That call (like the Israeli instance) confirms that society's persistent Covid problems cannot, popular hue and cry to the contrary, be blamed on the unvaccinated.

Dr. McCullough states that fifty percent efficacy threshold actually counts as only one of two traditional criteria by which to judge whether a vaccine meets the usual regulatory standard. The other pertains to duration. An acceptable vaccine, according to McCullough, should remain viable, without boosting, for at least a year; many reputable vaccines (tetanus, hepatitis B) remain effective for five or ten. That both pharmaceutical companies and the U.S. government are calling for boosters only six to eight months after rollout furnishes additional proof that the Covid vaccines are not meeting expectations. They are falling short, not only of the sky-high hopes originally pinned on them but of the usual standards of performance that typically qualify a vaccine for official authorization and public use.

This, however, is only half of the tragic story. The other is that, as a number of top scientists have long asserted, no amount of "boosting" is likely to prove at all effective. Indeed, on the contrary, it is likely only to additionally suppress natural immune capability and, by the mechanism of immune escape, to accelerate the development of vaccine-resistant variants. Delta, in fact, probably represents the first wave of such.

Dr. McCullough's relevant comments echo those (cited earlier) of Dr. Geert Vanden Bossche:

> The boosters are not adjusted for the variants. We know that Delta has considerably mutated the spike protein, and that's the only thing that is the antigenic target of the vaccines. The paper by _____ clearly shows that with Pfizer, for instance, there is antigenic escape. The antibodies from Pfizer can't adequately hit the spike protein that's produced by human cells after the vaccine is injected. There is antigenic escape. *So it doesn't matter how many boosters one gives, if it's missing the target, it is going to be futile*. In fact, ever since the booster program started, which was just a few weeks ago in Israel, there is already failure among those who have received the third shot.[236]

The whole issue of immune escape and vaccine (in)efficacy naturally figures centrally in the debate swirling around the relative value of vaccine-induced versus natural immunity. When Kennedy pressed Dr. McCullough on the apparent futility of the effort to combat the virus via booster shots, McCullough both ventured an explanation of the booster strategy and repudiated it while endorsing the unparalleled efficacy of natural immunity:

> The hope is to try to overwhelm [the virus] with a very large volume of antibodies, and we know that with the vaccines, the titers of the antibodies...are far higher than that with natural immunity, but those are antibodies directed against the spike protein.
>
> The natural immunity.... We have a full library of IGA since the respiratory illness starts in the nose and the mouth; then we have libraries of IgG against not only the spike protein in the natural infection...and many other antigens. We may have hundreds if not thousands of antibodies, and full T-cell, helper, T-killer cell and presenter-cell immunity. The natural immunity is robust, complete, and durable, and the vaccine immunity is, in a sense, an overshot on a very narrow library of antibodies directed against the spike protein.[237]

The upshot of all this?

> So what is happening is this antigenic escape, and trying to keep boosting the antibodies. But in a recent paper from Israel, they show that, month by month, the antibodies after vaccination drop by 40%. They are very high but then drop, drop, drop, drop. And then by six months, the natural immunity antibodies, which are only part of our natural immunity, exceed that of the vaccine immunity.
>
> So one of the things that is not supportable is any claim that vaccine immunity is better than natural immunity. It is just the opposite. Natural immunity is robust, complete, and durable.[238]

Dr. McCullough, like Geert Vanden Bossche before him, is not just spinning his wheels. A paper released out of Israel, "Comparing SARS-CoV-2 Natural Immunity to Vaccine-induced Immunity: Reinfection versus Breakthrough Infection" (August 25, 2021[239]), emphatically corroborates the superiority of naturally conferred immunity. Here is the *Science* magazine summary of the salient results:

> The new analysis relies on the database of Maccabi Healthcare Services, which enrolls about 2.5 million Israelis. The study, led by Tal Patalon and Sivan Gazit at KSM, the system's research and innovation arm, found in

> two analyses that *people who were vaccinated in January and February were, in June and July and the first half of August, 6 to 13 times more likely to get infected than unvaccinated people who were previously infected with the coronavirus*. In one analysis, comparing more than 32,000 people in the health system, the risk of developing symptomatic COVID-19 was 27 times higher among the vaccinated, and the risk of hospitalization eight times higher.[240]

In the no-nonsense language of the study itself:

> This study demonstrated that natural immunity confers longer-lasting and stronger protection against infection, symptomatic disease and hospitalization caused by the Delta variant of SARS-CoV-2, compared to the BNT162b2 two-dose vaccine-induced immunity.[241]

Alex Berenson, a science journalist, puts an exclamation mark on the results:

> Along with the other emerging data, this paper should end any debate over vaccines v[ersus] natural immunity.[242]

An August 28, 2021, *Zerohedge* piece by Tyler Durden that cites Berenson adds a graph of the disturbingly steep climb of cases in Israel, which has recently reached a *record level* of infections. That's right: despite its aggressive vaccination program, the number of new cases per day in Israel in late August 2021 (roughly 12,000) *exceeded* prior peaks of infection that *preceded* vaccination (peaking at around 9,000 in October 2020) or the rise of the Delta (a peak of roughly 11,000 in January to February 2021 declined to near zero in April 2021 before the steep Delta-driven ascent beginning toward the end of June 2021).[243]

This data seems to me a dramatic and frightening verification of Vanden Bossche's immune escape theorem and should give nightmares to everyone looking to mass vaccination for rescue from Covid. Durden gives apt expression to the phenomenon:

> As the first country to achieve widespread coverage by the vaccine, Israel is now in an unthinkable situation: daily case numbers have reached new record levels as the Delta variant penetrates the vaccines' protection like a hot knife slicing through butter.[244]

So much for Covid-19 vaccine efficacy, Mr. Cole and Mr. Mach (authors of the ACLU article in the *Times*). What about the other clause of the "safe and effective" mantra—a mantra that is beginning to sound hollow as a drum?

Believe it or not, the news on this score is even worse.

Let's begin where we left off: in Israel, in order to attend (as government officials here and abroad appear so loath to do) to signals of alarm.

Retsef Levi is an MIT professor specializing in data analysis relevant to public healthcare policy. Levi recently collected and collated data drawn from the records of Magen David Adom, the body responsible for providing emergency medical services in Israel. Vaccine rollout in Israel began around the first of the year in 2021. Levi compared data representing the profile of emergency calls during first five months of 2019 (and thus pre-pandemic) to the profile representative of the same period in 2021, during which Israel's vaccination program was in full swing.

One set of numbers stood out from the data. The incidence of calls for acute coronary syndrome in 2021 proved dramatically higher than the count for the same period in 2019. This is relevant because, according to well-substantiated scientific consensus, the symptoms of "acute coronary syndrome" are virtually indistinguishable from those characteristic of myocarditis and pericarditis, adverse effects associated with the mRNA vaccines.

The most dramatic increase occurred in the age group suspected of being most susceptible to this adverse effect. Calls for acute coronary syndrome involving ten- to nineteen-year-olds *doubled,* or increased by one hundred percent, from 2019 to 2021. Incidence in older age groups also rose significantly although not quite so spectacularly. Emergency calls prompted by acute coronary syndrome climbed forty-three percent for the twenty-to-twenty-nine age group; thirty percent for those thirty to thirty-nine; and just over twenty-four percent for forty- to forty-nine-year-olds. That such high increases did *not* register for persons over fifty only strengthens the presumptive association with the Covid vaccine as this adverse effect disproportionately impacts younger populations.[245]

Data from the Unites States' own Vaccine Adverse Events Reporting System (VAERS) recently examined by the Advisory Committee on Immunization Practices (ACIP) corroborates this line of concern. As of August 18, 2021, VAERS included more than 5,000 incidents of myocarditis. ACIP examined a little over half those cases in order to compare the expected rate of incidence of myocarditis within seven days after inoculation with an mRNA vaccine with the actually observed rate of incidence.[246]

Once again, the data analysis yielded startling—and startlingly disturbing—results. The gist is: once again, younger age groups proved spectacularly more susceptible to this adverse effect than older persons did. The number of *expected* instances for the latter exceeded that of the former; in actuality, *incidence among the younger population exceeds that of older persons many times over.* Young males, moreover, are far more susceptible than young females. The latter did experience *a marked excess of observed versus expected* cases in the younger (twelve to twenty-nine) age group; even so, incidence among young males was roughly five to ten times that of incidence in females. Moreover, in the most susceptible age group (twelve to twenty-four), the number of observed cases exceeded that of expected cases by a factor of anywhere from twenty to two hundred. Stating this very approximately, *males in this age group proved roughly fifty to one hundred times more likely to experience myocarditis than had been expected*—expected, I presume, by the vaccine makers and health experts, such as those sitting on ACIP who set public health policy.

In assessing, moreover, the raw numbers, one must also take into account that these are based on only half of the reported cases, and, in any event, the reported cases likely represent (as I have previously stated) only a fraction of the actual cases.

The officially reported numbers, in and of themselves, are disturbing enough—indeed, spectacularly so. This is all the more true if one reviews not merely incidences of myocarditis but the full range of VAERS statistics. *The Defender* reports in an August 2021 article titled "We've Never Seen Vaccine Injuries on This Scale—Why Are Regulatory Agencies Hiding COVID Vaccine Safety Signals?":

> In less than a year, more than half a million reports of injuries have flooded into VAERS following experimental COVID jabs, including thousands of deaths. Yet deafening regulatory silence has greeted this record-setting volume of adverse reactions, *which accounts for nearly a third of all reports accumulated by VAERS over its entire three-decade lifespan.*[247]

Dr. McCullough helps put a human face to these rather staggering statistics. In the aforementioned interview, Dr. McCullough gives a wrenching account of a largely healthy sixty-four-year-old woman who died as a consequence of blood clotting caused by vaccination. Dr. McCullough was not the first doctor to attend to this patient; she initially checked into a different hospital. Her symptoms, which she "absolutely" attributed to the vaccine, were severe from the first, and, despite treatment with anticoagulants, killed her in a matter of weeks. Dr. McCullough puts the onerous process of reporting such incidents in perspective in a manner that makes the staggering numbers of adverse event reports yet more impressive:

I went ahead and did the reporting, and it looks like my report was the first. This first event that landed her in the hospital; no one made the effort to report it. One would actually have to get the vaccine card, which I needed, and have the lot numbers, and carefully go through this, and I have to enter in all my medical information; who I am, my office location, the original hospital location. It took me about half an hour to do the entry. And I am telling you, the total number of these entries that have been certified by the CDC now, of Americans, is astonishingly 545,000. 545,000 times doctors took an effort to the level that I did, to enter in a vaccine injury, or now, a vaccine-related death. (I have to go back in now, and update the CDC that she has in fact died.)

This is astonishing. We have never had this. The total number, across 70 vaccines, on the US market, for about 278 millions shots [each year]—the total number of reports that go into this system per year is about 16,000. We are at 545,000 with the Covid-19 vaccine program alone.[248]

The number 545 is roughly thirty-five times great than sixteen, and the Covid vaccine program has been operating for only about eight months, or two-thirds of a year. That means that the *Covid vaccines are prompting VAERS reports at a rate roughly fifty times that of all other vaccines combined.*

And remember, for a whole host of reasons (which include not only doctors simply not bothering to take the time but also—according to multiple sources—officials failing to file submitted reports), VAERS numbers most likely represent a fraction of actual adverse events.

No few of these hundreds of thousands of reports, moreover, represent (as was the case with Dr. McCullough's patient) fatalities. Dr. McCullough states:

> We are at now 13,000 deaths that the CDC has told us has happened...and we have separate external analysis...by McGlocklin and colleagues out of London, that has shown that 50% of these deaths occur within two days of getting the vaccine; 80% occur within a week; most are seniors in their seventies or eighties who die, and 86% of the time there is no other explanation. Someone who was healthy enough to walk into a vaccine center, has died.[249]

Dr. McCullough continues to reference the CDC whistleblower's testimony:

> Separately, we know that [data from] the Center for Medicare and Medicaid Services, where they do know who has been vaccinated, and they do know when someone has died, has corroborated this and in fact extended the estimate: the number that have died is probably closer to 45,000 after a vaccine. About 186 should have been our tolerance for this, for the

> whole program, for the whole year. *So this is off the rails in terms of mortality, absolutely off the rails.*[250]

The astronomical mortality rate is, in and of itself and on the face of it, unacceptable.

Moreover, when the high vaccine-induced mortality rate is combined with the inefficacy of the vaccine and the generally low rate of Covid-caused mortality (cf. Ioannidis's work), the result—as born out by a six-month clinical trial study just put out by Pfizer itself—is that *the vaccine confers no mortality benefit; indeed, evidence indicates the contrary.* The vaccine does save a limited number of lives, but for every life it saves, two or three persons are dying from vaccine-induced blood clots and heart failure.

When Kennedy asked Dr. McCullough if he thought the vaccines were causing more injury and death than they were averting, the latter responded that, given the historic prevalence of Covid in the United States, it was difficult to assess that in the U.S. However, McCullough added:

> We can go to other countries where they are kind of on a nascent ascent of their Covid-19 curve. We can go to Australia, and the data is clear there. More patients are dying of the vaccine than of Covid-19 by probably a hundredfold or more. It's not even close.[251]

Yet people still believe the Covid vaccines are not only effective but safe. *Why?*

The answer to this, in large measure, of course, is that media outlets suppress accounts of injury and death, and government agencies repeat the "safe and effective" mantra over and over. But how can these agencies themselves justify, even internally, disregard of all the signs that the vaccines are *not* in fact safe at all but—by historic standards at least—extremely dangerous?

The Defender asks this obvious, urgently pressing question and references a source that begins to provide a kind of plausible—even if damning—answer:

> How is the absence of "early warning system" alarm bells possible? In a recent commentary, "Defining Away Vaccine Safety Signals," an experienced statistician [Mathew Crawford] suggested not only have safety experts' admonitions to get COVID vaccine safety monitoring "right" not been heeded, but CDC and other public health agencies have taken steps to intentionally hide safety signals.[252]

The mathematical details of the statistician Mathew Crawford's analysis are complex, at least to the eye of a non-mathematician. Yet its upshot is perfectly clear. On January 29, 2021, shortly after practical implementation of the

Covid mass vaccination program, the CDC updated its method for reviewing VAERS data for the purpose of safety review and evaluation. The *new* protocol revolves around a mathematically derived term called the PRR—the "proportional reporting ratio." It is this PRR that is supposed to sound alarm bells in the case that the frequency of adverse events for a Covid vaccine exceeds, by a statistically significant amount, that of the historic rates of such for other vaccines.

In light of the historically unprecedented rate of reported incidents of adverse events for the COVID vaccines, one would not think that an elaborate mathematical schema would be required to set off an ear-splittingly loud alarm. To be sure, a well-defined statistical method of analysis *could* be a valuable and even requisite tool for a host of borderline situations. It should most certainly *not* function, however, as a mathematical sleight of hand that denies the obvious, such as in the case of a clever magician who invites one or another adversely affected person up on stage only to make him or her entirely... disappear.

According, however, to Crawford's analysis, that is exactly what the official definition does. How? That critical PRR is mathematically so defined as to be *insensitive to the very variations it is supposed to measure!* Even for the statistically less savvy, Crawford's bottom line is easily understandable:

> One vaccine that kills and cripples 20 or 50 or 1,000 times as much as a very safe vaccine will show the same PRR... and no safety signal will be identified by the CDC. *By design*... even if I plug in some enormous number like 1500 [for incidence of Bell's Palsy or heart failure or *death* for a given vaccine], there is still no safety signal as per CDC definitions... Certainly, there are conditions that result in safety signals, but these are far at the extremes for the AEs [adverse events] that we most need to understand.
>
> Do you kinda get the sense that the PRR function is designed to hide signals of unsafe vaccines, not to identify them?[253]

Crawford does not hesitate to draw some strong conclusions from this sorry story of mathematical and administrative malfeasance:

> If my understanding of this situation is correct, the mass vaccination program should be immediately halted until the safety data is gathered, cleaned, and examined. *We cannot tolerate a misleading statement of "vaccines are safe and effective" in the face of regulatory agencies defining away the responsibility of performing the risk analysis needed to verify safety* (emphasis mine). The CDC leadership should be immediately

> replaced and investigated, and independent analysts should reformulate the task of tracking vaccine safety results.[254]

By the way, if you think Mathew Crawford is trafficking in *misinformation,* I would reply as follows: If you are mathematically expert and really can prove him wrong, by his own report he would love to hear about it.

> I really hope I've misinterpreted something. I stumble over ideas and make mistakes just like everybody else. Unlike the CDC, I'd like for you to share my numbers widely and invite critique. By all means, forward this to everyone you know. Maybe one of them can explain my error and set me straight.... I'd rather be a little embarrassed in the eyes of many if I'm wrong than to watch even one more person get sick or die and perhaps become another false COVID statistic.[255]

Crawford's elaboration of governmental malfeasance is mathematical. As he himself observes, though, this mathematics translates all too readily into a frightening human reality:

> What if it turns out that vaccines are killing and crippling millions of people around the world, but that those harmed are just well enough spread out that almost nobody saw sufficient signals to build an intuition about the problem. And what if the agency most responsible for examining safety signals defines their algorithm using a nonsensical mathematical formula that hides nearly all serious problems?[256]

So much for a statistician's counsel as to how numbers can lie and how the government has been manipulating them to do just that. Dr. Peter McCullough's conversation with Robert F. Kennedy Jr. provides corroborating evidence from the perspective of someone deeply familiar with appropriate processes of administrative and regulatory overview. In response to Kennedy's query about appropriate safety review mechanisms that are, or are not, in place, Dr. McCullough responded:

> The Vaccine Adverse Event Reporting System is the only source right now. Our FDA and the CDC, which are the joint sponsors of the public vaccine program—which *is* an investigation—they have no Critical (adverse) Events Committee; they have no Data Safety Monitoring Board; they have no Human Ethics Board. *This is an abrogation of standards of safety for participants in human clinical investigations.* It is the only time that I am aware of that we have not seen the Office of Human Research Protections (OHRP) step in on this.[257]

Dr. McCullough elaborates his theme by expounding upon what *should* have been:

> We should have had a Data Safety Monitoring Board, with the size of this program, doing monthly reviews of safety, and giving advice to the program as to whether or not it should continue, or whether or not there should be modifications in the program. There was no Data Safety Monitoring Board involved.
>
> Looking backward, we had a mortality signal with this program at 27 million Americans vaccinated on January 22 [2021]. The mortality was 186 patients and that would exceed a [standard level of] confidence [because it is] above the usual, expected [number] for the entire class of injections at 150 deaths. So on January 22nd, if we would have had a Data Safety Monitoring Board review the data, *the DSMB would have shut this down in February,* and they would have had to look at the deaths and say: "Where are they happening? Are they happening in Covid-recovered patients who shouldn't be receiving the vaccine? Are they happening in the frail, elderly [population]?" They would have asked some questions.
>
> Shockingly, we are in August, and our vaccine program sponsors, the FDA and the CDC, *have yet to have a single press briefing or a single report on comprehensive safety.* All we have is this self-queried VAERS report.[258]

Kennedy proceeded to ask Dr. McCullough for clarification about the number of deaths that would normally trigger exceptional concern and call for immediate review of a vaccine program. In his response, Dr. McCullough indicated that typically, pre-Covid, roughly 278 million shots are administered in the course of a year in the United States, and the number of deaths associated with those injections is not expected to exceed 150.

> If we have 150 deaths with 278 million shots, in the United States, and they are not temporally related to the vaccine—they get reported at different times—and now suddenly we're faced with 186 [deaths] at 27 million [shots] with the Covid-19 vaccine. Any high quality Data Monitoring Safety Board—and I tell you, I am in this business, I do this, I have chaired over two dozen of these; I chair them for the National Institute of Health; I chair them for Big Pharma—I can tell you, if I were chairing a Data Safety Monitoring Board, we would have had emergency meetings in January, and it is very likely, if we couldn't explain what was going on, we would have shut down the program in February.[259]

Kennedy proceeds to express his belief that the CDC is not overseeing any relevant autopsies or indeed *conducting any sort of systematic investigation into the possible causes of Covid-19 vaccine-related mortality*. Asked whether Dr. McCullough's understanding of the situation confirms that view, Dr. McCullough responds:

> On two occasions, the CDC has very casually put out on their website, one in March and one in June; they have put out a statement that the CDC doctors and FDA doctors have reviewed all the deaths, and *none* of them are related to the vaccine. *None*. Not a single one. That includes these immediate deaths that occur in the vaccine center, where the vaccine personnel are doing CPR, for instance.
>
> I tell you, at that point, when that first statement came out in March...that was probably the turning point for me. I was already behind on the mortality signal. That January 22 landmark—I missed it. Clinically, I just missed it. But when they made that statement in the middle of March, *I realized something was going on. It's the hardest thing for Americans to swallow this, but that's malfeasance. That's wrongdoing by those in the position of authority.*[260]

Dr. McCullough supports his allegation by sharing his professional knowledge of the kind of procedures that should have been (but were not) followed:

> The FDA and the CDC in no way could have reviewed 16,000 deaths. That takes *forever* to get all the hospital records, the death certificates, to review everything, to carefully look at when the vaccine was given; to have two separate reviewers. They have to review it for causality; they have to make a causality assessment. When they disagree, there has to be a third adjudicator. That takes forever. They could not have put that together. They could not have put together the review structures and do that type of due diligence.
>
> And there would have to be external experts because the CDC and the FDA, they are the sponsors of the program. These people's jobs depend on it. They are completely biased. They can't be the ones reviewing the deaths. There must be external experts. We do it in every single clinical trial. In fact, external experts were involved in the original registrational trials. So that the standards that were conducted, that were used for the registrational trials, for all three manufacturers, suddenly are thrown out, and *now there's absolutely no safety [oversight] paying attention to the public program.*[261]

Dr. McCullough concludes this discussion by citing yet still another enigmatically incriminating circumstance:

> You know, in October of 2020, there's a slide set that was produced by the CDC. And they had all kinds of plans for monitoring safety during the public program. They were going to use a whole variety of databases; they were going to be checking things, and quickly reviewing the safety events as they occurred. *None* of that was done. *None* of it. *None* of the safety standards. *Americans had absolutely no protection on safety during this program. It's a complete lapse of the regulatory standards for clinical investigation.*[262]

So here is what we have: tens of thousands of deaths, hundreds of thousands of injury reports, all of this exceeding many, many, many, many times over that of all other vaccines combined, and no, absolutely no, responsible oversight.

And so, Mr. Cole, Mr. Mach (of the ACLU), the last plank falls away into nothingness. Effective and...*safe?*

This is a castle in the air: no glorious Camelot, but rather a dark, murderous Mordor, a hypnotic illusion supported and sustained by a legion of credulous foot soldiers, commanded, perhaps, by some inner circle of insidious orcs or snaky Gollums greedily grasping the Ring of Power.

That ring may yet be precariously held in our—in We, the People's—hands; but how long do we Frodos and Sams have, still, to resist the pull of power and overcontrol, the seductive lure of the Rule(r) that promises security and an end of Fear at the cost of that pearl of great price: humility that *can* heal, human love, truth, and freedom?

PART III

INFLECTION POINT

Chapter 23

THE PRESIDENT VERSUS WE, THE PEOPLE

I want to talk to you about where we are
in the battle against Covid-19.[263]
—President Joseph Biden

On September 9, 2021, President Biden spoke to the nation for thirty minutes on the topic of Covid. After lauding the "progress" the country has made since the onset of the pandemic a year and a half earlier, President Biden declared:

> Even as the Delta [variant of] of Covid-19 has been hitting this country hard, we have the tools to combat the virus if we can come together as a country and use those tools.[264]

I agree with President Biden here. The crucial question, however, is the nature and character of those tools and their means of effective use.

President Biden then proceeded to identify what was in *his* toolbox. His inventory should have surprised no one:

> If we raise our vaccination rate, protect ourselves and others with masking, and expanded testing, and identify people who are infected, we can and we will turn the tide on Covid-19.[265]

At this juncture, that last promise rings regrettably hollow, because we have been—quite literally—the subjects of these tools, now, for months and months and months. Meanwhile, Covid-19, in its by now not-so-new Delta dress, remains rampant and all sorts of crippling restrictions remain still very much in place.

President Biden blames this unhappy predicament *not* on the deficiency of his chosen tools but on a certain subgroup of citizens—no insignificant minority, but the quarter or third or so of the country that remains unvaccinated because they do not trust his chief instrument. Afraid of being damaged, they decline to be jabbed, a refusal that triggers the President's ire:

> Many of us are frustrated with the nearly 80 million Americans who are still not vaccinated, even though the vaccine is safe, effective, and free.[266]

In light of what we have just discussed (and will further discuss) relative to the efficacy and the safety of the vaccines, President Biden's next statement resonates with the kind of unconscious irony (not to mention condescension) all too characteristic of the proponents of the controlling Covid narrative:

> You might be confused about what is true and what is false about Covid-19.[267]

This is true—*someone* here must be confused! I am not sure, however, it is those eighty million Americans, of whom I myself am one; indeed one, like eighty or a hundred million *others*, who will be directly affected by the restrictive mandates President Biden, standing on the same fault-riddled ground as the ACLU's David Cole and Daniel Mach, announced in his speech.

Let's go over some of that same terrain once more, referencing, when apropos, key moments in President Biden's speech. I begin, again, with the issue of vaccine efficacy.

Since I addressed this question some pages back, yet more evidence has emerged to confirm Dr. Peter McCullough's unambiguous conclusion: "The vaccines are failing." A study published on September 9, 2021 (the same day as President Biden's speech), by Dr. Nina Pierpont (MD, PhD) analyzes data from three high-quality studies employing diverse methodologies in three disparate locales: Massachusetts, Vietnam, and the United Kingdom.[268] The title of the paper, which is not so much an academic piece as a medical professional's expert review and practically oriented interpretation of relevant data, states its conclusion clearly enough: "Covid-19 Vaccine Mandates Are Now Pointless: Covid-19 Vaccines Do Not Keep People from Catching the Prevailing Delta Variant and Passing It to Others." The paper begins with a summary which, on account of the lucidity and concision of its logic, I share in full:

EXECUTIVE SUMMARY

I. Excellent scientific research papers published or posted in August 2021 clearly demonstrate that current vaccines do not prevent transmission of SARS-CoV-2.

II. Vaccines aim to achieve two ends:
   1. To protect the vaccinated person against the illness.

2. To keep people from carrying the infection and transmitting it to others.
   (a) If enough people are vaccinated or otherwise become immune, it is hoped that the disease will stop circulating. We call this herd immunity.
   (b) On the way to herd immunity, there is an assumption that people who are immunized can form safe clusters or groups within which no one is carrying or transmitting the virus.

III. Unfortunately, this last assumption (II.2.[b]) is no longer true under the new variant of SARS-CoV- 2, Delta (B.1.617.2), which now accounts for essentially all cases worldwide.

IV. Delta is more infectious than the Alpha strain (B.1.1.7) that prevailed in the UK from January to May 2021 (and in the US from March to June 2021), meaning that Delta is passed more readily person-to-person than the previous dominant strain.

V. New research in multiple settings shows that Delta produces very high viral loads (meaning, the density of virus on a nasopharyngeal swab as interpreted from PCR cycle threshold numbers).
   (a) Viral loads are much higher in people infected with Delta than they were in people infected with Alphab. Viral loads with Delta are equally high whether the person has been vaccinated or not.c. Viral load is an indicator of infectiousness.… The more virus one has in the nose and mouth the more likely it is to be in this individual's respiratory droplets and secretions, and to spread to others.

VI. Due to evolution of the virus itself, all the currently licensed vaccines (all based on the original Wuhan strain spike protein sequence) have lost their ability to accomplish vaccine purpose 2(b)above, "To keep people from carrying the infection and transmitting it to others."

VII. **Vaccine mandates are thus stripped of their justification, since to vaccinate an individual no longer stops or even slows his ability to acquire and transmit the virus to others.**

VIII. Under Delta, natural immunity is much more protective than vaccination. All severities of COVID-19 illness produce healthy levels of natural immunity.[269]

Pierpont's paper continues with a presentation of documentary evidence from the three relevant studies.

The first study (conducted by the Massachusetts Department of Health and the CDC and published August 6, 2021) derives from the well-known outbreak of Covid-19 in Provincetown, Massachusetts, in July 2021, an episode that transpired in the course of two weeks of densely attended public events.[270]

The gist of the findings is as follows: seventy-four percent of the cases in Massachusetts' residents (a total of 346 individuals) afflicted fully vaccinated persons (those who had received two doses of Pfizer or one of the Johnson & Johnson vaccine). As sixty-nine percent of Massachusetts residents were fully vaccinated at the time, the outbreak indicates that vaccinated persons were *just as susceptible* to the virus as unvaccinated persons. If the vaccines had offered significant protection, it would be expected that the percentage of vaccinated persons infected would have been significantly *lower* than the percentage of infected unvaccinated persons in the population. While the precise vaccination coverage of the attendees was not known, the relevant demographic (the class and culture of those attending) suggest that it was very likely equal to or greater than the sixty-nine percent state average.

We have already discussed the second study cited by Pierpont, the Chau study in Vietnam, and so will not offer further comment on it here.

The third study (released on August 24, 2021, and summarized in *The BMJ* [formerly *The British Medical Journal*] a few days prior to that) seems to me in many ways the most telling.[271] The study derives from ongoing, population-wide testing and analysis in the UK conducted with the express purpose of evaluating vaccine efficacy. The methodology entails PCR testing of randomly selected households across the UK, ignoring symptoms, vaccination status, and previous infection. Also, and this is a key point, it includes testing for viral load in both the periods of Alpha dominance (January to mid-May 2021) and Delta variant dominance (mid-May to August 2021).

During the period of Alpha dominance, 12,287 persons tested positive for Covid-19.

Eighty-eight percent of these cases occurred in unvaccinated persons who had no history of prior infection. Only 0.5 percent of the positive cases involved fully vaccinated persons, and 0.6 percent involved those with a history of Covid-19 infection. Clearly, both full vaccination and natural immunity from prior infection conferred powerful protection during the Alpha era.

The rise of the Delta variant, however, changed everything. Pierpont noted:

> During the Delta-dominant period, the sample was 1939 new positive PCR tests. Of these, 17% (326) were from unvaccinated people without prior COVID-19 disease, 1% (20) were unvaccinated with evidence of prior disease, and 82% (1593) were fully vaccinated. This is approximately the percentage of the UK population who were vaccinated by August 18,

2021—when 75–83% of UK residents were fully vaccinated and 84–89% had received at least one dose.[272]

Pierpont draws the logical, sobering conclusion from these numbers:

> Like the Massachusetts study reviewed above, this suggests that the new Delta variant infects vaccinated and unvaccinated people with equal probability. To go from 0.5% of randomly sampled new infections in vaccinated people (under Alpha) to 82% (under Delta) in several months as the populations is becoming more and more vaccinated—these are extraordinary numbers.[273]

I would note here, too, that we are here dealing with a relatively large sample size (thousands of persons) spread over a large geographic area including diverse demographics, and so are confronting results less open to incidental bias than the Massachusetts study. Yet, as Pierpont points out, the results only verify the striking fact-based scientific conclusion:

> If vaccination is still effective in preventing infection, we would expect the proportion of infections in a random population sample to be less than the proportion of the population vaccinated. If 82% of randomly obtained positive tests occur in vaccinated people, and about 82% of people are vaccinated, then vaccination is not reducing the likelihood of infection at all. Efficacy at preventing infection has become zero.[274]

In case the political implications of these scientific results are not transparent enough, Pierpont spells it all out in no uncertain terms (and the emphasis in the text below is hers):

> These three different studies in three countries with three population sampling methods produced the same results: *with the current, dominant Delta strain, vaccinated people become infected and carry just as much infectious virus in their upper respiratory tracts when infected as unvaccinated people. The reproducibility of this finding makes it a very strong finding.*
>
> The study in Vietnam shows clearly that *infected vaccinated people transmit the infection to others.*
>
> Under the current dominance of the Delta variant, being vaccinated or not has *no influence on a chief determinant of infectiousness: the size of the viral load carried in the nose and mouth of an infected person. In addition, both vaccinated and unvaccinated become infected in significant numbers approximating the ratios of vaccinated and unvaccinated in the population.*

> The *rationale for mandates*—that each individual has a responsibility to be vaccinated to limit spread of the virus to others—is hereby *seriously or even fatally undermined.* The decision to be vaccinated, under Delta predominance, has become *entirely personal, affecting only the future health and wellbeing of the individual* receiving the vaccine.
>
> Blaming the unvaccinated for the rapid spread of the Delta variant has no merit whatsoever, since both vaccinated and unvaccinated infected people are equally infectious to others, and vaccinated and unvaccinated people are represented in illness samples in proportion to their representation in the general population, showing they are equally likely to become infected.
>
> These findings also equalize vaccinated and unvaccinated in terms of quarantine, vaccine-based exclusion, or the wearing of masks.[275]

Pierpont published her paper, remember, on September 9, 2021, the same day President Biden delivered his speech in which he blamed the unvaccinated for the country's continuing ills and imposed several restrictive mandates. Clearly, the timing was not coincidental. Pierpont's paper represents a comprehensive rebuttal of the scientific premises underlying the President's policy and, by extension, the rational legitimacy of his policies.

Predictably, in addition to challenging vaccine efficacy, Pierpont continues to highlight two considerations of paramount importance: the real efficacy of *natural immunity* regardless of viral variation and the *unsafe* character of the vaccines. Her own final conclusion delivers a legal warning:

> Given all the above evidence, mandating others to take a vaccine is a potentially harmful, damaging act.
>
> Since the principal reason for COVID-19 vaccine mandates—protecting others from infection—has evaporated with the ascendance of the Delta variant, those who mandate COVID-19 vaccines may wish to seek legal counsel regarding their culpability and liability (including personal) for potential long-lasting harm to those whom they pressure into vaccination with threat of exclusion from employment or education or other public activity. Remind your attorney that if an unborn or nursing baby is damaged, liability persists until the child is age 23—plenty of time for discovery of the ways whereby vaccine producers and government regulators may have suppressed important information about harmful effects.[276]

We will come back to that matter of suppressed information shortly, but not before returning to Israel, the world's premier human vaccine laboratory, and adding still more recent evidence regarding vaccine inefficacy.

Before continuing, it is worth revisiting the reason why Israeli data deservedly plays such a central role in framing Covid policy decisions in the United States. Not only is Israel at or near the top of the list of most vaccinated countries in the world (as of August 19, 2021, seventy-eight percent of Israeli residents over the age of twelve have received at least two doses of the Pfizer vaccine and many by now have received additional booster shots), but Israel's early deal with Pfizer and aggressive mass vaccination enabled the country to achieve very high vaccination rates very quickly. Because of its fast start, Israel's vaccine program is effectively two to four months ahead of that of the United States. This means that the virus has had that much more time to adapt to—and potentially "escape" from—the vaccines in Israel, so that measures of vaccine efficacy there function as a kind of bellwether of what we are likely to see here in the United States two to four months down the line. Other factors, too, contribute to the special role played by Israel and its data in U.S. Covid policymaking. As *Politico* reports:

> The Biden administration has long relied on data from Israel, which has one of the highest vaccination rates in the world, to inform its Covid-19 response.... The administration's focus on Israeli data underscores the extent to which the U.S. is leaning on other countries' experiences to forecast the next phase of the pandemic here. That is partly because the highly contagious Delta variant swept through other parts of the world first, and partly because of better data tracking in countries like Israel that have national healthcare systems. The U.S. continues to struggle to collect and analyze reliable Covid-19 data because the federal government has long neglected the country's public health infrastructure.[277]

Since results of the vaccination program in Israel at this (mid-September, 2021) juncture can only be regarded as disastrous, that bellwether is looking more and more like a canary in a coal mine—and a dead one at that.

Just how bad is the news from Israel? It is so bad that, as mentioned previously, Israel is, in mid-September 2021, experiencing record number of daily case counts—even higher than it did in the early stages of the pandemic, before anyone was vaccinated. It is so bad that you are no longer considered "fully" vaccinated in Israel unless you have had not your second but your third shot. (Predictably, as Dr. Peter McCullough stated, such boosting does not seem to be helping.) It is so bad that Portugal and Sweden recently banned all Israelis, regardless of their vaccination status, from entry, a move the *Times of Israel* feared might be implemented by other European countries.[278]

The bad news pertains not only to case counts but also to incidence of hospitalization and death. This distressing fact undercuts the one potentially cogent criticism of the logic underlying Dr. Nina Pierpont's anti-mandate argument. The claim can and has been made that even if vaccination does *not* impede the spread of Delta-triggered Covid cases, it does help keep those vaccinated from becoming seriously ill, thus precluding hospital overload and making sure anyone who does need treatment receive appropriate attention. That, after all, has been the fallback position of the proponents of vaccination who have had to recognize that vaccination does not (as Pierpont argues) effectively prevent spread.

Kim Iversen, in a recent segment of her show, commented on *statewide* figures in Massachusetts. After confirming (and referencing the states' own health officials' confirm of) Pierpont's conclusion that vaccination does not impede spread, Iversen articulates this fallback position:

> If you have more cases today than you did at the same time last year, and yet the majority of your population is fully vaccinated, and it's a majority of them catching the virus, how can you square that and the idea that these vaccines stop the spread? You can't, and *our public health officials know this*. But again, it's not about spread, they finally admit, it's about overwhelmed hospitals.[279]

The problem with that argument is that in the Delta era, at least, its truth is eminently debatable. Like most everything in the Covid domain, the process of assessment is, first of all, vulnerable to the kind of data manipulation and misrepresentation characteristic of so many features of the controlling Covid narrative—such as government claims that ninety-nine percent of persons in the hospital are unvaccinated, despite these claims having been drawn from data for months during which most *everyone* was unvaccinated. Moreover, over the course of the last month or so, data from highly vaccinated countries including Israel strongly indicates that *it is not only the Covid vaccine's capacity to preclude infection and spread that wanes dramatically over time but also its capacity to prevent serious illness and death*.

Does it not stand to reason? As the virus gets better and better at evading the vaccine's defenses is it not likely, in time, to get that much better at doing so altogether, even precipitating ADE? Given that the vaccines do *not* build upon and strengthen the body's natural broad-based immunological defenses, but introduce an experimental mechanism that depends on targeting a narrow, moving target less and less likely to be hit, there is *no* guarantee that, ultimately, the overall immunological effect of the vaccine will be beneficial.

Already in mid- to late August 2021, by which date Delta had sufficient time to assume dominance, *nearly sixty percent of those hospitalized for Covid-19 in Israel were fully vaccinated.*[280] The ominous character of that fact was not lost on the chief information officer at Clalit Health Services, Israel's largest health maintenance organization. "This is a very clear warning sign for the rest of the world," declared Ran Balicer. "If it can happen here, it can probably happen anywhere."[281]

A month later, the news became even worse. Commentator Kim Iversen recounted how Israel, with the great majority of its population "fully" vaccinated with two doses of Pfizer by February, saw a dramatic surge in cases in the summer months.

> What they discovered was, the vaccine wears off. They saw a skyrocketing number of cases even after they hit the so-called herd-immunity threshold of 70%. They reached [that threshold] and suddenly saw massive spread.[282]

The news, though, was not all bad:

> ... but it looks like it might help against severe disease. [After] the early reports that came in from April, May, June... they were saying: "The people who are getting really sick are the unvaccinated."
>
> That *was* true, we do know that. But then, as time went on, the hospitals started filling up with fully vaccinated people. They saw more and more cases among the fully vaccinated, and more and more them becoming very severe to the point where the majority of their cases in the hospitals and in the ICU and those dying were fully vaccinated people.[283]

Iversen's data tracking has not, in fact, been limited to Israel but included, among other countries, Iceland, Chile, Uruguay, the Seychelles, and Saudi Arabia. She remarks:

> I have a whole list of countries that I've been monitoring on this. And it was really clear early on that the vaccine was not stopping the spread, but it did seem to keep people out of the hospital for a period of time. But then Israel found even that wears off.[284]

That discovery, continues Iversen, moved Israel to inaugurate an aggressive booster campaign. You are now not "fully" vaccinated in Israel—and so able to participate in any normal wise in society—unless you have had *three* shots.

The results?

They were encouraging, at first—but only briefly. After an initial dip, cases, hospitalization, and deaths climbed steeply, reaching new highs during the last few days of mid-September. Politico reports:

> The Biden administration's push to roll out coronavirus vaccine booster shots this month has largely been shaped by unpublished data from Israel's vaccination campaign, according to two individuals familiar with the matter. *The Israel data...shows that the Pfizer vaccine's ability to prevent severe disease and hospitalization is waning over time—as is the shot's protection against mild and moderate disease....* Although the CDC has published a series of targeted studies that suggest Covid-19 vaccines' effectiveness against infection is decreasing, particularly in the elderly, the Israeli data is more comprehensive and more alarming (emphasis mine).[285]

Believe it or not, none other than Dr. Anthony Fauci recognized the power of the data:

> Asked about the extent to which the Israeli data showed vaccine efficacy waning, Biden's chief medical advisor, Anthony Fauci, said it was "enough that you would be impressed. I would be very surprised if the U.S. data don't turn out to be ultimately very similar to the Israeli data."[286]

The following is Iversen's own sharp summary observation:

> The data shows (the vaccine's efficacy) significantly wears off, even against the most severe of outcomes. We're about four months behind Israel in vaccination. In August, they saw their hospitals and morgues filling up with fully vaccinated people. This means, the stats will shift. The fall and winter, we can begin to see the hospitals and morgues filling up with fully vaccinated people as the vaccines wear off. Fully vaccinated people today will essentially be unvaccinated in the coming weeks and months...
>
> Are we following science, or are we following fear? Are we really following the data, and making sound decisions based on that data? Or are we just pretending that we know it's going to work, and then demanding it of everyone?[287]

"Just pretending": isn't that what the Emperor, his court, and most of his country's people are indeed doing, and doing very well?

Yet the system is not entirely without checks and balances, a fact rather dramatically exhibited when, a little over a week after President Biden's speech, the FDA unexpectedly decided, by a resounding 16-to-2 vote, *against* approving Pfizer booster shots for the general population. The Israeli data undoubtedly played a role in that decision; a number of outside experts (each of whom were granted a three-minute comment period near the middle of the eight-hour FDA session) cited it in arguing forcefully against approving boosters. Retsef Levi noted:

> You already sent a presentation to the Israeli Ministry of Health that praises the efficacy of the boosters. I would like to caution against this premature celebration, and remind you that similar statements were made just six months ago, around February, on the two initial doses.... Covid-19 deaths in Israel, in spite of all the boosters, are on the rise, whereas in other countries, including in many states in the U.S., they seem to be on a downward trend.[288]

Immunologist Dr. Jessica Rose offered a cogent comment, calling attention to the positive danger of indiscriminate mass vaccination driving immune escape. Commenting on a graph titled "Evolutionary pressure on viruses to speed up mutation?" (one rather difficult to interpret in the few seconds allowed but clearly reflecting the gist of the data already cited), Dr. Rose states:

> Israel is one of the most injected countries and it appears from this data that this represents *a clear failure of these products to provide protective immunity against emergent variants and to prevent transmission regardless of how many additional shots are administered.* This begs the question as to whether these injection rollouts are driving the emergence of the new variants. There is clear and present danger of the emerging of variants of concern if we continue with these alleged booster shots.[289]

President Biden's assumptions regarding vaccine safety—a parameter both distinct from and (via cost-benefit analyses) related to vaccine efficacy—also ran into stiff resistance at the FDA hearing from Dr. Rose and many others. After observing that "safety and efficacy are the cornerstones of the administration of biological products meant for human use," Dr. Rose presented a very legible graph comparing the frequency of reports of both all adverse events and deaths for all vaccines combined over the last ten years and adverse events and deaths in 2021. Rose asserted:

> There's an *over 1,000% increase* in the total number of adverse events for 2021 [as well as comparable discrepancy in deaths], and we are not done with 2021. This is a highly anomalous on both fronts. The onus is on the public health officials at the FDA and CDC and policymakers to answer to these anomalies and acknowledge the clear risk signals emerging from the VAERS data and to confront the issue of COVID injectable products use/risk. In my opinion, the risks outweigh any potential benefit associated with these products, especially for children.[290]

Dr. Rose presented additional graphic evidence that, as of August 27, 2021, VAERS data showed that one of every 660 persons are "succumbing to and reporting immunological adverse events associated with COVID products," an historically high figure that Dr. Rose observed does not take into account the recognized *underreporting* of such incidence to the VAERS system. (We will return to the matter of underreporting in subsequent chapters in this part of this book.)

Steve Kirsch, founder of the COVID-19 Early Treatment Fund, called attention to "the elephant in the room." Drawing upon data from Pfizer's own six-month trial report, Kirsch alleged that the data clearly shows that the COVID vaccines do not reduce mortality rate, but—because of very low benefit and relatively high risk—do just the opposite. That is, more people stand to die from the vaccine than are saved from death by Covid by it. Kirsch stated:

> We were led to believe that vaccines are perfectly safe, but this is simply not true. For example, there were four times as many heart attacks in the treatment group in the Pfizer six-month trial report. That wasn't bad luck. VAERS shows heart attacks happen 71 times more often following these vaccines compared to any other vaccine. In all, *20 people died who got the drug—14 died who got the placebo.*[291]

My readers should know that many of those who offered testimony (including those whom I already cited) can hardly be blithely dismissed as "anti-vaxxers." Dr. Rose is an immunologist; Steve Kirsch is an entrepreneur who founded the COVID-19 Early Treatment Fund not because he opposed a vaccine program on principle but, on the contrary, because, in the early months of the pandemic, he recognized that the government was not funding desperately needed research in repurposed drugs and early treatment options. One of the most telling testimonies, moreover, was offered by Dr. Joseph B. Fraiman, an emergency medicine physician in New Orleans, who appealed to the FDA and other health authorities to do the work objectively necessary to prove—rather than presume—vaccine safety and efficacy, so that he could, in good conscience, answer the questions of the vaccine-hesitant. Because it puts a human face on a great deal fundamental to both the science and sociopolitics of Covid-19 in America, I give Dr. Fraiman's testimony:

> Where I work over 65% of the population is not vaccinated. I am here today to ask for help for those working on the front lines to help reduce vaccine hesitancy. For this, we need larger trials that demonstrate that vaccines reduce hospitalization without finding evidence of serious harm.

I know many think the vaccine-hesitant are dumb or just misinformed, but that is not at all what I have seen. In fact, typically, independent of educational level, the vaccine-hesitant I have met in the ER are more familiar with vaccine studies, and more aware of their own Covid risk than the vaccinated.

For example, many of my nurses have refused the vaccine, despite having seen Covid-19 cause more death and devastation than most people have. I ask them: "Why refuse the vaccine?" They tell me, while they have seen, firsthand, the dangers of Covid-19 for the elderly, the obese, diabetics, they think their risk is low. They are not wrong. One nurse showed me this Oxford risk calculator. A 30-year-old healthy female has about a 1 in 7,000 chance of catching Covid and being hospitalized over 90 days. [The displayed chart also shows the chance of COVID associated death to be 1 in 250,000.] She asked me, can I could assure her that the studies found her risk of serious harm from the vaccines is lower than her risk of hospitalization?

The truth is, I can't. Our trials weren't big enough. They weren't big enough to identify that vaccines cause myocarditis. Yet now we know they do.... A recent observational study suggests the risk of vaccine-induced myocarditis in young males is higher than their risk of hospitalization from Covid. Is this true? We don't know. It's based on observational data. To know it's *not* true, we need a large trial that proves that the vaccines reduce hospitalization more than they cause myocarditis in this age group.

The former FDA commissioner said, "The original premise of the vaccine was to reduce death and hospitalization, and that was the data that came out of the initial clinical trials." Except, as you all know very well, and, unfortunately, so did my nurse, the initial clinical trials did *not* find a reduction in death or hospitalization, likely because they were inadequately powered. Yet the former commissioner is correct. The initial trials should have been powered to find a reduction in hospitalization. We need your help on the front lines to stop vaccine hesitancy....

Without this data, we, the medical establishment, cannot confidently call out anti-Covid vaccine activists who publicly claim that the vaccines harm more than they save, especially in the young and healthy. The fact that we do not have the clinical evidence to say these activists are wrong, should terrify us all.[292]

Yes, Dr. Fraiman, I couldn't agree more. It *should* terrify us all...because those "anti-Covid vaccine activists" might just be right. After all, at this point (as you yourself admit), the *extant scientific evidence is all on their side.*

Why, then, have those studies Dr. Fraiman is calling for not been done?

In my opinion, the answer is relatively obvious. ***Relevant personnel fear that more substantial evidence, especially now, in the age of Delta, will only corroborate what we already know: The vaccines are neither safe nor effective.*** The chief means of maintaining the contrary view thus remain—not robust data sampling and honest transparency, conditions actually requisite for informed consent—but the opposite. That (at least as far as Big Pharma is concerned) is business as usual: disguise and dissimulation and vain pretense that literally capitalizes on the killing combination of people's fathomless fear, credulity, and Millgramesque faith in authority.

Yet let us get back to President Biden's speech. When we hear the President paternalistically imploring parents to vaccinate their healthy teenagers as a means of ensuring their safety, such arrogant nonsense must be reckoned especially tragic:

> Let me speak to you directly to ease some of your worries.... The safest thing for your child 12 and over, is to get them vaccinated....That's it. Get them vaccinated. As with adults, almost all of the serious Covid-19 cases we're seeing among adolescents are in unvaccinated 12- to 17-year-olds, an age group that lags behind in vaccination rates. So parents: please get your teenager vaccinated.[293]

This emotional appeal is based on what, at present, must be considered blatant falsehood. As Dr. Fraiman indicates, a recent study, titled "SARS-CoV-2 mRNA Vaccination-associated Myocarditis in Children Ages 12–17: A Stratified National Database Analysis," suggests that adolescents are two to six times more likely to contract vaccine-induced myocarditis than to suffer hospitalization from Covid. Here are the key results (CAE stands for cardiac artery ectasia, an abnormal widening of coronal arteries, a variation of CAD or cardiac artery disease):

> **Results:** A total of 257 CAEs were identified....For boys 12–15 without medical comorbidities receiving their second mRNA vaccination dose, the rate of CAE is 3.7 to 6.1 times higher than their 120-day COVID-19 hospitalization risk...and 2.6–4.3-fold higher at times of high weekly hospitalization risk...such as during January 2021. For boys 16–17 without medical comorbidities, the rate of CAE is currently 2.1–3.5 times higher than their 120-day COVID-19 hospitalization risk, and 1.5 to 2.5 times higher at times of high weekly COVID-19 hospitalization.[294]

It is true that the study shows CAEs to be *relatively* rare. The key word here, though, is "relatively" because Covid-caused hospitalization is *far more* rare—on the order of one to two incidents per 100,000 young adults. The problem is, of course, that any mass vaccination campaign involving the inoculation of millions or tens of millions (or more) turns "rarities" into a significant number of real-life casualties. In his response to President Biden's pitch, Del Bigtree puts the gist of the matter bluntly: "This idea that the greatest risk to your child is the virus over the vaccine: that is simply not true. *It is just not true*."[295]

Those adverse events statistics, remember, are not just numbers but real human stories, far too many of which are heart-wrenchingly catastrophic. Here, for instance, is the hospital-bed witness of one otherwise perfectly healthy young teenage male, John Stokes, suffering, like far too many others, from myocarditis:

> I am in the hospital right now with heart complications from the Covid-19 vaccine. I want to inform as many people as I can about the risks from taking the vaccine that I wish someone would have told me.
>
> I am a Division 1 athlete with no prior health issues. I got the second Covid shot Tuesday, and within four days, I had been diagnosed with myocarditis and was told that I probably won't be able to play my senior season now. It is a side effect from the Covid vaccine, and it is really not being reported or addressed, and it is a serious issue that we should all be informed about before making this decision.
>
> It isn't right for people to be forced to take the vaccine because there are actual side effects like this that could happen to you, and the NCAA should not mandate student athletes to get the vaccine because of what could happen to so many fellow student athletes…: Everyone should be informed of the side effects, and no one should be forced to take something that could cause what has happened to me.
>
> No one knows the long term effects, and what's possibly going to happen from this. It's uncharted territory because everyone else with the same heart issues from the vaccine…we're all being tracked, and monitored. We're basically like test subjects from the vaccine. It's a very serious issue [and the knowledge of this] needs to be spread. I've spoken with other student-athletes that have also had to have either heart surgery or have had heart issues from this, and it's very scary stuff. A lot of people in our age group are apparently at higher risk for heart issues from the vaccine and it really does need to be talked about.[296]

And so I ask this: to whom, Mr. President, are you listening? Are you listening to advisors willing to say and do most anything in the interests of the pro-vaccine agenda, or are you listening to Americans who are suffering the devastating consequences of what is, in fact, dangerous disinformation that you yourself spread and empower by executive action?

President Biden prefaced his appeal to parents with his own construction of right and wrong—and his own version of a voice from the hospital bed.

> My message to unvaccinated Americans is this: What more is there to wait for? What more do you need to see? We've made vaccinations free, safe, and convenient.... We've been patient, but our patience is wearing thin. And your refusal has cost all of us. So please, do the right thing. But just don't take it from me. Listen to the voices of unvaccinated Americans, who are lying in hospital beds, taking their final breath, saying, "If only I'd gotten vaccinated."[297]

What more do Americans need to see? Dr. Setty answered that question directly in his article months ago, and none of his conditions have been met. Dr. Fraiman, who could not stand up to his well-informed nurse, answered it again on September 17, 2021.

The problem with President Biden's own melodramatic fiction is just that: it is fiction, whereas that of John Stokes, the young American speaking quietly but courageously to the nation and the world from the hospital bed to which he is confined, uncertain and afraid of the future, is the heartbreaking voice of reality and of truth. Nor is Stokes' voice an isolated one—far from it. Many, many can tell similar or still more tragic stories. Yet the voice of those social sinners who failed to see the light and convert before it was too late to secure their own absolution and who, on their deathbed, whispered "If only..."—where are they?

The question is no merely rhetorical one. In fact, one ABC affiliate, WXYZ-TV Channel 7, aiming to bolster President Biden and his plea, put out a call that might enable us all to hear just these voices. This was the message published on WXYZ's Facebook page:

> After the vaccines were available to everyone, did you lose an unvaccinated loved one to COVID-19? If you are willing to share your family's story, please DM us your contact information. We may reach out for a story we're working on.[298]

Thus the call went out, loud and clear. And the response was deafening—albeit of an entirely different kind than had been solicited and expected. Rather than hearing from its target audience, the WXYZ Facebook page was flooded with responses from persons adversely, and tragically, affected not by Covid-19 ravaging a loved one but by Covid-19 vaccine-caused death and damage. The title of the September 13 *World Tribune* article reporting this story?[299]

Unexpected and Heartbreaking:

Thousands flood ABC affiliate's Facebook page
with vaccination horror stories

A call for stories by WXYZ went out Friday afternoon. By Monday noon, ABC had received 39,000 responses, most all of them "angry and heartbreaking," a great many lamenting vaccine-caused injury and death. Here's a selection:

> ***Lost my Mom*** *10 days after she got her 2nd Pfizer jab. She couldn't swallow or talk correctly the very next day…was hospitalized and basically never "woke up" again. Was sent home on hospice after 5 days in the hospital and died at home 2 days later.*
>
> ***My daughter 33 years old died*** *10 days after getting the shot. She had an enlarged heart and she had a terminal lung disease pulmonary hypertension! She shouldn't of gotten the shot! Pfizer only first shot.*
>
> ***My son's classmate lost her mother*** *from heart complications due to the vaccine.*
>
> ***No but I know a teenager hospitalized myocarditis*** *the day after the second Pfizer shot.*
>
> ***My dad flatlined*** *after his second dose of Moderna.*
>
> ***I have a friend that dies*** *after receiving the Pfizer. Went to the Er with unexplained tremors the day after. They got tremors to stop; released him. He died the next day.*
>
> ***It's about 4 weeks after the 2nd shot*** *for me. I have chest pain all the time. i'm terrified I'm going to drop dead of* ***a heart attack.***
>
> ***My daughter*** *got the first dose of Moderna then conceived a baby. My* ***grandson was stillborn*** *with heart and brain malformations that a Pfizer VP said could happen during the 20th and 22nd day of conception. But hey he is a crazy guy right. Hmm. Not. Also the FDA won't have full test results in regards to teratology until 2025.*

One respondent had several horror stories and expressed a common sentiment: disgust at lack of real media coverage:

> ***My parent's neighbor*** *woke up the next morning after the shot suddenly completely deaf. His doctor told him it's from the vaccine and if*

> *his hearing didn't return within a few weeks he will be permanently deaf. He **is now permanently deaf.***
>
> ***Our rabbi's mentor** (a very prestigious rabbi) was recovering from covid in a rehab facility. He was doing well, walking and about to be discharged home. The facility forced him to take the vaccine because it became their policy, even though he refused. He immediately developed paralysis in one arm. They then forced the second shot on him, he refused again but the facility insisted. After the 2nd shot he **developed complete, progressive paralysis and died.***
>
> ***Why do we not see these stories in the news?** Why are the journalists silent on the thousands of vaccine injuries leading to permanent disability and death? What happened to honest journalism? Please report these stories in the news!*

Reports of heart attacks and strokes were disturbingly abundant:

> ***My Dad** started having problems after his first shot. But was bound and determined to get second shot. He **died** 5 days after second shot of a massive heart attack. He had no known heart problems before!*
>
> ***My father in law** had the covid vax then had a stroke and **died.** They ruled out all the normal stroke causes. It was the vaccine and my husband will be reporting it to VAERS. Do a report on that!*
>
> ***No stories on that.** But a guy I knew got double shot and 2 days later dropped dead of a heart attack. Why don't you report on THAT*

Stories of non-lethal injuries are hardly less heart-wrenching.

> ***My daughters teacher** had immediate severe reaction (within the 15min observation period) after the first dose. She was diagnosed with **Guillan Barre syndrome** and now has to use a wheelchair. How about a story on vaccine reactions?*
>
> ***The VA in Palo Alto** gave my Father in law his THIRD booster?... He's wobbly and slurring his words, cant find words to communicate, etc. It's like he's a toddler again. **What the heck is in those viles?***
>
> ***No, but vaccinated friends lost their pregnancies** as a result of their covid shots.*

No few of the responses pushed back against the popular notion that the unvaccinated pose a greater threat to others than do the vaccinated:

> ***My fully vaccinated husband and I** just recovered from covid and **gave it to our unvaccinated children** who we were trying to protect by getting the shots in the first place!!! How about covering that story instead of producing more propaganda.*
>
> ***I am a physical therapist** with almost 30-years experience. In the nursing home/rehab where I work, we have had a higher percentage of residents with the shot than without the shot to contract the delta variant.*
>
> ***I know someone** who was FULLY vaccinated and **always wore their mask,** they were recently in the ICU and passed away.*
>
> A registered nurse had some particularly choice words:
>
> ***The vaccine has become so politicized** that even if it is useful for preventing serious illness or death from covid, they pretend that adverse effects don't exist and so they don't warn people and don't actually monitor people for them. My mother had a hypertensive crisis from the Moderna booster which could have caused a stroke, and now she has to be on blood pressure medication. I also developed high blood pressure after one dose of Pfizer.... We know a 22-year-old woman who also developed hypertension and tachycardia.... They are endangering people's lives by pretending the adverse effects don't exist. They know they exist which is why they don't want to give boosters yet. They think it will cause even more adverse effects.*

Reports of those who died after refusing the vaccine were, for the most part, missing in action. Instead, the following post represented the general tenor which includes, again, frustration with mainstream media:

> ***I know 5 people who have lost friends or family** members after being vaccinated.*
>
> ***Nope.** only deaths and injuries of vaccinated Very sad. Let people choose if it's right for them. Maybe they don't want to take the risk.*
>
> ***Crazy** that most of the comments here are the polar opposite of what WXYZ-TV Channel 7 was looking for to fuel more fear into the public. Why don't you report what is ACTUALLY happening?*
>
> ***Hey, Channel 7,** be a leader in journalism and start reporting what's really happening. Or can't you report **the truth?***

~

President Biden: please rehearse the ABCs of democratic governance. The WXYZ "poll" could be regarded as a kind of election. Given the phrasing of the question, the odds were stacked in your favor. Yet the results? The *other* side won—not by a landslide, but by an avalanche. On this world-important issue, is yours a government *of, by, and for the people*? The evidence, I think, is piling up against you—you, and those *vial* mandates.

Chapter 24

MORE SCARY: IN THE BELLY OF THE HEALTHCARE BEAST

We are not yet done with the all-important issue of safety. Nor have we shared the last word on the serious adverse consequences of draconian mandates, the justification of which is based not on evidence, science, and reason but on obfuscation and intimidation. As almost unbelievably bad as the official VAERS safety data is for the Covid vaccines, the scariest thing is that, in reality, it is undoubtedly unimaginably worse because the vast majority of cases of vaccine injury and death go unreported, *and do so largely by design.*

I have already recorded Dr. Peter McCullough's (uncontested) allegation that the agencies who should be responsible for robust safety monitoring of an experimental product, the FDA, CDC, HHS and relevant affiliates, have entirely dropped the ball. They are AWOL—derelict of duty. That fact, while in itself sufficient to discredit the claim that the vaccines are "safe," is not, however, the worst of it all. The powers that be, from the highest echelons of the CDC, FDA, and NIH down through state and local health officials, medical licensing boards, and hospital administrators, *systematically suppress the reporting of vaccine-induced injury and death.* This suppression entails a number of intimately intertwined elements:

1. Failure to provide *a functional system* of reporting that makes it truly practicable (in terms of knowledge, time, energy, and effort) for healthcare providers (doctors, nurses, physician assistants, etc.) to report adverse events.
2. Failure to *mandate* reporting of safety events or to enforce existing laws/mandates to report.
3. Failure to *educate* health providers so they know their obligations to report and are empowered both to initiate and complete the reporting process.
4. Active *discouragement* of the reporting of adverse events so as to avoid undermining the approved pro-vaccine message. The forms of disincentive run the gamut from gentler sorts of peer pressure and disapproval

to covert and overt threats of disciplinary action, including dismissal or loss of medical license. Also noteworthy in this connection is the ominous clause of the present protocol stipulating that the filer of a VAERS report is *criminally liable* for any report found to be false or erroneous.

5. Inadequate, sloppy, or even blatantly *skewed data-gathering procedures* that systematically distort medical reality so as to hide vaccine harm and support the pro-vaccine message.

Dr. Peter McCullough is himself a leading physician in a position of authority and the one deeply knowledgeable as to both the medical and administrative dimensions of filing a VAERS report. For him, the process of filing a VAERS report was, by his own admission, onerous enough. For the vast majority of less knowledgeable health professionals, it is no simple matter of setting aside an extra thirty minutes (bad enough for any busy doctor or nurse). It is also a largely thankless task, the completion of which requires surmounting daunting practical as well as sociopsychological barriers. No wonder a CDC-sponsored 2007 Harvard study found that *less than one percent of actual adverse events were actually reported.*[300] To obtain a more accurate picture of vaccine harm, then, we probably need to take the existing VAERS numbers and multiply them a hundredfold.

If you imagine I am making all of this up and that it is not the health authorities but I who am spinning tales to support some predetermined position, listen, then, not to me, but to *the voice of people.* Let's address the above five points, loosely, in reverse order, while doing just that.

On the one side, and pursuant to point #5 above, listen to a segment of a September 10, 2021, discussion between Carolyn Fisher, the director of marketing at Novant Health Center (a conglomerate of fifteen major hospitals headquartered in North Carolina), Dr. Mary Rudyk, an internist who also happens to be Novant's former chief of medical staff, and Shelbourn Stevens, the president of the New Hanover Medical Center.

Carolyn Fisher begins addressing the issue of public messaging vis-à-vis Covid and vaccination status:

> As far as how we get information out to the community, on meaningful numbers, on a weekly basis: that's on our website and we've been sharing that through social channels as well, particularly those graphics that show the number of patients and the percentage of them that are unvaccinated,

the percentage of unvaccinated in the ICU, and the percentage of deaths. So those are numbers we put out.[301]

Dr. Mary Rudyk, the former medical staff chief, responds:

> I guess my feeling at this point in time is maybe we need to be completely—a little bit more *scary* for the public.... There are many people still hospitalized, that we're considering post-Covid. But we're not counting in those numbers. So how do we include those post-Covid people in the numbers of patients we have in the hospital?[302]

After a brief exchange during which a slightly befuddled Fischer seems to balk at the notion of a questionable inflation of Covid numbers, Shelbourn Stevens enters the conversation, indicating that the patients to which Dr. Rudyk is referring are currently classed as "recovered" but might still be considered as Covid patients, and suggests continuing the conversation "offline" in order to deliberate how to package relevant data *before* taking it to the marketing department (to Carolyn Fischer). The captured video clip concludes with Rudyk saying the following to Fischer:

> I'm just going to say, Carolyn, I think we have to be more poppy, we have to be more forceful, we have to say something coming out, *"you know, you don't get vaccinated, you're going to die."* I mean, let's just be really blunt to these people.[303]

"These people," of course, refers to unvaccinated persons. This video clip, displaying hospital staff deliberately contemplating how to massage data so as to serve the Health Center's pro-vaccine policy, went viral, stirring outrage that in turn prompted Novant Health to issue the following statement defending its policy makers and their process:

> The team members involved in this excerpt of an internal meeting are seeing the highest level of COVID-19 hospitalizations and deaths so far in this pandemic—despite having safe and effective vaccines widely available. This was a frank discussion among medical and communication professionals on how we can more accurately convey the severity and seriousness of what's happening inside of our hospitals. Specifically, the data we have been sharing does not include patients who remain hospitalized for COVID-19 complications even though they are no longer COVID-19 positive, so it does not provide a complete picture of the total impact of COVID-19 on our patients and on our hospitals. We continue to be concerned with the amount of misinformation in our communities and consistently strive for more ways to be transparent and tell the whole story.[304]

Novant Health's response reveals the disingenuous doublespeak characterizing so much official Covid rhetoric. The very possibility that the vaccines may not be safe and effective remains automatically precluded from the first. Thus, caught in the act of compromising accuracy in the interests of ideologically informed public relations, the Health Center implies that all questioning of the official position amounts to naught but "misinformation" and—even while providing cover for conduct that covertly if not overtly suggests anything but total truthfulness—pretends to strive for transparency and full disclosure.

Even so, the cited conversation's chief value lies in the revelation of official *attitude* rather than concrete methodological wrongdoing. Because the argument can, perhaps, be made that the patients in question *could* logically be logged in the Covid column, Rudyk's proposed reclassification represents data manipulation far *less* patently egregious than other diverse forms of the same that are seemingly endemic to the sphere of Covid-related public health administration. I have, in the course of this volume, already pointed to multiple instances: Dr. Setty's exposure of the nonsensical, vaccine-friendly double standards employed in judging whether a patient does or does not have Covid; Dr. McCullough and Mathew Crawford calling attention to the various nefarious ways authorities deny vaccine-induced death, even reclassifying these as deaths caused not by the vaccine but by Covid; and, perhaps the most rampant abuse of all, the indiscriminate categorizing of test-positive patients as Covid cases whether or not the disease had anything to do with their reasons for hospitalization or death.

The magnitude of this act of deception is just to beginning to come to light. On September 13, 2021, *The Atlantic* ran an article titled "Our Most Reliable Pandemic Number is Losing Meaning." It reports on the results of a recent study by Harvard Medical School, Tufts Medical Center, and the Veteran Affairs Healthcare system.[305] After pointing out that case counts depend on the number of people tested and death counts lag and fail to account for serious illness, *The Atlantic* piece reveals that the number of hospitalizations—"our most reliable pandemic number"—is not so reliable after all but may, in fact, be grossly misleading.

The researchers analyzed electronic records for almost 50,000 Covid hospital admissions distributed throughout the hundred-plus VA hospitals spread across the United States. Employing blood oxygen level as a reliable means of assessing whether a patient suffered, on the one hand, moderate to severe illness or, on the other, from a mild or asymptomatic case, the study found this:

> From March 2020 through early January 2021—before vaccination was widespread, and before the Delta variant had arrived—the proportion of patients with mild or asymptomatic disease was 36 percent. From mid-January through the end of June 2021, however, that number rose to 48 percent. *In other words, the study suggests that roughly half of all the hospitalized patients showing up on COVID-data dashboards in 2021 may have been admitted for another reason entirely, or had only a mild presentation of disease* (italics mine).[306]

Such inflated Covid numbers—which undoubtedly appeared on the dashboards of hospitals outside the VA system too—clearly inflate, artificially, the perceived Covid threat and, concomitantly, exaggerate its impact on hospital resources. Evidently, however, that order of inflation did *not* suffice, in the medical staff's opinion, to make Novant Health Center's Covid numbers "scary" enough to get the pro-vaccine message across. So, instead of real transparency or any genuine effort "to tell the whole story," their former chief of medical staff deliberated additional means of hiking the Covid numbers while unconsciously voicing the pro-vaccine establishment's fantasy of total control and annihilation of the other, an end attained by getting in everybody's face and saying, straight-up, out loud: *"If you don't get vaccinated, you'll die."*

So much, for now, for people on the mainstream side of the Covid issue. Let's turn to persons on the dissenting side, addressing first briefly, once more, concerns about medical and scientific integrity and difference of opinion (cf. point #4) and then return to (cf. points #1, #2 and #3 as well as #4 and #5) the all-important issue of vaccine safety and how it is, or is not, tried, tested, and proven.

Dr. Peter Doshi, a professor at the University of Maryland and an editor of the prestigious *BMJ*, stood as yet another physician-scientist who offered telling testimony at the September 17, 2021, FDA meeting. Dr. Doshi spoke to the issue of how officially sanctioned positions and policy translate into active suppression of any professional words or deeds that threaten the party line:

> Last week, three medical licensing boards said they could revoke doctors' medical licenses for providing COVID vaccine misinformation. I'm worried about the chilling effects here. There are clearly many remaining unknowns and science is all about proving unknowns. But in the present supercharged climate—and I'll point out that many members on this committee are certified by these boards—what is the FDA doing so that members can speak freely without fear of reprisal?[307]

I think it a good bet that we know the answer to that question: *nothing*. Dr. Doshi's words suggest what may well be—so far as the expression of scientific opinion is concerned—the American equivalent of Dr. Byram Bridle's story. Yet, quite apart from question of any *research* scientist's freedom of inquiry and expression, Dr. Doshi's comments bear, too, upon the more mundane but absolutely fundamental matter of data gathering, specifically, *the filing or non-filing of reports documenting vaccine injury and death.*

Unbeknownst to many, there is here, on just this field of concern, a battle being fought—an epic, if unsung, battle. So far, it appears to have been a rather one-sided affair, with all sorts of heavy artillery backing up the official position, while, on the other side, we see a scattered army of citizen-soldiers armed with little more than the homegrown tools of common sense, conscientious concern, and the knowledge born of firsthand experience. To get a close-up look at this conflict, a perspective from the trenches, let us listen in to the story of one rebel hero, a medical professional devoted, *above all,* to the mission of the public health and to the fulfillment of the terms of true service: purity of heart, clarity of mind, and courageous will as well as the *honesty of deed* required to make sure that hospitals and health systems are not places of doing harm but of promoting healing.

Chapter 25

THE PEOPLE'S EYEWITNESS: DEB CONRAD AND THE VAERS SCANDAL

Deborah Conrad is a certified physician assistant in a local community hospital in New York State. A veteran of fifteen years of service, she has risen to a position of leadership in her care community and serves as advanced care director of her hospital's medical executive committee. As such, in addition to her extensive everyday care activities, she is instrumental in performing tasks such as formalizing and disseminating treatment protocol for specific conditions and other medically critical matters. A highly dedicated professional, Conrad exudes the human concern and ethical integrity that one would hope to find in every healthcare worker. In a recent appearance on Del Bigtree's *The Highwire,* Conrad, after describing her position and duties, affirms: "I *love* my job. I *love* my job. Being in the medical field, and knowing how important it is to make sure that we keep people safe...is (my) number one priority."[308]

As a physician assistant who works in a hospital, Conrad is responsible for inpatient care. She handles transitions between ER and hospital admissions, ongoing care in the hospital, and discharge and so is well positioned to know much of what is going on in the hospital, especially on account of her leadership role in the hospital community.

On the recent episode of *The Highwire,* the viewer first witnesses a video featuring Conrad providing an account of her personal experience as a healthcare worker during the Covid crisis. As her monologue is worth reading (or even better, listening to), I give the transcript here, more or less in full:[309]

> I have been pro-vaccine. My kids are vaccinated. We rolled them [the Covid-19 vaccines] out to...essential workers at first. There were many that were excited. I understand we were all looking for a way out.
>
> After rolling them out to the general public, the elderly, the nursing homes in the area, we would get elderly in with Covid. It was weird. A week after they would get their first dose, they would test positive for Covid. And then we started seeing patients, coming in, you know, [saying,] "I got my vaccination," and a week later, they're in for pneumonia.

I can say for sure, in 2021, this is the year of pneumonia. I've never seen people with so many pneumonias. Even in the middle of summer. All summer, that's what we would get in the hospital, pneumonia, pneumonia, pneumonia.

After the vaccine rollout, I definitely noticed an uptick in heart attacks, strokes, blood clots, gastrointestinal bleeds, gastrointestinal complaints, appendicitis. We even saw pancreatitis, recurrent cancers. It was noticeably increased. It wasn't just me noticing it. Everybody seemed to notice it. It became clear to me that there was something wrong.

I knew nothing of VAERS. I didn't know about our responsibility to report. It was never even talked about when these vaccines were rolled out. I mean, you would hear it in the news, here and there, but there was never this push to make sure providers were made aware, that if you are getting patients in the hospital with these issues...you got to go this website, and start reporting, and start paying attention. That was never educated to us, at all.

I went on the website...and the first thing I noticed was that it said, "Healthcare providers are required by law to report certain adverse reactions to VAERS." I said, "What do you mean? What law?" Then I looked further, and it had a whole section on exactly what you are supposed to report: specific things you are supposed to report to VAERS after the Covid vaccine rollout. (Here the relevant text is displayed:)

MANDATORY REQUIREMENTS FOR PFIZER-BIONTECH COVID-19 VACCINE ADMINISTRATION UNDER EMERGENCY USE AUTHORIZATION

4. The vaccination provider is responsible for mandatory reporting of the following to the Vaccine Adverse Event Reporting System (VAERS):

- vaccine administration errors whether or not associated with an adverse event
- serious adverse events (irrespective of attribution to vaccination),
- cases of Multisystem Inflammatory Syndrome (MIS) in adults and children
- cases of COVID-19 that result in hospitalization or death.

(The monologue continues:)

So that's when I started reporting patients on my own. Well, very quickly, that became a full-time job, in and of itself. I would say, within three weeks to a month I had already had 50 patients reported. And that was just of the providers that were willing to tell me about patients; [the ones that] recognized that there may be a problem.

So I went back to my administration, and said: "I need help. I can't do this all myself. It's overwhelming. I'm on the phone with the CDC all the time. I'm on the phone with these patients. I need more people to know about it, so that they can help me, and we can do the right thing."

But that was met then with resistance. Because that's when the vaccines were really starting to get pushed. Everybody's got to get vaccinated. This is how it is going to go. By me admitting that we need a report because there may be some issues, it would create vaccine hesitancy among the healthcare workers, among the other staff, among the patients.

Well, that's when things changed. Because I wouldn't be quiet about it. What I did was, I put envelopes in our emergency room, and told many of our providers: "Hey, if you got a patient who comes in, and they just got their vaccine, or you think something might be related in any way, go ahead and put their demographics in the envelope, and then I'll take care of it, call the patient, and get the report done." [I was] thinking it was only going to be a few reports a week.

No. Like I said, it turned into *a full-time job,* very quickly.

When you roll out an Emergency Use product that you are going to mass release on the population, wouldn't you assure that you have safety mechanisms in place? The first thing you would do is to assure that people were educated about side effects, what to report, who to report to, *before* you did that? That should have been the first thing. Educate your healthcare providers who are going to see these people in the hospital.

Well, then, how come we didn't get educated as healthcare providers?

I was told we were supposed to educate ourselves. That it's not their responsibility.[310]

At this juncture, Deb Conrad then called her hospital's president to ask why side effects were not being reported. She recorded part of the conversation:

Deb Conrad (DC): Why are we not wanting to report this?

Hospital President (HP): I don't know that it's a matter of not wanting to report it. I think the position the system is taking is that each provider has the responsibility to report on their own patient.

DC: But if the providers aren't provided education on what we're supposed to be reporting, and the importance of such, how do they know to do it?

HP: But I believe the providers should educate themselves when they're dealing with patients related to Covid vaccinations.

DC: They don't even realize that these are specifically the conditions that we're supposed to be reporting to VAERS. So when we had a ton of them, I mean, we get thrombocytopenia, blood clots. Just Tuesday, I think it was, we shipped out, I think, three cardiomyopathies; a blood clot. We got a guy on the floor and, well, he just died. I just pronounced him a second ago. [He] got his shot and literally two weeks later, the guy ends up with cancer blown out of nowhere. A portal vein…[We] get strokes. I had a lady that had a stroke within 48 hours of her vaccine. Fully on anti-coagulation. I had a lady have a bilateral T and she was on Eliquis after her vaccination. I know these are things that are reportable.[311]

Conrad continues to tell us that the hospital administration then spoke to its risk management team respecting her actions. The consequence? *She was no longer allowed to report on any patients other than those whom she personally attended.* She received a warning to that effect and an admonishment that she needed to support the vaccine effort. Here is the corresponding email:

Hi Deb:

Just a quick email to follow up after our call today regarding VAERS reporting. Thank you again for taking time to speak to us during your day off. First, I want to acknowledge you have our full support in reporting to VAERS as indicated. Per our discussion, moving forward you will only report adverse events you encounter on your patients. If another provider sends you patient information and requests you file a report you will advise them they need to complete the report with VAERS themselves. If you have concerns another provider is not completing a VAERS report when it is indicated you will either complete a Safe Connect and/or bring that concern to *(name redacted)* or myself.

Additionally, in your clinical role and as a leader in the organization you will support *(redaction)* approach to the vaccine which is following CDC and DOH guidance.

As mentioned, I will be meeting with…command leaders specifically to discuss the *(redaction)* approach to VAERS reporting. Currently, VAERS reporting is the responsibility of the provider caring for the patient. If any changes are made in this approach you and our medical staff will be informed.

Thank you for your ongoing efforts to ensure our patients get the highest quality care and ensuring we are doing our best to keep them safe.

Have a great weekend![312]

Conrad continued:

You know, during the pandemic, I received an excellence award for my patient care, and just how dedicated I was.

> Certificate of Recogntion
>
> 2021 Physician Excellence Nominee
>
> Deborah Conrad, PA
>
> In recogntion of your **passion** for your work and your intention to **improve quality** and facilitate **teamwork** while delivering **excellent, compassionate care.**
>
> Chief Medical Officer 3/30/2021

> Now I'm being looked at as this dangerous individual who is putting patients in harm's way.[313]

Deb Conrad then closed with these words:

> These patients deserve to be heard. These [vaccine]-injured, or…I have to say, potentially [vaccine]-injured, because we don't know, right? But they deserve to have a voice. They are being shunned, too. They are being told they're crazy, that they have anxiety, that it's not real. They don't have anybody fighting for them.
>
> There are injured patients out there. There are people whose lives are completely destroyed as a result of these vaccines. There are people who are now in the ground because of these vaccines. I have no doubt about it. I'm speaking out, because I want to be their voice. I hope others come forward, too. Because I know I am not alone. I know I am not alone.[314]

This monologue presents a highly condensed version of a long short story, many of the details of which Conrad fleshes out in live interview with Del Bigtree (host of *The Highwire*) after the playing of the videotape transcribed above. The structure and chronology of that story (the title of which I borrowed from *The Highwire*) can be broken down into four chief parts:

Deb Conrad and the VAERS Scandal

I: *Deliberate Ignorance: Unpreparedness and Early Warning Signals*
II: *Digging In: Deb Conrad, VAERS Reporter*
III: *Turning Point: The System Pushes Back*
IV: *Denouement*

Let's unfold Deb Conrad's story more fully, filling out each of its relevant chapters with material from her dialogue with Bigtree.

I: Deliberate Ignorance: Unpreparedness and Early Warning Signals

As noted in her monologue, at the outset of the pandemic, Deb Conrad, fifteen-year veteran physician assistant, was entirely unaware of VAERS. Del Bigtree found this a bit shocking and inquired how that might be, and if it were more or less the norm. Deb Conrad affirmed that in her experience, at least, indeed it was, in part because doctors and nurses caring primarily for adults (as opposed to pediatric personnel) did not routinely deal with vaccine-induced reactions.

She did emphasize, however, that this seemed to her *all the more reason* why, *before* the rollout of the vaccine, healthcare professionals should certainly have been educated not just about the *existence* of VAERS but about their *obligation* to report adverse events to the system—and *how* to do so as well. The total lack of any such information campaign seemed, in view of the relatively untested character of an EUA-authorized vaccine and the massive character of the rollout, nothing less than a travesty—official irresponsibility that willfully refused to do what was obviously necessary to put any sort of safety guardrails in place before racing the vaccine down the steeply curving public-health highway. Conrad noted:

> I was not aware of VAERS. When the vaccine was rolled out, that was not something we received education on. You would think we would have. I mean, you are rolling out at an EUA [Emergency Use Authorization] product with no long-term safety data, and very limited short-term safety data; you're rolling that out on the mass population, and people who had prior Covid, wouldn't you want to make sure that people were aware of what to do if you get a patient in the hospital or the clinic, in the ER, with some complaint after the vaccine? Wouldn't you put a system in place, or some sort of email to educate your providers: "This is what you need to do"?[315]

This issue of education does not even address the problem of the functionality of the system itself. Conrad emphasized many times on just how involved the process of reporting to VAERS is, even if one does know the ropes. On the one hand, the rigor does serve important ends, assuring that any VAERS-verified report represents a bona fide incident. When Bigtree asked Conrad about the rumor that VAERS numbers may be unreliably inflated because it's easy for anyone to file a report, she responded:

> No, it is a full-time job. Reporting to VAERS is a very involved process. I give kudos to VAERS...They really do try to get the information. Because

> of that, it is a very involved process.... Anybody can report to VAERS, but I believe very few patients actually report themselves, because they require so much data that a patient wouldn't know. They ask questions about bloodwork, your individual story, dates of the vaccine, lot number of the vaccines.... Most patients would go to their provider to ask them to report.[316]

On the other hand, the laboriousness of the process makes it largely impractical for the great majority of healthcare providers—including those well aware of the system—to initiate and complete the process of filing VAERS reports in the course of a busy schedule. The reporting system, moreover, is made even more onerous by unnecessary technical difficulties. Conrad noted that if you are in the midst of filing a report and, as often happens, are called away to attend to a patient, the system will not preserve the file and requires you to start all over. Even more exasperating, she reported, is the experience of finishing a report, clicking the "submit" tab, and receiving the following message: "Submission (or 'Authentication') Failed." In this case, the entire report is lost and must be redone.

Deb Conrad, however, refused to be defeated, in good measure, because soon after the vaccine rollout she did begin seeing warning signals: disturbing and even alarming signs of possible (or probable) vaccine-induced harm. Conrad stated:

> About in February [of 2021], I started noticing an influx of patients coming in with weird conditions. At first I thought, *this is just coincidence*. Just like everybody else, *this is just coincidence*. But it was odd enough that I kind of started to take notice. But then there was a specific patient that really kind of hit home for me, and I said, "No, this isn't a coincidence. There's something very wrong here." That's when I started to kind of look into things a little bit further, and started really to get concerned.
>
> This particular patient had been vaccinated just less than 48 hours prior, and he died...of a multisystem inflammatory syndrome. He had acute kidney injury, and bilateral pneumonia, and a heart attack, and sepsis, and died. It was really quite shocking. So shocking that the providers taking care of him notified me of his case. I had nothing to do with this patient's case personally, but the providers themselves were very concerned about it and so they came to me, and said this case needs to be looked at, needs to be reported. At that point, I had already started doing some reporting.[317]

As the days rolled on, Conrad became more and more convinced of just how important it was to be assiduous in reporting potential vaccine adverse effects to VAERS. Remember, though, that it is not the care provider's responsibility to determine whether or not an adverse event is in fact vaccine induced; that determination is made later by government health officials (which, as Dr. McCullough and others note, constitutes another corruption-prone moment in the whole system). As long as a given adverse event transpires within a certain period of time after vaccination, healthcare providers are technically, and legally, obliged to report it.

On account of all the aforementioned obstacles, however, as a rule, they don't—unless, like Deb Conrad, they are unusually dedicated, competent, and conscientious individuals.

In her incipient role as a VAERS reporter, however, Deb Conrad quickly discovered just how time consuming the job of reporting to VAERS really was. Believing that everyone, including her administrative superiors, would be intent on doing the right thing, Conrad initially approached hospital management to recruit assistance for the task she now recognized as imperative, even though most of her colleagues appeared entirely ignorant of the legal obligation to report. In her own words, she stated:

> I actually went to my leadership, and said, "Is anyone aware of this? We need to start doing this." And of course because it is such an involved process, nobody really wants to do it. We don't have the time… There's no time in your day to do it. They came back to me and said, "You know Deb, if you want to take this on, that's okay: go ahead."[318]

That's real managerial responsibility for you, isn't it? At least they didn't tell her *not* to try to make up, on her own, on her days off, what should have been the whole hospital's concerted effort to supply reliable safety data to experientially verify the as-yet unproven *assumption* that, when rolled out to an entire population (whole demographics of which had not been participants in any clinical trial) the Covid vaccines were *not* doing more harm than good. No, hospital management didn't go that far. Not yet.

II: Digging In: Deb Conrad, VAERS Reporter

As management initially more or less encouraged her to do what she could (on her own time, of course), Deb Conrad reached out to her colleagues to assist her in the task of making sure notable adverse events were reported, as both the law and good conscience required. Here is a memo she wrote to two colleagues at the time:[319]

From: Deb Conrad
Sent: Friday, March 12, 2021, 10:45 AM
To: ____________
Subject: Question on reporting vaccine reactions.

Hi to you both. In the last month or so we have been admitting a fairly large amount of patients who are having adverse side effects after getting their covid 19 vaccines. These are happening either the day of or the day after and sometimes 4–5 days after with pts reporting that they were sick all week but didn't know to come in. *None of these case have been reported to VAERS I checked with the ER and the pts they are seeing in the ER for the same and they are not reporting these either.* With an EUA where these vaccines are not fully licensed or approved full transparency [is needed] and all vaccine reactions are [should be] reported to VAERS. We have no protocol or guidance on how to do this for hospital systems. My sister who works in an ICU in Buffalo is seeing these same reactions and they are not being reported to VAERS as they are not told they have to and have no protocol either. Some of these have been quite serious—one with a brain bleed and one who died from multifocal pneumonia 2 days after her second dose. In the last month I have known of or taken care of 10–15 pts with issues related to the vaccines. I have called VAERS and emailed them with no response on how to proceed and make the process easier for hospital systems. Studies have shown that 90% of vaccine reactions go unreported. Give again that these vaccines are under EUA full transparency is imperative. *I am willing to take this project on myself and be the person whom providers from the ER and the hospital report cases to so I can get them reported to VAERS.* My very healthy best friend just suffered a severe autoimmune reaction after receiving the Johnson and Johnson vaccine so I have some interest in this project. As you all know *I am very passionate about always doing the right thing and putting patient care first* which is why I am so passionate about this project. *These are happening way too frequently for them to just be considered "coincidences."*

Thank you, I am interested in starting this right away as I have been keeping a log of some of the instances I know of.

Deb

In order to implement this initiative, Deb Conrad placed envelopes in the ER and fast-track system in the hospital so that doctors and nurses who encountered cases of potential vaccine injury could readily convey relevant preliminary information to her.

Some of her colleagues were sympathetic to her independent initiative; others were not. As Deb Conrad observed:

> Not all of my colleagues agreed with me because they didn't even really want to believe that these vaccines could even potentially cause any problems, plus we didn't even know what problems we were supposed to be looking for. So I had a lot of my colleagues not really give me any reports. But a lot that did.... [Well, that] volunteer position turned into a full-time job. My entire week off, that's all I was doing."[320]

When Bigtree further inquired if any of Conrad's colleagues warned her that her independent initiative might be frowned upon by her higher-ups, she responded:

> I never thought in a million years that anybody would be against this idea. Because, again, I have this belief that we are all healthcare workers, and we have a common goal of doing the right thing, and keeping our patients safe. That's what's drilled into us. So I never in a million years thought it would be looked at in any negative light.[321]

She added that some of her colleagues did say, "You're being too emotional about this. Deb, you always care too much; you're looking too much into this. Why are you wasting your time?" To this she replied: "Because it's the right thing to do."

In the interview, Bigtree then asked Deb Conrad for more specifics on the kind of ailments she was seeing in the hospital. He mentions that several oncologists he knew had told him about a disturbing trend among their patients. Oncologists know which of their patients are in remission, and they often have a sense of how long the remission is likely to endure. In recent months, however, he noted that these oncologists reported multiple cases of cancers returning suddenly and unexpectedly—in fact, more or less overnight. Eventually suspecting that the phenomena could be vaccine related, they began inquiring whether a given patient had recently been vaccinated, and, if so, when.

Bigtree then alludes to Deb Conrad's prior mention of an increase of cancer in her hospital. He inquires if the rise in cases was bad enough to represent a noticeable phenomenon—one that could conceivably be related to the concurrent vaccination rollout. Her answer:

> Very much so. One of the early patients I reported on was somebody whose cancer came back from remission, and rapidly killed the individual. It was kind of crazy. I don't know, the cancer's in remission; you're going about your life; then all of a sudden: *wham*, and its back. And it's back with a vengeance, to the point where you can't get the patient on treatment quick enough. And that's happened quite a few times. It's very noticeable.

> And not just myself. Even our oncology colleagues.... I actually called one of our oncologists about this particular patient and he agreed, "Wow, this could really be possibly related." This was very early in the VAERS reporting, and very early in this recognition. *Since that time, that's unfortunately a very common thing we see.*
>
> We are also seeing new cancers come out of nowhere. Very weird things.... Solid organ tumors that we can't get biopsied before they kill the patient. They just progress so rapidly, you can't even get these patients a biopsy to find out what kind of cancer it was. So the families are left with either a biopsy, to determine what kind of cancer it was, or unknown [cause of death].[322]

Bigtree proceeds to ask about another syndrome linked to the vaccines:

> What about thrombocytopenia? This is something we've heard a lot about with AstraZeneca, first in Europe, and then Johnson & Johnson here.... We're seeing that Pfizer, Moderna seem to have the same problem. Blood clots, thrombocytopenia, Have you seen any of that?[323]

And Deb Conrad replies:

> Very much so. Very much so. Heart attacks, cardiomyopathies, thrombocytopenias, strokes, are big ones; blood clots. Interestingly enough, 2021 is the year that our blood thinners no longer work. It's amazing. We've had quite a few patients that have developed pulmonary emboli as well as blood clots in the legs on full anti-coagulation. Full blood thinners. And we just look at ourselves. I actually had a colleague tell me the other day, "Well, you know, drugs aren't 100%." It's interesting. In 2021, *a lot* of our drugs don't seem to be 100% anymore.
>
> And we're seeing some Bell's palsy. I did report a couple of cases of Bell's palsy. A lot of odd neurologic complaints. Seizures, people with these weird tremors. They can't control their body. I had a patient recently with that complaint. A lot of falls. GI complaints; gastrointestinal complaints; brain bleeds.
>
> One of things we saw early on was elderly people passing out after the vaccine. They would get their second dose. Then go home. They were feeling fine. Then the family would find them on the floor the next day, passed out [having hit their head]. To the point where I said: "Maybe we should be telling people at these vaccine centers: if you are taking in an elderly patient, stay with them that night because you might find them on the floor the next day." We were seeing a lot of that.
>
> Pneumonias. A lot of pneumonias. Sepsis...[324]

As Deb Conrad's level of concern mounted, she reached out to federal and state health authorities for assistance in her effort to make sure that vaccine adverse events were in fact being reported as technically required by law. Here is the transcript of a phone conversation between Deb Conrad (DC) and a representative of the New York State Department of Health (NY):

> DC: We talk about New York State numbers and that the vaccine is safe and effective. How do we know that? Because if no cases are being reported to you guys of fully vaccinated patients who are coming in with Covid, then how can we make that claim? Because I can tell you, we just lost a guy the other day to COVID pneumonia. He died, and he was fully vaccinated in March, and came in with severe COVID pneumonia and died in our ICU. So I mean, that wasn't reported to you guys. So how can you claim as a state that they're safe and effective when hospitals are seeing this, and you guys aren't made aware because there's no mandate to be made aware?
>
> NY: Right. That's not a state claim, though. It's federal...but that's why it is important. We do want people, we do want all of the providers to be able to report this, even if it's not mandated...because that's the only way that, like you said, this would be able to be found out.
>
> DC: There is no education. The only education we're receiving is how we're supposed to be pushing the vaccine. But there's no education about what to do when a patient has a problem.
>
> NY: Deb, I feel you, and I really do appreciate your work, and I hope you continue doing it.... Because even though it's not something I can say at this moment, that I know for sure that it's mandated...unless they're an actual vaccination provider that was giving out vaccine; achh.... The enforcement is not there.[325]

It must be cold comfort to New York healthcare workers, such as Deb herself, to know that it is not the State of New York that is claiming that the vaccines are safe and effective but only the federal government. This must be all the more disturbing, given that the same state that cannot (as the unnamed official regretfully confesses) muster the will and energy to effectively enforce reporting requirements so as actually to confirm (rather than assume) vaccine safety, nonetheless feels perfectly entitled to require its healthcare personnel to submit to a vaccine that its own officials cannot possibly know to be safe.

When Del Bigtree inquired what Deb Conrad had expected, and how she felt after this conversation, she responded:

> I was frankly just floored. I couldn't understand why.... Again, if you are going to release an Emergency Use product [for which] we don't have any really long-term, short-term safety data, on an entire population of people that were not represented in the clinical trials, why wouldn't you assure that that safety reporting was done? That the people who would be potentially seeing injuries would be educated? Hey, we're rolling out these vaccines....These are some of the conditions we might see. Make sure this is what you do. This is what you do: you report to VAERS.... Wouldn't you want that?
>
> It was mind-boggling to me. It's funny, I tell one of my colleagues all the time, whenever I see her, I think I'm going crazy. Why doesn't anybody else see this? Is it so difficult? It just seems like it's the right thing to do. We are healthcare providers. Our first duty is to *do no harm*, and to assure safety for our patients in our communities. That's what we do.[326]

That said, this New York State official had at least listened to Deb Conrad, and had offered a sympathetic, if singularly unhelpful, response. Meanwhile, Conrad continued:

> I knew what was happening was wrong, and needed to be heard, and told. Because my duty is always to my patient, and doing the right thing. So I wrote a couple of emails to the FDA, alerting them to what was going on, you know, thinking they were going to get back to me, and we would have some solution to this problem.[327]

Is it naive to believe that federal health authorities—not to mention the pharmaceutical companies themselves!—are genuinely and proactively interested in taking effective measures to guarantee public health and safety? Is it naive to think that they are committed to taking all necessary steps, including a functional VAERS, to make sure they are not approving and championing dangerous products?

Evidently it is.

Anyone, moreover, who acknowledges this and nonetheless supports any mass vaccination program, and most especially, vaccine mandates, can hardly be considered to be thinking rationally. The FDA and other responsible administrative agencies do not actually have to take practical steps to ensure a *functional* system for the reporting of vaccine adverse events in order to *know* vaccines are safe and effective: No, all they need do is flourish a needle in the air, wave their magic wand, and—as the eyes of the fear-stricken population glaze over—repeat *"Safe and Effective... Safe and Effective...Safe and Effective..."* and then stand by and watch in satisfaction as their hypnotized subjects man the media channels, halls of congress, and city streets, parroting, as programmed, "*Safe and Effective… Safe and Effective…*" while the toll of vaccine injuries and deaths inexorably, yet more or less invisibly, mounts.

The FDA's response to Conrad's inquiries? Silence. Deafening silence.

Increasingly exasperated (or "disgusted," to quote Conrad), she penned (or typed) the following at the end of April, 2021:[328]

> To: paul.richards@fda.hhs.gov
> Sent: Friday, April 30, 2021 10:33:43 PM EDT
> Subject: concern surrounding transparency of injuries potentially due to covid 19 vaccination
>
> To whom it may concern:
>
> I am writing with great concern about the lack of full transparency surrounding adverse reactions possibly related to covid-19 vaccines. Since my last email I have experienced great frustration with the VAERS reporting system and the reporting system set up with moderna, pfizer and johnson and johnson. They have made it impossible to report the many patients coming into my hospital with possible serious side effects and deaths following their vaccines. Considering these vaccines are under emergency use and are not fully approved I cannot understand why a better reporting system was not enacted to make the process more simple.
>
> Moderna, Pfizer and j and j told me that they have nothing to do with VAERS and want me to submit individual reports on their website for each patient. I have reported over 50 patients in the last 4 weeks who were admitted to my hospital and 6 deaths and it is impossible to go back on these reports to now submit separate forms to the vaccine manufacturers. I do not get paid to report and am the only medical provider reporting in my entire hospital as no one wants to take responsibility, has no guidance on what to report or do not have the time to do it. I have spent countless hours on behalf of these patients on my days off already and I now have over 50 emails from VAERS wanting updated information. This is an impossible task.
>
> *I am disgusted with what I consider to be a purposeful lack of transparency to the American people. I am sick of hearing my colleagues tell me that the strokes, heart attacks, new arrythmia, covid-19 infection, pneumonias, blood clots, bleeds, seizures and deaths are just coincidences. It is not our job to determine a cause and effect, it is the job of the FDA to protect the American people from potentially harmful products. How can the FDA do their job if there is no transparency?*
>
> These patients have been injured and they want answers of which I have none. I have seen no movement from the CDC, VAERS, the FDA or

the vaccine manufacturers to help hospital systems report and deal with the massive influx of potentially injured people as a result of taking these unapproved products. *All I see is massive campaigns to continue to push people to get vaccinated with no accountability or compensation when someone is injured.*

Thank you for your time,
Anonymous medical professional

III: Turning Point: The System Pushes Back

Inevitably, the conflict between Deb Conrad, the people's hero, and the establishment that employs her finally came to blows—not physical ones, to be sure, but blows nonetheless. The turning point came when Deb took independent initiative to make sure that an insufficiently detailed official communiqué pertaining to a possible vaccine side effect—thrombocytopenia—would not lead medical staff to act in manner that might result in needless injury or death. For if that condition does manifest, certain measures normally employed to deal with blood clotting in *non*-vaccine related instances might be dangerously inappropriate if the event were in fact vaccine induced. In the latter case, usual blood-thinning agents can be counter-indicated because of already low platelet count associated with vaccine reaction.

The official communication did not spell the relevant information out clearly enough. Deb Conrad had independently researched literature on vaccine-induced thrombocytopenia and accordingly sent an email to healthcare staff clarifying exactly what should and shouldn't be done if the condition seen was suspected to be, in fact, vaccine induced.

It was the kind of clarificatory health-treatment protocol that Deb Conrad had, in her leadership position, disseminated before. One might imagine that the hospital administration would have been grateful for this important—indeed potentially life-saving—elucidation. On other occasions, they probably would have been. This time, however, was different.

Why? Because Deb Conrad was now encouraging colleagues to keep a sharp eye out for what was, or could be, vaccine-induced injury. She had, to be sure, addressed kindred concerns before, but never quite so tangibly or directly. Whatever the specifics of the internal dynamic were (the effects of Deb's personal campaign were no doubt cumulative), this action figured as the straw that broke the camel's back. It could, after all, contribute materially to vaccine hesitancy among staff and, eventually, patients.

Del Bigtree put the matter succinctly enough: "You're discussing something that happens from vaccine injury. You're talking to the entire staff about it. So they are looking out for it. The people above you were not very happy about that."

No, they were not. Deb Conrad got called to the hospital equivalent of a principal's office that same day. The following is the transcript of the conversation between Deb Conrad (DC), the hospital chief medical officer (CMO), and the hospital director (HD):

> CMO: I know you sent out an email to staff this morning, and I wanted to make sure we had an opportunity to talk about this sooner versus later.... Listen, Deb, I absolutely understand your concerns about the vaccine, and I absolutely believe that your heart is in the right place with, you know, with wanting to make sure we are doing our due diligence and reporting the adverse events. That said, the email that went out this morning really needed to be discussed, but I think that we really need to make sure that we're providing a consistent message to our team, and we need to make sure that's also in alignment with what our health system is asking us to do. There's a risk to the organization from a perspective of both under-reporting and over-reporting. So how do we make sure that we're sending the right message out to our providers and that they have the information that they need to be doing this correctly, because I share your belief that it's important that we get these reports in. But I think we have to be thinking a little bit more about the process and *what's sort of expected here*.
>
> From what our risk team is telling us is that really you can only be reporting on the patients that you are providing direct care for, and so you cannot, and I know you've been volunteering and trying to be helpful, but we need you to kind of dial it back and focus on the patients that you are directly responsible for. And then if folks do reach out to you because you've been saying, hey, reach out to me, they need to be directed to VAERS, and they need to do the process themselves. For the patients that they think need a report. Okay?
>
> DC: I have been telling them to do it. And they don't do it. The reason I took this on is because nobody else wants this respons[ibility]. I mean, it's brutal. Because you then will be getting phone calls from the CDC every single day as a result. I mean, the FDA really is the problem here because they did not advise hospital systems what we're supposed to be doing.

CMO: The approach has been that this is the responsibility of the individual provider who believes that they have identified a potential adverse event. I know this is frustrating but you can't control whether or not someone else is going to put the report in. You can control what you do for your patients, and then I think if you're concerned that folks are not reporting on their patients, you're welcome to put in a safe connect. You're welcome to talk to Peter, myself and we can kind of address those with providers.

DC: But like I said, I brought this stuff up back in February, and I see no, no response. I mean that's my frustration.... We are not doing these patients a service. And again, the FDA, they did not tell us, and they still will not tell me what conditions are we supposed to be reporting. They are vague. They don't know because they never got the clinical trials. They never did them. *We are the clinical trials. That's basic.*

CMO: I don't want us to go down any kind of rabbit hole here, but I think the thing we have to be clear about.... I'm just going to be frank with you because that's the only way I know how to be, Deb. But I will tell you in reading the few emails that you sent me and then reading the email that went out to the provider, it does come across a bit, very—not very, but it comes out quite, almost, anti-vaccine. Right. And clearly as an organization, as a health system, right? And as an organization that's working on following CDC guidelines, and following the guidance of the Department of Health, we are very much advocating for patients to receive the vaccine, and we're very much working on.... There's tons of efforts out there to try to reduce vaccine hesitancy.

I have some concerns that the tone that you have with this a little bit is certainly being felt on the floor. Right? And being felt by your colleagues. We need to be a little bit careful about that. Right? I support your mission and goal of wanting to make sure that we are following the law and that we are reporting adverse events. But I also want to make sure that as a leader in the organization and as a provider within the organization, that you understand, we want people to get the vaccine. Right? *We want people to understand that on the whole, this is a very safe vaccine.* Right? And that the science supports that.

DC: I appreciate that. I do. But I can't understand why as a whole.... In the world, people are acting like everything is grand. It's not. It's clearly not.

CMO: I think we may have to agree to disagree on what's happening, you know, kind of globally with the vaccine. I do think that we're seeing... yes, just like other vaccines, there are folks who are going to be negatively impacted, but certainly on the whole, we've seen a tremendous benefit to the vaccine. You and I are not individual providers, we're employed providers. *We toe the company line. That's part of our responsibility...to be supporting the mission of the organization.*

DC: So even when we're getting COVID-19 patients who are positive and fully vaccinated in the hospital, we're going to leave it up to the individual provider to report? Because I'm telling you, they're not reporting. That should be reported every time. And it's not. I can tell you, I know of patients because I finally reported them because the provider didn't.

I have yet to see one double-blinded, randomized controlled clinical trial, that shows that these vaccines are going to be effective long-term after six months, whatever. We don't know that. *And if we're not reporting hospitalized patients who are coming in fully vaccinated with COVID, that's an atrocity. It's an absolute atrocity.*

HD: What we do see, though, and I know it's an FDA-approved thing, but we see people with Pneumovax come in with pneumonia all the time, and people with the flu shot come in with the flu all the time. Just because the vaccines, whether they're COVID or they're flu or Pneumovax, they're not perfect vaccines.

DC: I agree. We have no long-term studies right now. The CDC is saying that these vaccines are only effective for six months, but yet we're telling people take off your masks and run around if you're vaccinated. But at the same time, the CDC is saying, you're not. I mean, it's crazy. It's just crazy.

CMO: This is new to all of us. This is certainly a different thing than we've seen. Just to be clear again, I absolutely support your work and making sure that you're reporting these events. You *cannot* report for other folks and so just direct them to report on their own. You're a leader, and your voice carries a lot of weight with the team and it seems to be very widely known that you're extremely skeptical of this vaccine.

You have every right to your personal belief and your personal opinion, Deb. But we just need to be careful as providers and leaders, that we are also trying to be consistent with the mission and the message of the organization.

DC: From now on, if somebody comes up to me, I'm just going to tell them, look, you got to do your own research.

HD: Whenever you take a new medicine, even though obviously it's a vaccine, it's a risk-benefit decision, it's a little bit unknown, but, at the same time, the CDC and the Department of Health are recommending it for everybody. I think that many people know, yes, there's risk, but yes, there are benefits. Currently, *the national sort of people are pushing to have these things done.* You can look at your own research or things like that, but I just want to be careful that we don't discourage people in a time when we're really trying to get the population vaccinated and get the disease under control.

DC: I'm mad at our governing organization in this country because I do not feel that they prepared us providers with this rollout for what we are supposed to be doing. We have no guidance. We have no answers. And when I try to call the drug companies for answers, they give me the same song and dance about how everything's under experimental use, and we don't have any answers. We can't advise you. *I wouldn't buy a damn, you know, dryer from a company like that who won't stand behind their product. I mean, it's unbelievable.*[329]

A dryer. A damn dryer. Would you buy a dryer from a company that could not guarantee that it would actually dry your clothes rather than leave them thoroughly damp, no matter how many times you ran them through? Or, even worse, might burn, shred, or otherwise destroy them? A company, moreover, that—*if* such things happened—could not be held legally liable, and would take *zero* responsibility, but instead tell you that it worked really well for most people so they could hardly be faulted for your personal failure to share in and recognize the great public value of their vaunted machine?

I doubt it. Remember that next time you consider getting a Covid-19 shot. Or insisting someone else get one. Because it's not your clothes that are getting tossed around in that dryer, but you. Your body. Or your child's.

And: *(HD):* ***"The national sort of people."*** What sort of people are these? People like Anthony Fauci or Rochelle Walensky, putative "doctors" and agency heads who don't treat people but tell practicing physicians what they can or cannot do? People like Albert Bourla, CEO of Pfizer, who dabbles in deals that look suspiciously like insider trading, signs coercive contracts, and dreams of never-ending revenue streams from never-ending boosters? Jeff Zients, communication director of the White House Covid Response Team, who touts the administration's "relentless" effort to get shots in arms no matter what the cost? Senator Gary Peters, who imagines vaccines as agents of redemption but doesn't have the common sense or courtesy to listen to passionately committed world-renowned scientists and physicians speak about medicines that actually work?

Those "national sort of people," I'm afraid, aren't my sort of people. In fact, I am not sure they qualify as fit representatives of *We, the People* at all, because that *We,* as the philosopher Plotinus tells us, differs essentially from the merely collective *Ours* that tends toward exclusionary mobbishness. That *We,* wise Plotinus tells us, represents *the authentic human principle*—that inviolable core of true humanity, that immortal spirit in each and every one of us, and characteristic of *We, the People* as a whole—*when* that whole consists of a diversity of individuals living and acting in untarnished simplicity, principled integrity, heartfelt compassion, and freedom.

Like Deb Conrad.

A dryer. A damned dryer. Stick to your figurative guns, Deb, and others, untold others, will gain the courage to stand and deliver.

IV: Denouement

The conversation between Deb Conrad and her superiors makes the true story behind the "safe and effective" label transparently clear. Even though the product (the Covid-19 vaccine) is minimally tested (despite hollow assurances to the contrary) and experimental (under EUA authorization only), healthcare providers are essentially commanded, from on high, to act—*pretend*—that it has been conclusively proven to be safe and effective and to conduct business in a manner that bears out that assumption no matter what the actual evidence is or may be, even if the only way of sustaining that assumption entails precluding, by administrative fiat and disciplinary action, any nurse's, doctor's, or researcher's words or deeds that might effectively challenge or undermine that premise. This profoundly dishonest, not so much *un-* as *anti-*scientific posture, serves as the real basis of the claim that the vaccines are "safe and effective," which is thus in no wise rational or evidence based but the product of destructive political and medical voodoo.

Let's return to the as yet unfinished Deb Conrad saga. Reined in by her superiors, no longer permitted to perform service above and beyond the call of duty, Deb was compelled to restrict her efforts to her own patient base. Even so, by that time, she'd already completed well over a hundred reports and had quite a few more in process, many of which, unfortunately, would now never see the light of day. Asked by Del Bigtree if any of her colleagues moved to pick up the slack by following through and filing reports, Deb shook her head.

"No," she replied. "Because it's such an unbelievable task. They just can't."

Turning to a distinct yet closely related subject, Bigtree inquired about Deb Conrad's "frontline" perspective on the oft-heard contention that it is the unvaccinated that are filling up the hospitals, soliciting her personal estimate of the percentages of cases coming into the hospital (especially the ER and ICU) that involved vaccinated versus unvaccinated persons.

> That is something I've actually been tracking for a couple of months. Specifically in July [of 2021], I had a particular day when we had 35 patients on our in-patient hospital census, for our group. 30 of them were fully vaccinated. Of those, all seven patients in the ICU were fully vaccinated, and nine of those [35] patients were listed initially as unvaccinated. But I went back and talked to the patients, and they were actually vaccinated, so I updated the system.[330]

Bigtree naturally inquired how that discrepancy occurred. Conrad explained that patients are not asked their vaccination status upon entry to the hospital. If you received your vaccination somewhere in the hospital's wider healthcare system, your status would automatically be registered, but if you were vaccinated at a local pharmacy or any other out-of-network venue, that vaccination would not be electronically registered unless you asked for it to be so. If you did not, you would remain classified as unvaccinated.

Here, I, along with Del Bigtree, would like to express my astonishment that vaccination status was not requested upon admission to the hospital. One might believe this was a laudable respect for privacy, if we were speaking of any institution other than a hospital. As we are, however, speaking of such, it should be obvious that a lack of such knowledge can not only lead to disastrous health outcomes but also make data collection conducive to reasonable accurate vaccine safety and efficacy assessments nigh impossible. One could be sure that, without Deb Conrad's intervention, nine of the thirty-five patients on the dashboard that day—over twenty-five percent—would have been logged in the wrong column, yet another means of falsely (whether with or without deliberate intent) inflating the number of "unvaccinated" patients occupying the hospital.

Regardless, Deb Conrad's account contributes to turning the usual "pandemic of the unvaccinated" story on its head.

> So…I updated the system and found that 30 out of 35 patients [including all 7 of those in the ICU] were fully vaccinated. At that point, our county vaccination rate was about 45–46%. And yet, who is in the hospital sick?[331]

Although Deb Conrad does not explicitly state as much, her testimony implies that she did not regard this day, or these numbers, as anomalous but generally indicative of the more or less typical "state of the union." Doing a little simple math, the percentage of vaccinated individuals in the hospital that day was just over eighty-five percent—the precise reverse of the official narrative claiming the vast majority of the persons in hospitals were and are unvaccinated. Moreover, the percentage of vaccinated persons in the hospital was almost *twice* that of vaccinees in the general population, suggesting that, in this locale at least, not only did vaccination offer no protection from Covid, but (if one were to judge from this admittedly small sample) also dramatically *increased* one's likelihood of hospitalization.

Deb Conrad did bring this disturbing truth to the attention of her colleagues. Here is the response she received, and her own assessment of the merit thereof:

> I was told, well, a lot them are elderly, and things like that, and they are more likely to be vaccinated. There are a lot of things that could affect those numbers. But it's still odd, right? Every patient in the ICU that day was fully vaccinated. Where are our sick unvaccinated people?
>
> We do get them, don't get me wrong, but compared to our vaccinated patients.... They [the vaccinated] are in there, and they are sick. And I'm not saying just from Covid; I'm talking about all these other weird conditions. And many of these vaccinated people are actually on their third, fourth, fifth admissions after the vaccine.[332]

So much, once more, for the truth of the official Covid-19 narrative. But the denouement of Deb Conrad's own personal story? On this day, September 27, 2021 (you will understand the significance of that date shortly), I will let her (with an assist from Del Bigtree) finish that story in her own words.

> DB: There are nurses and doctors protesting, taking to the streets now, all across this nation, because of vaccine mandates in their hospitals....I have never met nurses and doctors that don't believe in vaccines, or don't...take the vaccine if they are told to get the vaccine. Now there's this crazy anomaly taking place. I can only assume that, for a group of people that sort of just normally believe in vaccination, to be walking away from their jobs—they've obviously seen some of the things that you've seen. They've seen something that's scaring them, and making them really nervous about the vaccine. So under these circumstances, in New York, I have got to believe the pressure is on. After what you have seen, are you going to get this vaccine?
>
> DC: Absolutely not. I'm terrified. I'm more afraid of this vaccine than I am of Covid.
>
> DB: How is that working out with your hospital?

DC: Well, my last day is going to be the 27th of September. I will be let go from my position.

DB: Just because you won't get the vaccine?

DC: Correct. I understand it is supposed to be a voluntary termination, but I am not volunteering to leave. I love my job. I want my job. My community needs me. But...I'm scared. I'm scared because of what I've seen.[333]

As it happens, I am transcribing these words, which conclude this section of Deb Conrad's story, on September 27, 2021, the last day, for the time being at least, of Deb Conrad's career as a healthcare professional. Despite, or because of, her manifest excellence, her story at this juncture hardly features a happy ending:

DB: When you think of your career....These are your friends, this is your community; the thought that these may be your last days getting to do your job, what do you reflect on, in your career, coming to this moment?

DC [broken voice]: It's very difficult because I am very well respected in my community. I haven't just been at the hospital. Before I had my kids, I always worked two and three jobs. I worked in urgent care. The community knows me. I love my community. I serve them well, and the fact that I'm not going to be able to do that, devastates me. [Softly] Just devastates me.

Because when I leave, who is going to be their voice? Who is going to be these people's voice? When they come in, because they are going to come in, with their vaccine injuries, after I'm gone. And who is going to be their voice? No one.

That is what devastates me. They deserve a voice. They deserve to be heard. Many of them can't work anymore. They are on disability; they're dead. They have children. They have lives. Many of them don't have disability insurance, and they got hospital bills mounting. They don't have a voice, because they are being told they are crazy. That is what devastates me the most. I'll give up my career, and many will. I have many on my side that are walking away from careers that they love, because they are so scared.[334]

And that's...the truth.

Chapter 26

A DIRTY, NOT-SO-LITTLE SECRET: AMERICA'S IMPENDING HEALTHCARE CRISIS

So this, Mr. President, is what your vaccine mandates are doing to Americans, to *We, the People*—the real, not "the national sort" of people in this country: driving many of the best and the brightest, the most competent, conscientious, committed, and compassionate, from their jobs, from the communities that they love and need, and the communities that love and need them. For what? Sophisticated snake oil, and an illusory *idée fixe* of what constitutes the public good.

This is a travesty, and bodes ill for the country. The phenomenon of experienced professionals leaving longstanding jobs is no joke. In the field of healthcare, it threatens an impending staffing crisis.

Now, allow me to share a "not so little"—and barely hidden—"secret."

As the numbers of those healthcare workers unjustly forced from their jobs mounts, the attrition itself constitutes a public health crisis, one that threatens to deprive patients of urgently needed care. On August 19, 2021, a young registered nurse posted a clip on TikTok that reads as follows:

> As a registered nurse, I'm going to let you in on a little secret. Do you know why there's not enough beds in the hospitals with the Delta variant? Because a lot of nurses aren't getting the vaccine, so therefore they are being released from their employment.
>
> There's something called ratios. One nurse to X amount of patients. There has to be a cap somewhere, even if they break those ratios. So hospitals, if they do not have enough staff to care for patients, will then turn patients away or say: "We don't have enough beds." Because "beds" are not just based on how many beds are actually in the facility, it's how many healthcare providers you have capable of taking care of those patients in those beds within the ratio.
>
> So in San Antonio, Texas, the hospitals aren't "overrun," they just don't have enough staff, because they are leaving, in masses, due to not wanting the vaccine.[335]

Recent news confirms that this nurse's words are no exaggeration. It is also worth nothing that this problem is not, by any stretch of imagination, limited to Texas, or indeed any given state, but represents a nationwide phenomenon that one commentator frankly termed a "breakdown" of healthcare in America.[336]

Already on August 26, 2021, two weeks before President Biden's speech expanding the reach of vaccine mandates, one could read this headline in Cleveland-area news: "[University Hospitals], Cleveland Clinic CEOs worry COVID-19 vaccine mandates could lead to staff reduction, endangering patient care." The article states:

> Healthcare workers who would rather quit or be fired than get the COVID vaccines are a concern for the Cleveland Clinic and University Hospitals, leaders of the two hospitals systems said.[337]

Then, on September 10, the day after President Biden's speech, one could read in the fierce healthcare news: "AHA [American Hospital Association] concerned federal vaccine mandate could exacerbate severe worker shortage." The article reads:

> An impending federal requirement for all healthcare staff to get the COVID-19 vaccine could exacerbate massive workforce shortage issues that are plaguing the hospital industry, a key industry group said.[338]

The CEO of the AHA stated: "As a practical matter, this policy may result in exacerbating the severe workforce shortage problems that currently exist."[339]

A few states imposed their own vaccine mandates well in advance of President Biden's September 9, 2021, address. The California Department of Health, for instance, announced a mandate for healthcare workers in the state on August 5, requiring first doses by a September 30 deadline. On August 29, three and a half weeks after the announcement, one could read this headline on the CalMatters website: "Nurse shortages in California reaching crisis point." The article states that Lois Richardson, attorney for the California Hospital association, affirmed the following: "Hospital administrations say the state's new vaccine requirement is compounding the shortage.... All of our hospitals are saying staffing is a big problem."[340]

Officials are awaiting the impending September 30, 2021, deadline with trepidation, fearing an exodus of healthcare workers at or near the deadline.

New York State, which announced mandates on August 16, 2021, which become effective September 27 (Deb Conrad's last day on the job), faces similar issues. On September 10, one could find this headline from KIRO 7 news: "NY hospital to pause baby deliveries after staffers quit over vaccine mandate." Evidently, six of the staffers at this hospital's maternity ward quit; seven remained unvaccinated at that time, as did over one-quarter (twenty-seven percent) of the whole hospital staff.[341]

What this hospital's staffing situation may be now, as I write this, a day after the mandate deadline, I do not know. I *do* know, however, that New York State intends to call out the National Guard to help alleviate healthcare worker shortages.

What *isn't* wrong with this picture? If you were sick and ailing on account of Covid, or anything else, in New York State, would you rather be taken care of by some fill-in from the National Guard with who knows what medical expertise, or by a fifteen-year-certified physician assistant, like Deb Conrad?

By edict, though, of those "national sorts of people," Deb Conrad and her ilk have been deemed *unfit to serve.*

She might be able to serve, though, if she wants to move to Nebraska. Nebraska's two largest hospitals jointly announced vaccine mandates on August 16, 2021. Evidently, though, the fiat did not play well with staff. Ten days later, on August 26, you could read these headlines in (of all places) *The New York Times:* "Nebraska is recruiting unvaccinated nurses to plug a staffing shortage."[342] It doesn't stop there, however. Evidently, the staffing issue is so acute that Nebraska hospitals are now not only offering $5,000 hiring bonuses but prominently advertising the *absence* of any Covid vaccine requirements. As per the language on one state hiring site, "No mandated COVID-19 vaccination" counts as "one of the many great benefits" offered by the position. "Join our team," the ad states, "and *continue* to serve your community as a nursing professional."[343]

The reference here is clearly to those *masses* of healthcare workers who, like Deb Conrad, are being denied that right.

On *The Highwire,* Del Bigtree puts in his two cents on the national picture:

> [President Biden] is literally passing a law that is clearing nurses and doctors by the thousands across this nation out of hospitals, leaving them unable to care for patients, and then when they get overrun, it will be the unvaccinated that did it.[344]

And who are these unvaccinated? Sick persons like those *5 out of 35* patients who were *unvaccinated* in Deb Conrad's hospital that day in July 2021, *none* of whom occupied a bed in the ICU?

Although healthcare workers clearly are on the frontline of this problem, the issue itself cuts across all walks of life, and nurses are naturally not the only ones being asked to choose between their professional livelihood and their own convictions about what is right, good, and in their own private interest as well the public interest. The list thereof includes teachers, firemen, soldiers, policemen, therapists, prison guards, athletes, artists performing in restricted venues, airline employees, and bus drivers. President Biden's edict (just one clause of his executive action) orders mandates by all employers supervising at least a hundred persons, and so the list goes on, and on, a Whitmanian catalogue of Americans of diverse kinds:[345]

> The pure contralto sings in the organ loft…
> The policeman travels his beat…
> The fare collector goes through the train…
> The conductor beats time for the band…

As Whitman's own lush inventory remains very nineteenth century, we could update it by adding on diverse contemporary professions:

> The nurse undoes the bandage, tenderly dresses the wound…
> The hoopster charges the rim, leaping high for the rebound…
> The guard by the exercise yard, taciturn, marks all who pass in or out…
> The pilot in the cockpit, calm at the controls…
> The trooper in the patrol car, eyes scanning the street…
> The counselor, listening carefully, concern lining her face…
> The fireman in action, battling the dragon of flame…

Whitman's "Song of Myself" is the iconic poem of American democratic inclusivity, the ground of which is and always must be not autocratic and coercive violations of individual autonomy but the sovereignty of the individual and their physical and spiritual freedom. Whitman knows very well that the boundaries of the Self of which he sings do not stop at the limits of my or your person. No sooner does he begin his "Song of Myself" by declaiming, "I Celebrate myself, and sing myself," than he adds, "And what I assume you shall assume, / For every atom belonging to me as good belongs to you."[346]

In singing the Self, Whitman is not celebrating any simple or limited egocentricity. On the contrary, he is giving expression to that central core of the human being that allies it, before and beyond any all differences, with that same essential humanity that indwells every person, that "common heart" (Emerson) that binds us all together in fellowship and in love, and which—grounded in freedom—can be neither commanded nor coerced.

The dynamics of democracy were established to guard against two cardinal evils: (1) the tyranny of a king or any kind of autocratic regime, and (2) the tyranny of the majority, that is, the oppression of a minority by prevailing opinions that nonetheless violate inalienable human rights. The preservation of democracy demands protection against *both* forms of oppression.

In considering vaccine mandates, we are in a sociopolitical arena that demands recollecting the foundational principles of democracy. I would contend that such mandates represent a type of tyranny that combines the two kinds of oppression just named. In this instance, moreover, a potent synergy of the two lends a dangerous appearance of legitimacy to measures that, if either one of the two kinds (autocratic governance or popular opinion) were lacking, would undoubtedly be much less powerful.

Yet what justifies me to speak of "oppression" in the first place? Why do vaccine requirements not merely represent forms of governance duly legitimized by the kind of popular mandate characteristic of governance "of, by, and for the people"?

The answer to that is relatively simple. From the first, a *veneer* of scientific truth supposedly established by "expert" opinion has justified illegitimate and indeed unconstitutional violation of the right to free speech. The systematic censorship of differing scientific views, even when such views are expressed by persons often far more highly credentialed and qualified than the official "experts," represents an unpardonable sin within the precincts of a supposedly democratic society.

In the absence of any fair press law, moreover, the censorship of scientific opinion extends into the sphere of media, both regular news outlets and social media. The suppression of speech exercised in most relevant domains of society infringes on the liberty not just of select scientists and doctors but of the whole universe of dissenting opinion. Without a modicum of freedom and fairness in the space of public discourse, no prevailing opinion that demands sacrifice on the part of a minority can claim democratic legitimacy, because the very train of thoughts, words, and deeds that likely engendered that prevailing opinion has proceeded along avenues that are singularly both unscientific and undemocratic.

If the path to your opinion is paved with the gravestones of democracy, you cannot claim your conclusion to represent good governance or your end to be a thriving Athenian grove. In the wake of Covid, what might Alexis de Tocqueville have to say about *Democracy in America*?

Chapter 27

JOINING THE RANKS

On September 15, 2021, I wrote another letter to President Cambray of Pacifica Graduate Institute. I kept it brief and addressed some updated points from my previous letter, including a few words on vaccine inefficacy, vaccine safety or lack thereof, mortality risk from Covid, thoughts on early treatment, and more—summaries of many of the points presented in this book.

A few weeks after I sent this letter, Pacifica Graduate Institute announced its policy for the reopening of its campus in the winter term of 2021. That policy, answerable to President Biden's edict, mandates vaccination for all persons who wish to set foot on Pacifica's campus. Additionally, all staff and students must register with an agency so that they can present electronic proof of vaccination upon entering and wear face masks at all times on campus.

As I am unwilling to comply with these strictures, I will no longer be teaching at Pacifica unless and until these restrictions are lifted.

As I reflect on this, I find myself recalling that James Hillman, a guiding spirit of Pacifica, a devotee of the *anima mundi* and a quintessentially American personality, taught that the soul lives, dwells, and speaks not only in the interior depths of the personal psyche (as per the classical Jungian teaching) but just as much in the *polis,* the space of social and political community. Today, the current of events has mercilessly stripped away the flimsy scrim separating the inner and outer, the personal and political spheres of existence—boundaries Hillman sought always to trespass and dissolve. He would undoubtedly hear with appreciation the words from Eleanor Roosevelt with which I shall close this chapter of our story, one recognizing and honoring the unit of force underlying democratic society: the rightful prerogative and power of you, and I—of We, the People:

> Where, after all, do universal human rights begin? In small places, close to home—so close and so small that they cannot be seen on any maps of the world. Yet they are the world of the individual person; the neighborhood he lives in; the school or college he attends; the factory, farm or office

where he works. Such are the places where every man, woman and child seeks equal justice, equal opportunity, equal dignity without discrimination. Unless these rights have meaning there, they have little meaning anywhere. Without concerted citizen action to uphold them close to home, we shall look in vain for progress in the larger world.[347]

PART IV

ENDGAMES

Chapter 28

MOUNTAINS OF POWER: FROM ROME TO SLAB CITY

The worldwide campaign for mass vaccination has been premised upon, and continues to stand propped up by, a widespread and indeed global subordination of science and medicine to politics: suppression of the intellectual freedom and impartiality requisite if science is to be science in fact as well as name, and—as Deb Conrad's story so vividly illustrates—the correlative compromising of the art and science of Medicine to the detriment—the *catastrophic* detriment—of public health and welfare.

Despite increasingly rigid governmental control of the healthcare system, innumerable doctors are in fact not only aware of these truths but morally appalled as well as practically stymied by them. Accordingly, as reported by *The Desert Review,* "an international alliance of physicians and medical scientists met in Rome, Italy, on September 12–14 [2021] for a three-day Global COVID Summit to speak truth to power about COVID pandemic research and treatment."[348] The summit featured a statement called "The Physicians' Declaration," which Dr. Robert Malone read out in Rome, and the text of which I give here[349]:

The Physician's Declaration

We the physicians of the world, united and loyal to the Hippocratic Oath, recognizing the profession of medicine as we know it is at a crossroad, are compelled to declare the following:

WHEREAS, it is our utmost responsibility and duty to uphold and restore the dignity, integrity, art and science of medicine;

WHEREAS, there is an unprecedented assault on our ability to care for our patients;

WHEREAS, public policy makers have chosen to force a "one size fits all" treatment strategy, resulting in needless illness and death, rather than upholding fundamental concepts of the individualized, personalized approach to patient care which is proven to be safe and more effective;

WHEREAS, physicians and other healthcare providers working on the front lines, utilizing their knowledge of epidemiology, pathophysiology and pharmacology, are often first to identify new, potentially life-saving treatments;

WHEREAS, physicians are increasingly being discouraged from engaging in open professional discourse, and the exchange of ideas about new and emerging diseases, not only endangering the essence of the medical profession, but more important, more tragically, the lives of our patients;

WHEREAS, thousands of physicians are being prevented from providing treatment to their patients, as a result of barriers put up by pharmacies, hospitals, and public health agencies, rendering the vast majority of healthcare providers helpless to protect their patients in the face of disease. Physicians are now advising their patients to simply go home (allowing the virus to replicate) and return when their disease worsens, resulting in hundreds of thousands of unnecessary patient deaths, due to failure-to-treat;

WHEREAS, this is not medicine. This is not care. These policies may actually constitute crimes against humanity.

NOW THEREFORE, IT IS:

RESOLVED, that the physician-patient relationship must be restored. The very heart of medicine is this relationship, which allows physicians to best understand their patients and their illnesses, to formulate treatments that give the best chance for success, while the patient is an active participant in their care.

RESOLVED, that the political intrusion into the practice of medicine and the physician/patient relationship must end. Physicians, and all healthcare providers, must be free to practice the art and science of medicine without fear of retribution, censorship, slander, or disciplinary action, including possible loss of licensure and hospital privileges, loss of insurance contracts and interference from government entities and organizations—which further prevent us from caring for patients in need. More than ever, the right and ability to exchange objective scientific findings, which further our understanding of disease, must be protected.

RESOLVED, that physicians must defend their right to prescribe treatment, observing the tenet FIRST, DO NO HARM. Physicians shall not be restricted from prescribing safe and effective treatments. These restrictions continue to cause unnecessary sickness and death. The rights of patients, after being fully informed about the risks and benefits of each option, must be restored to receive those treatments.

RESOLVED, that we invite physicians of the world and all healthcare providers to join us in this noble cause as we endeavor to restore trust, integrity and professionalism to the practice of medicine.

RESOLVED, that we invite the scientists of the world, who are skilled in biomedical research and uphold the highest ethical and moral standards, to insist on their ability to conduct and publish objective, empirical research without fear of reprisal upon their careers, reputations and livelihoods.

RESOLVED, that we invite patients, who believe in the importance of the physician-patient relationship and the ability to be active participants in their care, to demand access to science-based medical care.

IN WITNESS WHEREOF, the undersigned has signed this Declaration as of the date first written.

As of October 8, 2021, more than *11,400* doctors and scientists had signed the Rome Declaration. The number continues to climb *despite the risk incurred by those who do so.* That means that *well over ten thousand* doctors and scientists the world over have expressly and publicly recognized that their professions are currently subject to what amounts to a (largely corporate controlled) government takeover of science and medicine, a potentially fatal corruption of this foremost plank of humankind's interest in and care for its physical and psychical wellbeing.

This is, or should be, news indeed—a cry in the wilderness of public opinion sounded in the historic power center of the West, the city at the heart of its religious heritage, and the place where political and spiritual empires have, in the past, most spectacularly conflicted and converged. And yet (further evidence that media, too, has suffered profound corruption) where did I find report of this momentous event, this urgent Covid Call to Humanity? Not in *The New York Times* or *Washington Post*, nor in the *Chicago Tribune* or *San Francisco Chronicle*, nor on any YouTube feed gone viral, nor under the heading of any easy-to-find Google search. If you search for "Rome Declaration," or "Covid Summit," or the like, entirely different content will headline your screen. The only place I could find it was in *The Desert Review.*

The Desert Review? This is fitting enough, to be sure, for a voice crying in the wilderness, but obscure enough for all that. Research informs me that, contrary to my guess that the paper hearkens from some semi-desolate locale in Utah or Arizona, the "award-winning" *Desert Review* represents a region in my home state of California, namely, Imperial County, located east of San Diego on the Mexican border. Lest mention of the Golden State conjure illusions of grandeur in your mind, Imperial is the least populous of all counties in Southern California, featuring a total of roughly 175,000 persons, concentrated in metropolitan areas such as Brawley, Calexico, and the county seat of El Centro, the largest urban center, featuring roughly 40,000 citizens.

Unremarkable as all this may seem, if you do ever find yourself in Imperial County, once you've sated your eyes on the austere, cactus-blooming beauty of Anza Borrego, you might consider heading over to one of the county's other chief attractions: Salvation Mountain, a hillside environment piece of visionary folk art constructed of adobe bricks, discarded tires, automobile parts, and thousands of gallons of paint located northeast of Niland near the Slab City squatter art commune. Local Leonard Knight created the mountain, beginning work on it in 1984, though the collapse of the original project five years later required a second, more soundly engineered version that lasts, and remains maintained today, some seven years after Knight's own death. Knight designed the mountain to broadcast a Christian message of universal love, and the most prominent face of the mountain features a version of the Sinner's Prayer, with these words enclosed in a huge red heart visible for great distances in the desert waste: "Say Jesus I'm a Sinner Please Come Upon My Body And Into My Heart."

The Sinner's Prayer originally emerged (so runs one chief account) as a Protestant reaction against Roman Catholic dogmatism and the insufficiently feeling doctrine of justification of merit by good works. Perhaps, then, we can view *The Desert Review's* printing of the Rome Declaration as a reconciliation of sorts: a figure of the cooperation of the Pope and the People—formidable centers of power found both in Italy's Imperial City and California's Imperial Valley. To be sure, the salvation of the world today may indeed depend on its leaders, and the populace at large, hearkening to the message sent both by the eminent doctors and scientists who authored or signed the Rome Declaration, as well as the simpler, equally heartfelt message written in blood, sweat, tears, and thousands of gallons of paint by Leonard Knight, our folk-art Baptist-John, who, crying in the wilderness, pleads for salvation by inviting not a pathogenic spike protein but the healing power of Love to enter the vital core of our being—to *"Come upon My Body and into My Heart."*

Since having penned the above words a few hours ago, I believe I have solved an enigma: the question of why it is that Imperial County's *Desert Review*—virtually alone among newspapers in the United States—covered the Rome Covid summit in detail, printing The Physician's Declaration in full. I have discovered that Dr. George Fareed, who testified at the November 2020 U.S. Senate Hearing on Early Treatment (covered in chapter 2), works in Imperial County, maintaining a medical practice in Brawley. Not only have Dr. Fareed and his staff taken extraordinary care of thousands of Covid-19 patients in Imperial County, but Dr. Fareed himself took the road less traveled to Rome to participate in the September Covid Summit there. Dr. Fareed's own short address at the summit paints, in local color, the picture of what a good doctor can do and has in fact done to treat Covid-19 and how irrational government restrictions are, more and more, suppressing the means and methods proven most effective for treating Covid-19. I would like to share Dr. Fareed's text in full[350]:

> **Distinguished Senators** and Dear colleagues, friends, ladies and gentlemen, it's a great honor for me to address you today.
>
> My name is Dr. George Fareed. I practice medicine in a rural town called Brawley, California, that sits on the Mexican border. This small community became the epicenter of COVID-19 in California, and I, who continue to treat patients in both the outpatient and hospital setting, found myself in the "eye of the storm," treating very sick and contagious patients—not a place I thought I would be at age 76.
>
> However, my training in biochemistry and virology, along with my degree from Harvard Medical School, prepared me well for the battle ahead, a battle that I have been fighting now for the past 18 months.
>
> I, along with my colleague Dr. Brian Tyson, are winning the battle against COVID-19 for one simple reason: *we follow the science!*
>
> COVID-19 is a disease that can be easily treated in its early stage, but comes very difficult to treat as the disease progresses.
>
> As scientists such as Drs. Didier Raoult, Vladimir Zelenko, and Peter McCullough have taught us, the first stage of COVID involves viral replication resulting in symptoms such as flu-like symptoms of cough, fever, malaise, headache, and perhaps loss of taste and smell—if a patient is left untreated, this may progress into "cytokine storm" where oxygen saturation drops, and then into the thromboembolic stage where blood clots occur that can be fatal.

I've treated patients in all three stages—delaying treatment in an elderly or high-risk patient, those with co-morbidities such as asthma or diabetes, is nothing short of cruel as the disease predictably progresses—many then die. The standard "wait and see" approach to COVID-19 has been the greatest medical failure I have seen in my long career because *deaths are preventable*—but you must treat early!

NO ONE NEEDS TO DIE FROM COVID-19

Eighteen months ago, in March 2020, I, along with my colleague Dr. Brian Tyson, began treating COVID-19 patients early in the course of the disease with a combination of medications, initially primarily hydroxychloroquine [HCQ] and azithromycin or doxycycline, and nutraceuticals including zinc, vitamin D and C.

As Dr. McCullough explains, medications such as hydroxychloroquine act as ionophores to allow zinc into the cell to interfere with viral replication.

As time progressed, so did our treatment, and we added drugs such as ivermectin, fluvoxamine, and monoclonal antibodies, as well as aspirin and budesonide (steroid) to treat the other aspects of the disease.

We became part of an international network of physicians, including groups such as the American Association of Physicians and Surgeons led by Dr. McCullough and leaders such as Dr. Jean-Pierre Kiekens from Covexit.com—all engaged in one singular goal—saving lives through early treatment.

I developed my own protocols which vary slightly from patient to patient—depending on their clinical situation.

So—what do our results look like?

We have now treated over 7,000 patients, and there has not been a single death in patients treated within the first 5 to 7 days of the onset of symptoms. NOT A SINGLE DEATH. This includes patients with multiple co-morbidities as well as patients in their 90s!

As a medical director at a nursing home, while other nursing homes in the area suffered major losses, we saw very few deaths from COVID in our residents because of early treatment.

To put this in perspective, our County has seen around 30,000 COVID cases and there have been 750 deaths. We have treated over 20% of the patients, and have seen just a few deaths, and NONE when we have treated early.

Moreover—we are called on a daily basis from patients all over the US who are desperately seeking early treatment, and we have helped hundreds—the letters we receive from thankful patients are incredibly gratifying.

What is the proof that our treatment is "scientific"? Our results have been *duplicated* all around the world, and there are now hundreds of peer reviewed publications on early treatment. I have been honored to be on a few of these publications, including on Dr. McCullough's seminal paper on early treatment.

What is going on that COVID patients cannot get the treatment they need from their own physicians?

Perhaps the major reason is that our own health agencies such as the FDA and CDC have come out against these medications—even making false claims that they are dangerous.

First, we were told that HCQ was cardiotoxic based on sham study in the Lancet that was eventually retracted. Now we hear that Ivermectin is a "horse medication"—ignoring the fact that it is recommended by the CDC and WHO and millions of doses have been given to humans to treat parasitic infections—the propaganda against early treatment is then echoed in the media.

I and other doctors who treat COVID early have come under attack by our local health departments, hospitals, and even state licensing boards. With increasing frequency, my prescriptions are now being denied by pharmacies. Even as it becomes more evident that vaccines by themselves are not the answer, patients are finding it increasingly difficult to get treatment.

Moreover, there is censorship...my own YouTube videos regarding early treatment have been taken down and labeled misinformation...in the US, we say it is like the book "1984" or McCarthyism.

Censorship is never good in a free society, but especially damaging in medicine where patients benefit when physicians exchanging ideas. Rather, we depend on a few "experts" who don't even treat COVID patients.

The results, as we have seen, have been tragic!

CONCLUSION

When I began working in my rural community in 1990, I never dreamed that I would one day be speaking in the United States Senate and then in an international conference...but because I have seen first-hand how early treatment of COVID-19 saves lives, I feel an ethical and moral obligation to speak out and fight for not only my patients, but for the many around the world who continue to die unnecessarily.

This is a time that calls on the greatest of human attributes—courage. Everyone here must understand that we are in the greatest fight of our lives—when doctors are prevented from treating their patients with life-saving medicine, we know that something sinister is going on.

I thank you all for being here, and applaud your courage for standing up for your patients and the rest of humanity.

Thank you.

Dr. Fareed's speech paints a complete picture. First, in the foreground, we see the spectacular success of early treatment (which, if properly administered, as in Dr. Fareed's practice, reduces Covid mortality to ZERO); then—darkening the landscape—the campaign of disinformation resulting in censorship of scientific inquiry and proscription of the means of life-saving early treatment by way of government edict and commercial restriction. These latter *morally* if not *legally* criminal acts are sanctioned by press and media outlets that, rather than offering any kind of objectively balanced view of Covid news, obediently uphold this inhuman regime—one, by now, *directly* responsible for hundreds of thousands of unnecessary deaths and debilitating illnesses across the face of the globe.

We were just speaking of papal power, regarded by some, in accordance with dogma, to be perfect to the point of infallibility. In the world at large today, neither religion in general nor the Pope in particular truly wields that absolute authority. For the majority of persons, *science,* bearing reason's scepter, occupies that sovereign throne, delivering unto us *Logos,* the Word, so that what *science* holds as *truth* acquires an air of infallibility. Even as a person of faith will often be described as a "follower" of one or another prophet or school, today we speak (as Dr. Fareed spoke), of "following the science," invoking what qualifies today as the supreme court of public opinion.

The Rome Covid Summit, however, should urgently call our attention to the truth that the legitimacy of scientific, no less than religious or spiritual, authority depends wholly on the integrity of the human institutions that uphold that high office. Just as, first, Czech theologian and religious reformer Jan Hus and, later (a hundred years after Hus was burned at the stake), Martin Luther saw that the spiritual authority of the Catholic Church had been seriously impugned by mercenary practices (chiefly, the granting of indulgences) that served not ethics flowing from God but secured monies flowing from Mammon, so today in the precincts of the Vatican City we hear thousands of physicians declaring that *science* can no longer rightfully command the allegiance of the disciples of Enlightenment reason if her institutions and officers are bought and sold, and traffic not in the spirit of freedom and impartial inquiry but in the tainted coin of falsehood, illusion, censorship, and arbitrary fiat. Just as the very viability of the Christian religion, increasingly hollowed out from within, stood at a point of catastrophe at the dawn of the Renaissance, so too today does science—especially the venerable art and science of medicine—teeter on the brink, as the massive weight of Big Pharma and all the vested interests entangled in its manifold machinations tips the kingdom of truth toward an abyss of ignorance and deceit, and so a fall that bodes material ill for all. It is difficult to fathom the sheer magnitude of the crimes against humanity indicted in the Rome Declaration and—more humbly, yet more concretely—Dr. Fareed's own folkloric narrative.

It is difficult to comprehend, too, the intricate machinery that has managed to portray so effectively saints as sinners and sinners as paragons of virtue and truth. It is certainly not Dr. George Fareed or the thousands of patients he has so nobly and courageously served, who had better beat a path toward Salvation Mountain, but those engineers of evil responsible for denying effective treatment to untold persons afflicted by Covid-19, and who—if they mind at all the fate of their souls—should quickly hightail it toward Slab City, chanting the Sinner's Prayer all the while.

On second thought, even that would scarcely suffice—unless and until they make public confession of their wrongs, and do all within their power to set our present errant course right. If they do not do so, merciless hounding by ghosts of Covid past, present, and future must surely be all they can reasonably expect.

Chapter 29

ABBOT OF UNREASON, LORD OF MISRULE

Dr. George Fareed, a seventy-six-year-old, Harvard-educated family physician and a recent recipient of the Greater Brawley Chamber of Commerce's Branding Iron Award for his tireless service on front lines of Covid-19 care,[351] hardly fits your stereotypical image of the suspicion-ridden conspiracy theorist spinning webs of dark delusion. He is, however, courageous enough to state the obvious: "*When doctors are prevented from treating their patients with life-saving medicine, we know that something sinister is going on.*"

Is it really plausible to imagine that the concerted, systematic, ongoing effort to block early treatment for Covid-19 is *not* directed by *some* sort of cabal who display little or no regard for human health and welfare?

No. The conspicuous facts of the case make that an untenable notion, one inhabiting the very sort of irrational, fact-free zone many ascribe to the vaguely defined field of "conspiracy theory" itself. The real question is not: "Is there conspiracy at the heart of the Covid-19 story?" but instead: "What kind of conspiracy are we party to here? Who is behind it? Why? How does it operate?"

Big Pharma clearly plays a central role in this film noir, but Pfizer's ravenous appetite for cash is only half of the story.

I confront these questions head-on in the second volume of *Reset or Renaissance.* In the meantime, it is worth noting that conceding the conspiratorial element influencing official Covid policy effectively *explodes* the controlling Covid narrative. That narrative takes the essential independence and integrity of our public health agencies for granted. Correlatively—since health officials rely on Covid science to formulate policy—it presumes that these agencies are conducting business in a manner that respects and builds upon science, rather than corrupting and undermining it.

Science aspires to objective, impartial truth *not* grossly discolored by any given programmatic agenda. It is that repudiation of intellectual prejudice and partisan opinion that grants science its almost God-like sovereignty; authorizes it to stand for a truth above and beyond the realm of any personal or political interest.

The Rome Declaration, however, makes formal and public a truth that has been evident almost from first sloppy mathematical model of Covid deaths and wildly unreliable Covid tests: that, in the case of Covid-19, it is not politics that is following science, but it is science that is being kicked and beaten into submission and dragged along behind politics. Robert Malone puts the gist of the matter succinctly:

> **We're operating in a way that is independent of science.**
> **The science no longer matters, really. It's public policy by fiat…**

A science that no longer really matters is no real science at all. That is why the significance of the Rome Declaration transcends the particulars of the Covid-19 pandemic as it strives to defend not only the integrity of the art and science of medicine but also the *broader universal intellectual, moral, and political freedom* that art and science both depend on and tangibly represent.

Whatever the goals of the special interests groups shaping the controlling Covid narrative may be, one can say with a degree of surety that there has been a deliberate and orchestrated effort to influence Covid-related science so that it delivers results commensurate with those aims. I have detailed innumerable transgressions of scientific protocol; documented diverse sins of both omission and of commission; and data manipulation and obfuscation, the doing of "science" marred by methodological irregularities and faulty test design.

The catalog of these trespasses is so long and varied that I abandoned a preliminary attempt to offer something along the lines of a summary list. If your memory needs refreshing on this score, most all the prior chapters of the book will serve that purpose one way or another.

As we begin to move closer to the end of this book, I would like, however, to call attention to what may or may not be judged to be more a matter of misunderstanding than deliberate distortion.

By now, I hope the reader shares this writer's opinion that the safety issues associated with the mRNA Covid vaccine are so serious that—efficacy or lack thereof notwithstanding—these vaccines should no longer be marketed (let alone mandated). That said, the argument against the vaccination program can only be strengthened by presenting a convincing case that—even if, for the sake of debate, safety concerns were to be set aside entirely—a program of mass vaccination does *not* promise any kind of solution, or even amelioration, of the worldwide Covid-19 problem. An alternative vaccine-free approach, however, can indeed do so.

The next two chapters attempt to make this case rather more systematically than so far has been done in this book. The rest of this chapter (re)introduces that enterprise in a somewhat dramatic fashion.

Near the beginning of a recent (September 25, 2021) interview, Dr. Phillip McMillan asks Geert Vanden Bossche if developments on the Covid front over the last six or so months bear out the predictions Vanden Bossche ventured in his March Covid Call to Humanity. Vanden Bossche felt entitled to answer in the affirmative:

> Honestly, yes, it is what I expected. Of course, it is always very very difficult to predict exactly when what is going to happen. But *that we would have massive surges of the infection rates, especially in those countries that have a very aggressive mass vaccination strategy,* like in Israel, like in the UK, like in the United States: I think we are seeing this already… I think I also predicted that it first would primarily affect the more vulnerable people, the elderly, but then the virus would come back and hit also, increasingly, younger age-groups, which is what we are seeing right now…Overall, this is the picture I was expecting.[352]

Predictably, it was the scientist who thought most deeply about the relevant scientific principles at play in a highly complex and ever-evolving immunological situation who most accurately predicted what we have in fact seen unfold in Israel and other highly vaccinated countries (such as the United Kingdom and the United States). As discussed in prior chapters of this book, despite some short-lived alleviation of Covid distress, these countries continue to suffer elevated plateaus of infection and even worsening pandemic conditions. In the face of these harsh realities, have public health authorities been moved to revisit their thinking and strategies for success?

In response to this question, one may be tempted to ask. ***What thinking? What strategy?*** As the informed scientific discourse of the likes of Byram Bridle, Robert Malone, Geert Vanden Bossche, and other contemporary *personae non grata* make clear, the mass vaccination campaign unfolds not only in a largely fact-free but also in a largely *thought-free* zone—one that not only deliberately turns away from the phenomenon of vaccine injury but also neglects to give sufficient consideration to the complex evolutionary parameters essential to formulating a rational, well-informed vaccine (or no vaccine) policy.

As Vanden Bossche especially makes clear, such consideration indicates that mass vaccination with a leaky vaccine in the midst of the pandemic will impede rather than accelerate humankind's attempt to put the plague of Covid behind us. Scientifically speaking, Fauci and his cohort shoot from the hip, in the dark, scattering precious immunological ammunition as they go.

On the frail basis of a few preliminary and sorely inadequate clinical trials as well as willful blindness to any and all contrary evidence, public health policy now—with popular opinion in tow—apparently takes as more or less ***axiomatic*** that the vaccine can do only good.

If not great and wonderful good (eradication of the disease), then much good, nonetheless; if not much good (because of waning efficacy), then still some good. Authorities seem to see no need to consider alternative approaches or take serious account of possible ill effects. Their answer instead seems always to be shots and more shots—more and more of the same.

And those who resist the program? Should they not be *compelled* to comply with the regime by way of mandates, economic and social coercion, and even brute force?

Like the infamous French Reign of Terror, such dictatorial nonsense still cloaks itself in the royal garb of reason and science.[353] America's own Lord of Misrule, our Abbot of Unreason, Doctor Tony Fauci, hath (in answer to those who spread rumors of—gasp!—his nakedness) once proclaimed:

> If you are trying to get at me as a public health official and scientist, you're really attacking not only Dr. Anthony Fauci, you're attacking science.... You'd have to be asleep not to see that. That's what's going on. Science and truth are being attacked.[354]

As these words imply, this is very grave business, involving attack and counter-attack—a great deal of figurative swordplay. The historical scene also features some who are asleep and some whose eyes are—supposedly—wide open. The question is: Which is which, who is who, and what, really, is going on?

The titles I applied to Dr. Fauci above stem from English or Scottish mummers' plays, traditionally staged at Christmastide, which humorously dramatize St. George's slaying of the dragon as well as a resurrection of one or another antagonist fallen into the sleep of death. Congruent with this theatrical perspective, the spectacle we are watching play out on the world stage today would indeed be comical *if* it weren't such tragic farce. Doctor Anthony Fauci, our Lord of Misrule, as science and truth itself?

Still, perhaps I have somewhat miscast him. While it is true he cuts an excellent figure as (here, using the Scottish appellation) the Abbot of Unreason, he may be still better suited to perform another part in our own modern version of a mummers' play. After all, according to tradition, a doctor does appear and play a lead role in the story. After either George or one or another antagonist (there are many variants) falls in battle and lies slain on the stage, a doctor is duly called for to cure and raise the dead to life again.

Soon, a physician appears. Today, he might well be costumed in a white lab coat, for he is indeed a highly distinguished doctor—a far cry, to be sure, from any sort of charlatan!—as the text of the traditional Darlington Mummers' play amply attests. If we were to attend a performance of such today, we might witness and hear something along these lines:

("P" stands for a prince whose knightly son has just been slain in battle, either by St. George or (in other versions) a dragon. "D" is the doctor)

P: Thou dread beast, what hast thou done?
Gone and slain my only son.
Is there a Doctor anywhere to be found
That can cure this corpse sleeping on the ground?

D: A Doctor am I; my Mind the only one
Whose brilliance outshines the morning sun.

P: O good Doctor, what is thy fee?

D: Ten guineas it is, but I'll have ten *pounds* from thee.

P: *(eagerly)* Take it, Doctor, be my honored guest.
But tell me now, what illness canst thou best?

D: I cure the ague, the palsy, and the gout;
The fearful plague now roving here about.
A broken arm, or leg—I'll soon ease the pain.
And if you're well, just wait.... I'll make you sick again!

P: A noble doctor thou art, if this be true!
I stand in awe of everything you do.

D: I'm not one of those little mountebanks
That go about the streets
And tell as many lies in one half-hour
As pollsters do in seven weeks!
But what I do I do in front of your very nose
So if you don't believe your eyes, look with your toes!

P: Doctor—O my good Lord—now see here!
(gestures toward his fallen son)
What can you do to allay my fear?

D: I have a little vial called Covid vaccine. *(kneels for injection)*
One shot in this man's arm, two more in his spleen;
If he rises up again, he'll sleepwalk like me.
But if now he's gone for good, I'll triple my fee!

Chapter 30

LOSING STRATEGY

On a more serious note (if anything can possibly be more serious than this play), we need look, objectively, at where we are, and where we are going, with respect to Covid-19. While I expect this or that individual may serve with integrity and conscience, the current public health regime has shown itself to be incompetent if not corrupt and corrupt if not incompetent. How might we address the ongoing Covid crisis more rationally and effectively?

To move toward that end, we need to understand not just why the various components of the present agenda are flawed but *how these defective components fit—or do not!—together to make an even more completely dysfunctional whole.* We need, that is, to comprehend in depth the *strategic* as well as *tactical* deficiencies of the current Covid-19 campaign.

Let's take a moment to elaborate on these two crucial complementary terms. Formulation of a winning military *strategy* requires clear overview of all the factors determining the complex dynamics of a campaign and the development of a long-term, comprehensive plan to achieve specific ends. Few wars are won in one fell swoop. Accordingly, good strategic planning typically entails identifying a number of clearly defined preliminary objectives which precede and lead toward achievement of the ultimate aim—success, or victory, which itself may be variously defined (surrender of the enemy; usurpation or reclamation of territory; peaceful truce).

Tactics, on the other hand, involve the means of achieving prescribed ends. Strategy thus concerns itself with goals and tactics with the method by which these goals may best be attained. Whereas the former may be viewed as a matter of intellectual vision, the latter counts primarily as one of technique. Every successful strategy thus *matches well-defined, realistically attainable goals with appropriate and sufficient tactical means.*

Good strategy further requires that the distinct aspects or features of the plan *cohere* and so *cooperate* in working toward accomplishment of the *ultimate* aim. Even if specific tactics may bring about desired results, no strategic plan will succeed in the absence of synergistic coordination of its various measures. This may be construed as the systematic or *cybernetic* dimension of strategic planning.

Last, good strategic planning revolves around a key idea that identifies and maps effective use of a governing agency: some original source of power and operative intelligence that drives the whole system of action. *What* that source is, *how* the strategy proposes to draw on it, and the power of its agency *when actually put into execution* figure crucially into ultimate success, or failure.

In human and sociological (as opposed to mechanical or biological) systems, such governing agency proves most viable when it includes a sound spiritual element. For instance, in traditional warfare—which cannot be fought with heartless drones—fighting spirit or morale plays a key role. No strategical or tactical acumen can ultimately make up for serious deficiency on this score. An army or navy that does not believe in the ideals for which it is fighting loses power and often will eventually break down.

To summarize what we have understood so far of good strategic planning, this entails (or, at its peril, neglects):

1. A clear definition of attainable objectives, including a series of provisional, limited objectives that lead logically toward an ultimate goal or end;
2. A good fitting of appropriate and efficient tactical means to those ends;
3. A coherence and cohesion of the whole system, or cybernetic integrity;
4. A strategic gist or key idea that effectively organizes the whole system around a viable source of agent power and intelligence.

I present these aspects in this order for ease of understanding. Conceptually speaking, however, the last idea should perhaps be placed first, as it is the nucleus around which all else builds.

How does all apply to the annals of the Covid-19?

You will remember that, in his November 2020 Senate testimony, Dr. Peter McCullough presented a diagram depicting what he termed "the four pillars of pandemic response." Here, once more, is his outline:

1. Contagion control (stop the spread);
2. Early home treatment (minimizing hospitalization and death);
3. Late-stage treatment (in-hospital safety net for survival);
4. Vaccination (herd immunity).[355]

The scaffolding of this scheme provides a general framework that may serve as a good point of departure for formulating *any* comprehensive pandemic strategy. It is worth noting that the design implicitly includes a certain temporal flow, even if imperfectly. The event of illness and its demand for treatment occupy the *central* positions, while preventative measures head the schema and the putative population-wide aim ("herd immunity") concludes it. Note, as well, that, at each step, McCullough first names a *tactical means* and, consequently (in parentheses), the associated aim or *strategic goal* that action is supposed to accomplish.

McCullough's scheme, while universally applicable in general outline, is not so applicable in all particular details. Most especially, its formulation of the first and fourth pillars reflect planning initiatives *specific* to the official public health policy currently in force in most of the developed world, including the United States. They do not represent the only possible conception of means and ends at the first and fourth positions.

Despite McCullough's sharp criticism of our country's defective attention to the second pillar, the *general* validity of the outline as a whole, together with its *particular* formulations of the first and fourth pillars, do qualify it as a fit model for use in a qualitative analysis of the *strategy* informing present U.S. Covid policy and indeed that of much of the world. We can initiate such an analysis by reviewing salient aspects of the history of Covid and the success, or failure, of the U.S. response.

The reader will of course remember that from the moment the world heard of Covid-19, the prospect of a tsunami of death suffered at the hands of a sinister unseen enemy struck terror into the hearts and minds of untold persons. Not knowing how lethal the disease might be, the populace, inflamed by speculative mathematical models and zealous public health officials, initially assumed the worst and acceded to previously unheard-of contagion control measures (lockdowns, social distancing, ubiquitous masking, testing, contact tracing, and quarantining) in order to meet the first stated objective of our pandemic response: "stopping the spread."

Ever since then, the strategic and tactical dimension of that initial, panic-stricken pandemic response remains firmly in place as the first pillar of Covid policy, without consequential reexamination by governing U.S. agencies of the place of such measures in any comprehensive Covid strategy, much less the role they may reasonably and realistically be expected to play in contributing toward the ultimate objective of ending the pandemic. Instead, measures instituted on a temporary basis, with a specific limited rationale, persist as permanent features of our human landscape long after that original rationale has long been exploded.

What was the original purpose of lockdowns, distancing, masking, testing, tracing, and quarantining? All these steps were undertaken, initially, with the *limited* objective of "flattening the curve." But why try to flatten the curve? Strategically speaking, the tactics employed to "flatten the curve" were not conceived as a set of measures intended to *permanently* reduce the incidence of serious illness and death. Rather, these steps were originally taken as temporary, stopgap measures to minimize serious illness and thus allow hospitals to function effectively (the third pillar) *until* such time as a real solution to the pandemic might be found—a solution that would, ideally, eliminate the source of the problem altogether. That definitive solution was, from the first (and long before anything concrete materialized on this score), imagined to be the development and delivery of Covid-19 vaccines. No other means of bringing an end to the pandemic was ever conceived or seriously considered, at least in the realm of official discourse.

As we attempt, therefore, to comprehend the logic underlying of our Covid strategy as a whole, it is fair to maintain that the limited objective of the first pillar (contagion control measures to limit spread) was originally implicitly, if not explicitly, tied to the fourth pillar (a tactical program of mass vaccination), the strategic aim of which was to achieve herd immunity and thus end the pandemic.

As of the time of this writing, well over a year and a half into the pandemic, this tactical and strategic coupling remains in place—and indeed in essentially unmodified form, even though the intervening course of events has revealed the entire overall "plan" predicated on these joint initiatives to be one of complete and total failure. After nine months of an intense campaign that has resulted in the vaccination of roughly two-thirds of the country, Americans nonetheless remain restricted by fear, still don masks inside and sometimes out, often avoid group gathering, and continue to live in a cloud of unknowing as to whether the future will bring clearer skies or further storms of illness and death. We are increasingly subjected, moreover, to coercive mandates that tear at the social fabric of an already divided people and are engaged in fighting what often appears to be a losing war against Covid-19.

Our present failure was predictable, as is future misfortune—*unless* we rethink our policy from the ground up and change course.[356] Why, and how, could we readily have foreseen systemic failure of our Covid-19 response, and so gain the perspective necessary to amend it?

If comprehensive strategic planning depends on the four outlined criteria, our current policy fails, miserably so, *on all counts*. As Dr. Geert Vanden Bossche declared emphatically enough, "There is no strategy! Only tactics."[357] We are waging a campaign that is *strategically* as well as *tactically* sorely deficient. We have no *coherent, overall plan* that fits *technically sufficient means* to well-defined, realistically *attainable objectives*, the eventual accomplishment of which progressively builds toward a satisfactory result or *recognizable success*. Instead, we have a frayed patchwork of seriously and even drastically defective means keyed to a mishmash of ill-defined, unpalatable, or impossible goals.

Most crucially, the key idea or principle initially organizing our whole Covid strategy—herd immunity, *redefined as a certain threshold of vaccination*—has revealed itself to be inherently and irrevocably fatally deficient. Even the most avid vaccine proponents long ago conceded "herd immunity" to be an unattainable goal, so that the purpose of vaccination has now been downgraded to that of personal protection. Meanwhile, however, the shoreline of any conceivable end to the pandemic has dipped below the horizon of visible sight. *Even so*, an inflexible commitment to the vaccine agenda has effectively precluded any substantive reevaluation of the strategic premises of our official Covid response. Instead of such course correction, the government has chosen merely to *double down on deficient measures* in a manner that not only further compromises public health but—owing to the unprecedented coercion involved—threatens to destroy democracy.

Unsurprising, it all hearkens back to *the current pro-vaccine agenda's displacement and usurpation of the protective agency supplied by our own natural immune system*. That this displacement has always been and continues to be the nuclear gist of America's official Covid policy manifests in the persistent, arbitrary, and aggressively anti-scientific repudiation of the very *existence* of natural immunity as a biological reality.

As previously mentioned, this folly found its signature inscription in the *erasure* of the very idea of natural immunity from the scientific lexicon and its approved definition of "herd immunity." The controversy triggered by that maneuver has, however, visibly entered the public domain by way of Senator Rand Paul's repeated confrontations with public health officials (and sometimes other legislators) intent on denying natural immunity. As of the time of this writing, the most recent confrontation consisted of a pointed exchange on

September 30, 2021, between Senator Paul and U.S. Secretary of Health and Human Services Xavier Becerra, an exchange that foregrounds, as clearly as any episode in the history of Covid, the bald-faced nonsense that passes itself off as science during the current administration.

If, at this point, you remain skeptical of my claim that the *corruption of science* has both driven and (falsely) legitimated public policy, perhaps you may be better persuaded after reading Becerra's statement and subsequent dialogue with Paul.[358]

On September 21, nine days before his exchange with Senator Paul, Secretary Becerra delivered these remarks to the Howard L. Bost Memorial Health Policy Forum:

> Get vaccinated. Take steps like mask-wearing indoors. And encourage family and friends to do the same. We do these things not because they are fun or second nature, but because they work. They are based on science and evidence. They save lives. Call me crazy, and I guess some people really do, but truly, this does not require a rocket science degree, if there is such a thing.
>
> My friends, the earth really is round. How round is it? Well, more than 600,000 Americans have died from Covid-19. And because some flat-earthers, especially those in places of influence, choose to pedal fiction, we're losing more of our loved ones today than we were a few months ago.
>
> Flat-earthers, meet Delta. The Delta variant besieging our nation is faster, stronger and more contagious. It spreads more than twice as easily as the original Covid virus. It went from accounting for 1% of Covid cases in May, to be the beast behind the vast majority of cases today.[359]

A little over a week later, Becerra appeared before the Senate to offer testimony relevant to the issue of reopening schools during the Covid pandemic. Senator Paul had some questions for him:

> **Rand Paul:** Mr. Becerra, are you familiar with an Israeli study that had 2.5 million patients, and found that the vaccinated group was actually seven times more likely to get infected with Covid than the people who had gotten Covid naturally?
>
> **Xavier Becerra:** Senator, I'll have to get back to you on that one. I'm not familiar with that study.
>
> **RP:** I think you might want to be [familiar with the study.] If you are going to travel the country insulting the millions of Americans, including NBA star Jonathan Isaac, who have had Covid, recovered, look at a study

with 2.5 million people, and say: "Well, you know what? It looks like my immunity is as good as a vaccine, and maybe, in a free country, maybe I ought to be able to make that decision." Instead, you've chosen to go around the country calling people like Jonathan Isaac, and others, myself included, "flat-earthers." We find that very insulting. It goes against the science. Are you a doctor, a medical doctor?

XB: I have worked for over thirty years on health policy…

RP: You're not a medical doctor.[360] Yet you presume, somehow, to tell over 100 million Americans who have survived Covid that we have no right to determine our own medical care? This is an arrogance that is coupled with an authoritarianism that is unseemly and un-American.

You, sir, are the one ignoring the science. The vast preponderance of scientific studies, dozens and dozens, show robust, long-lasting immunity after Covid infection. Even the CDC does not recommend measles vaccines if you have measles immunity! The same was true for smallpox. But you ignore history and science.

You should be ashamed of yourself and apologize to the American people for being dishonest about naturally acquired immunity. Do you want to apologize to the 100 million Americans who suffered through Covid, survived, have immunity, and yet you want to hold them down and vaccinate them? Do you want to apologize for calling those people flat-earthers?

XB: Senator, I appreciate your question, and I appreciate that everyone has their opinion. We follow the facts and science at HHS, and we rely on what is on the ground showing us results…

RP: Except for the dozens and dozens of studies—in fact, most if not all of the studies show robust immunity from getting the disease naturally. The CDC says if you've had measles and have immunity, you don't have to be vaccinated. The same was true of smallpox.

You are selectively doing this because you want us to submit to your will. You have no scientific background, no scientific degrees. You want to mandate this for all of us. You're going to tell us, if I have a hundred employees, you're going to put me out of business with a $700,000 fine if I don't obey what you think is the science. Don't you understand that it is presumptuous for you to be in charge of all the science? Have you ever heard of a second opinion?…You are not willing to consider natural immunity?

XB: Our team has reviewed every study that is out there on Covid. 660,000 odd Americans, or more, have died because of Covid. We trying to do everything we can to save as many as possible. We're using the facts. We're following the science....

RP: Nobody is arguing the severity of this, but you are completely ignoring the science on natural immunity. So is Fauci. So is the whole group....

Think of the nurses and doctors and orderlies who all bravely took care of Covid patients. There was no vaccine for a year and a half. They took care of people; risked their lives. They got it, survived, and now people like you are arrogant enough to say: "You can no longer work in the hospital because, though you've already had the disease, we are going to force you to take a vaccine that science does not prove is better than naturally acquired [immunity]." That's an arrogance that should be chastened.[361]

What, exactly, is wrong with the idea of substituting the vaccination-only model for the traditional understanding of achieving "herd" (or, as I prefer to call it, "population-wide") immunity, which includes natural immunity as a central component? As Geert Vanden Bossche—standing on the bridge of time and, like some modern-day figure out of Munch, forming his mouth into an unheard scream of horror—continues to shout out to all the world: *it doesn't work*. It has not worked, cannot work, and—no matter how much "coverage" you attain or how much you "boost" your vaccination program—*will* not work.

Shall we rehearse the essential argument again? It will not work because the Covid-19 spike protein-specific mRNA gene therapies do not exert lethal pressure on the virus. Such vaccines merely drive the evolution of variants, some of which may well be more contagious or even more virulent. Short-term gains in reduction of serious illness and death wane relatively quickly, and in no wise offset the long-term compromise of the human immune system affected by an indiscriminate policy of universal vaccination, most especially one that includes and even targets young adults and children. Over the long term, repeated boosting does not improve the situation, but rather exacerbates it, and presents the prospect of a wholescale degradation of the strength and resiliency of humankind's natural immune system and ensuing debacle.

In line with this, Dr. Robert Malone, the inventor of mRNA transfection technology, spoke in an interview in late September 2021 about a key, related point that amplifies this picture. He detailed a mechanism whereby the vaccine's capacity to reduce incidence of symptoms of severe disease while, at the same time, *not* precluding transmission, can turn the vaccinated into "super-spreaders." He stated:

> The vaccinated are actually at higher risk for becoming super-spreaders because they're replicating virus at the same or higher levels than the unvaccinated, but they feel better. That means they are more likely to be out in the community. We're in an environment now, where both vaccinated and unvaccinated are at risk of infection, because the ability of the vaccine to protect against Delta is relatively modest.... You have people who are feeling relatively good, moving out into the community, highly infectious—infected and producing virus in high titers in the nose and oral pharynx, and that could well account for some of this surge.[362]

It is disturbing to recognize that our Covid "strategy," as presently conceived and implemented, offers *no* rational path toward the ultimate aim: an end to the pandemic. This simple truth effectively collapses the whole inherently faulty structure of our (and indeed, most of the world's) Covid response like a flimsy house of cards. Let us look, for a moment, at the impact of this fatal deficiency on *the cybernetic dysfunction of the whole ill-conceived "system" of our official Covid regime.*

As stated, the original justification for contagion control measures (the first pillar) was always implicitly, if not explicitly, linked to the idea that these measures would limit Covid-inflicted damage until such time as a successful vaccine would effectively eradicate the virus. Confronting reality and surrendering this delusive hope immediately put in question the underlying rationale supposedly justifying lockdowns, social distancing, masking, and the like, because the preliminary objective originally associated with these measures—"flattening the curve" for a *limited* period of time—no longer makes any sense. At the time of this writing, no one still speaks of flattening the curve, and the tactics of contagion control thus *no longer bear any intelligible relation to any comprehensive strategic plan or viable endgame.* In the absence of such, these restrictive measures threaten to become features of a life permanently caught and held in a state of unwilling suspension.

Another critical point pertaining to that first pillar of our pandemic response deserves attention as well. From the outset, significant confusion has reigned as to the real objective associated with contagion control measures and what is or is not realistically attainable by these most unappealing means. In certain places, such tactics have been pushed to the limit in order not merely to flatten any curve or perform damage control on Covid-caused illness but in order to exclude and preclude Covid contagion altogether. Island nations, including New Zealand (which instituted a "zero tolerance" Covid policy), have been particularly prone to this course of action.

Such a radical application of contagion control measures may appear to offer a viable, alternative strategy to vanquish the pandemic in a given area of concern (be it a country, region, or city). Instead of eradication of Covid by means of vaccine-induced herd immunity, the key idea here is wholesale exclusion and extinction of the virus from the territory in question. This strategy necessarily combines exclusionary tactics (travel bans) with the imposition of rigorous testing and tracing, and, in the inevitable case of persons who do contract the virus, quarantining. The goal requires not only keeping Covid from migrating into the region from outside but also acting aggressively to preclude any major in-house reemergence and internal spread.

As a matter of fact, both the psychology and tactics associated with the aim of not just limiting spread of the virus but precluding and effectively stamping it out altogether (like firefighters both manning containment lines and racing to extinguish all spot fires that jump it or spontaneously flame up underfoot) remain very much in force across the globe, *despite* the fact that experiences show, again and again, that *the goal associated with this strategy and these tactics is no more realistic than eradication by means of mass vaccination.* Australia represents another country that has embraced an extreme form of this policy, going so far as to confine test-positive persons in internment camps at that person's, or that family's, own expense. All this, however, has proved to be of little or no avail. Despite both its relatively high vaccination rate and these radical measures, Australia cannot boast of any notable success in extinguishing Covid-19. It can, however, brag of effectively transforming a country that still imagines itself a "liberal democracy" into what can only be called a police state.

Such sociopolitical horror arises, in part, out of faulty strategy and a failure to clearly match adequate tactical means with realistically attainable strategic objectives. Contagion control measures of various sorts *may* be competent to achieve the limited goal of reducing spread, though even this premise remains debatable. What is *not* debatable, however, is that such measures, even when taken to the most humanly intolerable extremes, are *not* capable of accomplishing the end of excluding and extinguishing Covid, no matter where the relevant jurisdiction lies or how geographically or demographically isolated it may be. New Zealand, for instance, has recently retracted its zero-tolerance policy, and—with the kind of candor all too rare among the leadership of nations—openly admitted the policy to be impracticable because it directs energy and resources toward an unattainable end and thus represents a "mission impossible" justly consigned to the trash heap of political history.

New Zealand notwithstanding, confusion as to the real objective of contagion control measures remains the general rule throughout most of the world. Because such tactics are not an intelligible part of any comprehensive strategy that includes a clearly conceived endgame, the aim of such measures—what they are, and are not, supposed to accomplish—remains persistently blurred and ambiguous. Instead of functioning as a stopgap means (flatten the curve) contributing to an ultimate end to be attained, primarily, by other means (vaccination), the deficiency of the latter tends continually to shift ever more of a strategic burden onto contagion control measures, *and vice versa.* Measures to "stop the spread" were never, originally, supposed to be a chief means of ending or even, ultimately, controlling the pandemic.

The inherently deficient means and correlative ill match of means to ends at both the first and fourth pillars of our pandemic response lay bare *the cybernetic deficiency of the system as a whole.* In a well-functioning cybernetic system, various components are not only logically connected in a coherent and cohesive energy flow, but they synergistically enhance, by way of positive feedback loops, mutual performance. Correlatively, if one or another component encounters resistance that decreases performance, performative power built into the system as a whole can often compensate for difficulty at that point.

Such are the basic operational principles of cybernetic integrity, whatever kind of system may be in question, including systems of governance. Indeed, the Greek root of the word cybernetics means "to steer," and the English Oxford Dictionary states that the term's French form, *cybernétique,* denotes "the art of governing." Governance consists chiefly of "steering" a complex organ of power (a cell, a biological organism, a machine, a system of communication, a body politic, or people) toward desired ends.

The "system" of the world's Covid response, schematically depicted in McCullough's diagram of four pillars, represents the epitome of *cybernetic dysfunction:* a machine designed *neither* to cohere *nor* to flow logically toward desired ends, but rather to suffer repeated failure at multiple points and thus perpetually break down and in fact "steer" toward increasingly negative outcomes. The system does include a major feedback loop, but this is a negative rather than positive one, magnifying deficiency rather than efficiency in the system as a whole and, in the worst case, eventuating in the sociological equivalent of the multisystem inflammatory syndrome sometimes ignited by adverse vaccine reactions.

The cybernetic dysfunction of the system revolves around the lacuna at its very center: the disconnection between initial input (the first pillar) and final output or outcome (the fourth pillar). Predictably, *it is the neglect of early treatment (the second pillar) that proves critical,* for this lack—this black hole in the heart of the whole—disrupts and blocks whatever constructive flow could conceivably transpire between input and output—between, that is, what individuals do up front, before the event of symptomatic illness, and the ultimate consequences for the population as a whole of the presence of the SARS-CoV-2 and our human response to it.

That dark void in the center of the system carries two principal cybernetic implications. First, it means that—unlike an approach based that recognizes natural immunity—*the event of illness itself can in no wise be constructively integrated into the system.* The event of illness can play no positive role—cannot effect a positive transference of energy and resources through the system of human response.

As a consequence (and this qualifies as the *second* principal implication), strategic aims are *discontinuously* identified with *either* the input level (what is done before illness, including contagion control) *or* the output level (here, the population-wide level of immunity). Correlatively, if the means employed at either the first or the fourth pillars prove deficient, no other part of the system compensates for that failure, and the crippled system engineers a dysfunctional response: *persistent and often intensifying iteration of deficient response mechanisms.*

This clearly does transpire at both the first and fourth pillars and, moreover, sets up *the destructive feedback loop* between them. In concrete terms: the more a government's contagion control measures prove deficient and thus fail to impede spread, the louder the call not to rethink these tactics, but instead both to intensify them and to insist on more and more vaccination coverage. Correlatively, the more mass vaccination proves deficient and fails to stop transmission and even illness and death, the more emphatic and self-righteous the calls for both more and more vaccination and, too, more stringent masking, social distancing, and even lockdowns.

Thus, the defective *bipedal* nature of the response system functions to mask the patent deficiency of each of its two principal pillars—the first and fourth.[363]

Meanwhile, the negative feedback loop works back and forth, *never in fact advancing the systemic response toward the ultimate goal of ending the pandemic, the very idea of which gets lost or forfeited* amid the vicious circle of ever-intensifying deficiency.

It should go without saying that an indefinite extension of the present status quo is not a viable end game, except perhaps for the likes of Albert Bourla, Pfizer's CEO. It is not illogical to suspect that Bourla likes to fondly imagine a future in which all human beings are dependent on his company for their very existence and addicted, as we all would thus become, to the next annual (if not biannual) Covid shot, and the next after that. To quote him:

> Within a year, I think we will be able to come back to normal life. I don't think that this means that variants will not continue coming, and *I don't think that this means that we should be able to live our lives without having immune... without having vaccination, basically.* Because the virus has spread all over the world. We will continue to see new variants that are coming out, and also we will have vaccines....
>
> They will last at least a year. I think the most likely scenario is annual vaccination.[364]

Make no mistake: the envisioned return to normality, enabled by vaccination, represents a classic bait and switch. Why should we believe a regime of mRNA Covid vaccination will, under any future circumstances, suffice to return life to normality, if it has not done so already? The situation, according to scientific principle, is, on the contrary, likely to get worse, not better, despite—*or rather precisely because of*—rampant vaccination.[365]

The wholesale cybernetic dysfunction of the U.S. system of Covid response, including the critical negative feedback loop, devolves from the intrinsic deficiency of its organizing principle or key idea: the central agency on which the whole depends as its ultimate source of power and intelligence. The problem with replacing natural immunity with vaccine-induced immunity goes far beyond a mere technical deficiency. The difference here is not merely one executive means versus another comparable one, as if we were comparing the power of one computer language, or one make of automobile, to another. We are speaking here, instead, of a fundamental and irreducible difference of kind.

In the case of natural immunity, the agent source of intelligence and power is, ultimately, Nature, as embodied in the human organism as it has evolved over untold eons of time. In the case of vaccine-induced immunity, the source is entirely unnatural. It is human intellect: the ability of certain members of our kind, by way of science and technology, to isolate and repurpose natural substances and processes for our—or their—own ends.

The primary source of natural immunity is inherently organic, continuous with the source of life itself, the mysterious processes of the sustenance, growth, maintenance, maturation, and reproduction inherent in organic system. It is no accident that the field of cybernetics developed in conjunction with the study of biology. A living organism, by definition, involves the complex coordination of multiple parts that enables both homeostatic equilibrium of the system and the functional resilience that enables it to respond appropriately to ever-varying environmental circumstances. These organic capabilities are, too, inherent in the human being's innate immune system, a dynamic and intelligent agency plugged into not one power source among others but the source of all life-giving and sustaining power: (Mother) Nature herself.

If, in accord with that enlightened philosophy underlying America's own Declaration of Independence, we understand Nature as not some kind of improbable machine oiled by naught but chance and necessity—or the Darwinian equivalent of a stochastically acute supercomputer—but the immanent expression of an intelligence and power far surpassing, and indeed the very origin of our own, and if, too, we conceive the independent sovereignty of America herself to be grounded in that same intelligence and power as it is known under the aegis of "the Laws of Nature and of Nature's God,"[366] perhaps we may begin to comprehend why, for so many Americans, and for so many people the world over standing shoulder to shoulder with us as we face the future, *the freedom to refuse vaccination represents a prerogative that could not be more deeply and intimately tied to those* natural *or unalienable rights of religious as well as political freedom that are our very birthright as American citizens and sovereign individuals.* These are rights for which we are prepared—in the name of that immortal spirit of truth, love, and freedom forever whispering in the ear—to fight, with all the formidable strength lent by just and righteous cause, even unto death.

CHAPTER 31

BIODYNAMICS VERSUS VACCINE DISTANCE

Conceiving a strategy that will allow us to move, intelligently and practicably, toward the end of the Covid-19 pandemic need not be an exercise in your proverbial rocket science. The problem, to be sure, is complex enough, nonetheless, all the elements of a successful solution are ready at hand and have been featured and elaborated in the body of this book. The task of formulating an overall plan, however, entails not only accurately identifying its necessary components but, as well, fitting these various pieces together into a coherent whole, and so developing a conceptual framework that outlines a comprehensive system of Covid-19 response—one that might furnish an alternative to the course we are currently following down the long, lonely road to nowhere.

To be effective, this alternative system of response needs to be, unlike our current dysfunctional model, *cybernetically efficient.* As per the aforementioned criteria, it would entail the following: good strategic planning, adequate tactics, synergistic coordination of its distinct features, and a viable primary source of intelligence and power.

Let us see, then, if we can put hearts and minds together and draw up a sketch of such a plan, a sitemap charting a path toward the end of the pandemic and a more human future.

To pick up where we left off in the previous chapter, we know that the immunological capability provided by Nature herself, "natural immunity," will serve as the alpha and omega of our system, which may be understood as an essentially *biodynamic* rather than technocratically engineered system of response. But how do we translate the agent source of power and intelligence inherent in natural immunity into a viable *strategic* principle, one capable of organizing and lending coherence to our thinking about a complex network of means and ends?

We can take our cue here from Dr. Geert Vanden Bossche. For Vanden Bossche, any effective answer to the pandemic begins and ends with the aim of *reducing infectious pressure*—lessening, that is, the probability that any given individual will not only become infected but, consequently, suffer serious illness. Vanden Bossche explains, too, in detail, why mass Covid vaccination does *not* reduce infectious pressure and suggests that the only really effective means of so doing involves *capitalizing on* and *building up our natural immunity*—empowering our immune system's innate ability to overcome infection either *before* any illness even manifests or after only minor, non-threatening incidence of the disease. The aims of *building natural immunity* and *reducing infectious pressure* are thus effective operational equivalents.

We know too, moreover, that if we succeed in *reducing infectious pressure below a certain threshold,* we can achieve population-wide (or *herd*) immunity, and so the end of the pandemic. Consequently, we can move toward that ultimate end by way of *a comprehensive strategic plan, all aspects of which cooperate toward the goal of reducing infectious pressure.*

We can begin to rough out a sketch of this biodynamic response system by making recourse, once more, to Dr. Peter McCullough's general framework, but modifying it to fit this very different strategic plan. In order to pursue this end, we may begin by reviewing and deepening an understanding of the schematic foundation of McCullough's four pillars. To repeat a final time, his four pillars are:

1. Contagion control (stop the spread);
2. Early home treatment (minimizing hospitalization and death);
3. Late stage treatment (in-hospital safety net for survival);
4. Vaccination (herd immunity).[367]

You will recall that earlier I alluded to a certain temporal flow intrinsic in his scheme. Interventions *prior* to any event of illness and correspondent necessity of treatment head the framework at the first pillar. Illness and the correspondent call for treatment occupy the second and third pillars. The fourth pillar refers, finally, to a population-wide goal or end state—namely, herd immunity, associated in this scheme with the tactic of mass vaccination. To facilitate the formulation of an alternative model, it will be helpful to recognize that, biodynamically considered, the essential structure of the model actually consists of three principal distinct moments.

The first pillar in the original model pertains to actions and interventions at the level of asymptomatic human persons, body and soul, including those (such as travel bans) that dictate the behavior of whole groups of persons. The first pillar thus pertains primarily to the realm of human behavior; volitional acts (including those of governing bodies that constrain human activity) as such affects the immunological capacity of individual human beings.

By contrast, the fourth pillar may best be construed to refer to the immunological condition of *the population as a whole* and the evolutionary dynamics relevant to entire populations. These do, of course, work back on the immune capability of individual persons (cf. the first pillar), but nonetheless require distinct conceptualization, as exemplified in the very concept of "herd" or population-wide immunity.

In between, at the second and third pillars, we encounter the effective center of system of response, namely, the event of illness, the consequent call for treatment, and medical engagement (or lack thereof) with the disease itself.

This elucidation should make clear that vaccination—which is not itself a strategy but a tactic—actually belongs, in this theoretically more refined scheme, not at the fourth pillar but at the first. It is, after all, an intervention at the level of the individual and, indeed, itself represents a "contagion control" measure designed precisely to "stop spread," albeit ideally in a more decisive fashion than masking and social distancing. The real difference here lies in the nature of the relevant means: masking, distancing, and the like address the spatial relation to others, whereas vaccination operates on the interior of the individual body by directly altering the biochemistry of a single person's own immune system.

Before elaborating a new model of Covid response, I believe it will be instructive to inquire as to how the measures of our present official system stack up with respect to the strategic aim we have identified as the crux of this initiative: the building of natural immunity and correspondent reduction in infectious pressure. Three chief points may be made in this connection:

1. It should be obvious that social distancing interventions of all types in no wise represent acts that enhance our natural immunity. Their point of application remains entirely external to any individual's natural immune system. Indeed, such measures tend to reduce natural immunological learning by diminishing the environmental exposure necessary for maintenance and growth of natural immunological defenses.
2. Vaccination does directly impact that system, yet we have seen that it does so in a manner that tends to compromise rather than strengthen natural immunity.

3. For treatment to produce substantial benefit for our immune resistance, it had best be early and effective, before the debilitation and risk of death represented by hospitalization. Yet such treatment is sorely lacking in the present model and indeed (as has been discussed ad infinitum in this volume) positively suppressed.

None of this, of course, is at all surprising. As the current system is based on the displacement of the very idea of natural by vaccine-induced immunity, it stands to reason that none of the measures associated with it work to build natural immunity, but, in fact decrease it.

In conceiving a new biodynamic system of response, the aim, therefore, must be to replace measures that defeat the building of natural immunity with ones that serve to build it. If our new model is to be cybernetically efficient and therefore practically effective, it needs do this in a manner conducive to a constructive synergy operating throughout the dynamic flow of the whole system so that interventions at the first pillar, as well as the second and third, cooperate in building the strengthened natural immunity that (at the fourth pillar) result in a population-wide reduction of infectious pressure and therefore a prospective end to the pandemic.

Is this possible? Yes, indeed. It is not only possible, but quite natural, because we are here contemplating tapping into an essentially organic system of response—one consonant with, rather than manipulative of and even antagonist to, Nature herself.

The key to cybernetic efficiency of the biodynamic system may be understood thus: because natural immunity derives from the fount of organic life itself and thus represents a force and an intelligence *native and internal to* the human body, the energy and knowledge it draws upon can indeed, like a river moving through a variegated landscape, flow continuously through the system as a whole, building strength as it does so. This presents an entirely different situation than a system built around a technological intervention (such as vaccination) that does not derive from an essentially inexhaustible organic source inherent to the body and its innate wisdom—an organic intelligence that, in turn, participates in the whole earth system, the biosphere itself.

Thus, given all we have discussed so far, it is not difficult to see how the various parts of our biodynamic pandemic response system can fit together, especially when we recognize a second key to its efficacy—*actualizing the possibility of continuous flow throughout the system by filling the black hole at the second pillar (and, by extension, the third pillar) in such a way that energy does in fact maintain a constructive flow through the central node pertaining to the event of illness itself.* If that can be accomplished, contracting Covid-19 itself need not automatically spell disaster for the individual or the collective but can be constructively integrated into the overall system of Covid response and, indeed, materially contribute to progress toward the ultimate goal.

At the same time, action at the first pillar, and so preliminary to the event of illness itself, must also clearly be of such a nature as to be consistent with the overall strategic plan of building natural immunity. Consequently, the essential formula for transforming our dysfunctional Covid-response system (which I designate as vaccine-distance) into a cybernetically efficient biodynamic system of response (which I will label *biodynamic*) can be described as follows:

1. Replace vaccine-distance interventions at the first pillar (vaccination and all contagion control measures, including masking) with measures that will enhance the immunological capability of our natural immune system. This would include three general classes of actions, between which there is some overlap:
   a) General yet vital good health measures, such as good diet, hydration, exercise, and all actions that enhance physical as well as psychological wellbeing;
   b) Covid-19 targeted nutraceutical health measures, including supplementation with vitamin D, Zinc, and others recommended by appropriate protocols designed by competent physician-run organizations such as the FLCCC;
   c) And, if desired, Covid-19-targeted pharmaceutical prophylaxis, including ivermectin.
2) Fill the abysmal void at the vaccine-distance second pillar with effective early outpatient treatment measures that should be readily and universally available and educate the public as to the critical importance of seeking such treatment upon contraction of the illness.
3) Replace existing dysfunctional hospital protocols with the full gamut of effective available treatments, many of which are appropriate (at different intensities) in both outpatient and inpatient settings.

To visualize the whole of our Biodynamic response system more clearly, we can revise Dr. McCullough's basis scheme so as to reflect these fundamental changes. The new biodynamic schemata, pairing, as in McCullough's original, tactics and associated strategic goals, would look something like this:

The Pillars of Pandemic Response (Revised Biodynamic Model)

1. Good health praxis and prophylaxis (disease prevention/amelioration)
2. Early outpatient treatment (overcoming illness/disease defense)
3. Inpatient hospital treatment (safety net/disease defense)
4. (Reduction of infectious pressure) (population-wide immunity)

The beauty of this biodynamic system inheres in precisely the kind of cybernetic integrity lacking in the vaccine-distance system. The integrity (as previously discussed) manifests in a few closely related attributes:

1. The components of the system are continuously and coherently connected and cooperate synergistically to maximize positive output.
2. Compensatory action inheres in the systemic relationships.
3. Feedback loops in the system are positive, not negative.

This second clause above means that deficiency or imperfection at one point neither disrupts energy flow altogether nor tends to be *magnified* by the system as a whole. Instead, deficiency at one point is compensated for at other junctures—and indeed even transformed into a positive contribution toward the ultimate objective.

This third-listed feature qualifies as uniquely characteristic of cybernetic efficiency in general. When the feedback loops in a system of relationship are negative, the increasing deficiency tends ineluctably toward breakdown of the system as a whole. When, in an efficient system, such loops operate positively, their presence transforms what might otherwise be a linear model into the kind of extraordinarily strong and stable circular systems characteristic of organic entities (such as the human body).

Remaining, for the moment, within the context of the linear model borrowed from Dr. McCullough, we may find it easy enough to see how the different components of pandemic response work together toward achieving the ultimate end. Good health practices directly contribute to building natural immunity, as do appropriate forms of nutraceutical supplementation. (Let us leave aside, for now, pharmaceutical prophylaxis with, for instance, ivermectin, noting only that it does not—unlike vaccination—diminish natural immunological strength and resiliency.) If an individual does contract a symptomatic case of Covid-19, appropriate early treatment can, in the prohibitive majority of such cases (recall Dr. Fareed's results), cure the disease, avoiding hospitalization or death, thereby *dramatically strengthening that individual's natural immunological strength and resiliency,* conferring robust, enduring, and versatile resistance to not just any one strain of Covid-19 but to all strains.

Thus, what had been the catastrophic center of the vaccine-distance system, becomes, as necessary, an engine of healing and strengthening of the whole system of natural immunity in the biodynamic one. *If* hospitalization is required, many similar measures can be employed to stave off deterioration and death and, once more, return the individual to active life with the benefit of a dramatic and enduringly strengthened resistance to Covid-19.

The consequence of this is a model that integrates the usually readily curable incident of illness itself into a pattern of response that systematically works toward achievement of the ultimate aim: *reduction of infectious pressure and thus the end of the pandemic.* Far from being prone to dysfunction that can result in recurrent breakdown and therefore uncontrollable surges of the disease (liable to occur when vaccine-induced immunity wanes because of gradual dilution of antibodies and the emergence of strains that escape the vaccine's narrowly targeted defense mechanism), the biodynamic system's tolerance of a certain incidence of disease and the system's positive feedback loops effectively block any out-of-control spiraling of disease and death because the system as a whole works to dampen and modulate rather than to increase and accelerate negative outcomes. Rather than systematic *deficiencies* synergistically magnifying each other as in the Vaccine-Distance system, in the biodynamic system it is the cooperative *efficiencies* that now do so.

You will note that, in my revision of Dr. McCullough's scheme, I have put both terms occupying the fourth pillar (reduction of infectious pressure and population-wide immunity) in parenthesis. Why so? As previously declared, these are really two essentially equivalent *strategic* goals or outcomes. Neither qualifies (as does vaccination) as a tactic. Indeed, theoretically, because at the fourth pillar we are speaking not of measures applied to individuals or groups but of the population dynamics and the evolutionary implications consequent on the response system as a whole, no particular measure regulative of human behavior directly affects this (even though all do so indirectly). Nor, in the biodynamic system, is any sort of additional intervention at this level (even if such were conceivable) required, because the design of the system as a whole inherently builds toward producing the desired outcome, that is, the increase of natural immunity and the decrease in infectious pressure.

It is, however, crucial to recognize that a positive feedback loop *does* operate between the fourth pillar and the first pillar. This has dual constructive effects. The more that infectious pressure is reduced in the population as a whole due to overall strengthening of natural immunity, the more that accomplishment eases the task of disease prevention on the part of individual persons. Additionally, in the longer term, individuals with strong natural immunity pass that capacity onto their offspring, further bolstering the natural immune systems of more and more human beings.

The true efficiency of the biodynamic system cannot be adequately represented in the linear format borrowed from Dr. McCullough's scheme. A more accurate portrayal requires a model akin to the more circular forms featuring relevant feedback loops, one of which, a visual representation of a rudimentary cybernetics system, I will share here:

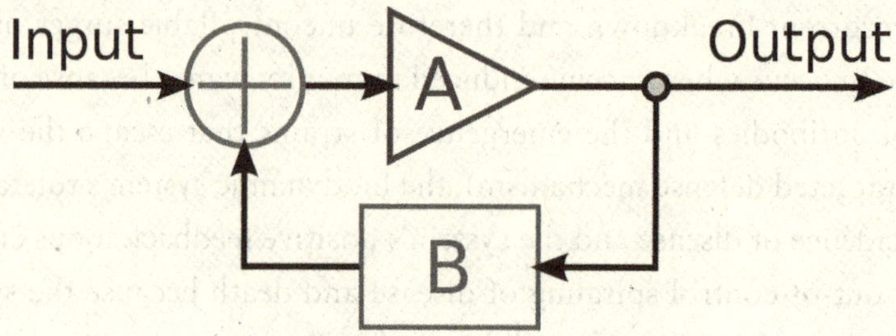

We can adopt our biodynamic Covid response system to this model by plugging in our first-pillar interventions as "A," and treatment options—*especially early treatment*—as "B." We will then regard the cybernetic "node" represented by the little circle marking the junction from A to B as *the event of illness*. As not all persons will contract the illness, for our purposes we can visualize that node as being placed just below its present position, indicating that only persons who do contract disease will undergo treatment; all others will continue to affect the population-wide level of resistance (at the Output point) more or less directly by whatever health and prophylactic measures (A) they enact or do not enact.

Those, however, who do contract Covid-19 and are successfully treated create the positive feedback loop that continually strengthens their natural immunity and thus increases the natural immune strength figured as the Input to the system as a whole. Moreover, as just detailed above, another positive feedback loop should also be envisioned connecting Output (the immunological resources of the population) back to Input, because population-wide immunity, even while built up from individual persons' immunological defenses, will, over time, reciprocally enhance the natural immune capabilities of individuals, representing Input into the system at the first pillar.

If we try, in a similar fashion, to employ the diagram as a basis for visualizing our present vaccine-distance system, we will quickly realize that it is not possible. The vaccine-distance system, in eschewing early treatment, guts the heart of the system as a whole, eliminating the positive feedback looping flowing from the event of illness through box B.

At the same time, however, the feedback loop between output and input operative in the biodynamic system applies here in the vaccine-distance system as well, except that, if we are evaluating natural immunity, this functions as a disastrous *negative* feedback loop, as ongoing mass vaccination, including boosters, depletes the strength and resiliency of the natural immunity originally disregarded in the very concept of the vaccine-distance system.

The original concept of the vaccine-distance system—as indicated by McCullough's fourth pillar—postulates a positive feedback loop between Output and Input, as mass vaccination achieves population-wide vaccine-induced immunity that effectively protects all individuals from the event of illness. This model, however, remains viable only *if* the interventions at A—vaccination, primarily, but also contagion control measures—prove almost *perfectly* effective, thus averting altogether the event of illness and so the path that, in the vaccine-distance system, dead-ends at B.

If, however, vaccination and other contagion control efforts prove seriously flawed, the cybernetic dysfunction of the system causes general failure and a demoralizing lack of steady progress. That is in fact the situation we find ourselves in at the time of this writing, twenty months after the onset of the pandemic, when—after both dehumanizing "contagion control measures" and millions of vaccinations, forced as well as unforced—we remain in a state of suspended animation, increasingly deprived of freedom and health of body and of soul with no visible end in sight.

PART V

POST-MORTEM

Chapter 32

WHO WILL HELP US?

Perhaps it will go down in history as Black Tuesday. Following FDA approval in late October, on November 2, 2021, all fourteen members of the CDC Advisory Committee on Immunization Practices (ACIP) voted to approve Emergency Use Authorization (EUA) for the Pfizer-BioNTech COVID-19 vaccine for children five to eleven years of age. According to the official statement issued by the agency and its director, Dr. Rochelle Walensky:

> The CDC now expands vaccine recommendations to about 28 million children in the United States in this age group and allows providers to begin vaccinating them as soon as possible.[368]

This reckless action calls to mind Geert Vanden Bossche's emphatic declaration:

> First of all, we have to stop this mass vaccination. The worst thing ever, the worst ever that we do is to vaccinate younger age groups.[369]

The *rational* justification for the committee's decision? Objectively speaking, there is none. As has already been amply documented, healthy children are at negligible risk of serious harm from Covid-19. On the other hand—even if we leave aside Vanden Bossche's concerns pertaining to viral evolution[370]—what of the risk of injury incurred as a consequence of vaccination itself?

According to the CDC statement sanctioning the vaccine:

> COVID-19 vaccines have undergone—and will continue to undergo—the most intensive safety monitoring in U.S. history.[371]

Is it possible to imagine a bigger fib?

Any close look at the facts belies the CDC's assertion. The list of transgression is long, and would include: scant, insufficiently powered studies, the evident inadequacy of which are acknowledged even by vaccine proponents (cf. Dr. Fraiman's public comments); the refusal to make many relevant results public at all and misleading interpretations of the data that has been published; the dropping of control groups; the complete void of information pertaining to long-term effects (a category especially relevant to children); statistical sleight of hand intended to suppress safety signals (cf. Matthew Crawford's analysis); the total absence of any data safety monitoring board or safety review (cf. Dr. McCullough's remarks); the deliberate exclusion and erasure, from the record, of adverse events, and the refusal to conduct autopsy analysis of persons suspected of decease on account of the vaccine.

The only way one can make sense of the official statement is to construe it—not in relation to any *objective truth*—but as an all-too-familiar public relations strategy. The agency relies on hyperbole ("the most intensive...in history"), especially *oft-repeated* hyperbole, to produce the impression of impeccable authority pronouncing unimpeachable truth. It evidently does so in order to *preempt* the very possibility of valid question; a strategy naturally suited to support a claim that has no substance, and the force of which relies on *sheer pretense.*

Sometimes, however, matters are arranged so that this world of scientific make-believe, this fantastic "see no evil, hear no evil, speak no evil" pharmaceutical Eden where the jab of a vaccine needle is as harmless as the kiss of a butterfly, slams up against the hard historicity of the real world—that world in which real people get the shot and suffer debilitating harm: ruinous, tragic, life-destroying injury, or death.

Of course, you are not necessarily *compelled* to witness the nightmarish juxtaposition of the testimony offered during Senator Ron Johnson's Panel on Federal Vaccine Mandates and Vaccine Injuries, also convened on November 2, 2021, and so unfolding even as ACIP's fourteen members prepared unanimously to approve Emergency Use Authorization of the Pfizer Covid-19 vaccines for children ages five to eleven. If you happen to be a Big Pharma executive or government official (Rochelle Walensky of the CDC, Janet Woodcock of the FDA, or any of numerous others, including Anthony Fauci himself), you can choose to continue to do your job the way you have been doing it for so long now, and simply ignore Senator Johnson's explicit invitation to attend the panel and actually *listen* to what Americans who followed your advice and believed in your assurances may have experienced.

Prior to the testimony of the vaccine-injured themselves (as well as the testimony of some relevant medical and legal experts), Senator Johnson offered introductory remarks that rehearsed and updated—factually as well sociopolitically—many of the major themes elaborated, again and again, in this volume: lack of transparency in government, the sabotage of early treatment options, neglect of natural immunity, vaccine inefficacy, and the irrationality and the socially disastrous consequences of mandates. Let us listen to the whole of Senator Johnson's prefatory comments[372] before turning attention to the witness borne by the vaccine-injured themselves:

> Telling the truth in today's cancel culture is not necessarily easy. You can pay a pretty heavy price for it. I really appreciate everybody participating…their willingness to tell the truth.
>
> It is a real shame that we are having to hold this round table. Had government officials, the heads of our healthcare agencies—had they been doing their job, had they been honest and transparent with the American public, we wouldn't be here today.
>
> The very sad fact of the matter is, they haven't.
>
> We are billing this as a discussion about the vaccine mandates, which is the current policy response to Covid, one that will rob us of freedom and take an enormous toll on human beings and on our economy. I think every American really needs to ask themselves a question: Since the beginning of this pandemic, have the policies followed by the U.S. government (you can ask this of the governments of the world, but we are going to focus on the U.S.), have they *worked*? Have the shutdowns worked? Have the mask mandates worked? Have the vaccines and are the vaccine mandates going to work?
>
> I am sure we have all hoped and prayed they would have. But the fact is, we have close to 750,000 Americans who have now been reported as having died with or from COVID. 750,000! In the U.S., we rank 23rd [that is, we have the 23rd highest fatality rate] out of more than two hundred nations. That is a bad ranking, in terms of number of deaths per 100,000. We are at 220 per every 100,000 persons that have died from COVID. Sweden…. Remember, everybody attacked Sweden. Personally, I think they approached this rationally. They protected the vulnerable. They isolated the sick. And they let the rest of the society carry on as safely as they possibly could. We are at 220 per 100,000. Sweden is at 145 dead from COVID.
>
> One of the huge blunders of our government response is that we not only ignored, but the higher-ups in the agencies sabotaged, early treatment. To this day, the NIH guidelines for treating COVID are basically to do nothing. Now, as far as I know, in medicine, with any disease, we are always talking about how early detection allows early treatment and produces better results. This makes perfect sense. Why didn't we do that with COVID? The only treatment prior to hospitalization that is recommended right now is monoclonal antibodies, and it is difficult to get those.
>
> So, the fact of the matter is, when we turn our attention to the vaccines, I don't think that there is a person here that is anti-vaccine. Obviously, those that have been injured by vaccines, were very pro-vaccine. But we have to ask ourselves: did the vaccines work? I have one chart behind

me, which combines a timeline of percent of Americans being vaccinated (and you can see we have approached over 60%), and the average number of daily cases. You can see that we had a huge surge toward the tail end of 2020. Even before the vaccines could even kick in, that surge was winding down. At that point, I think we were all hoping and praying that the vaccines would just stomp this thing out for good and we could move on with our lives.

Now, had the vaccines been effective, had they done that, you would see a tailing off of that curve basically to infinity. But that's not what we see. We see a whole new surge, a surge of a variant called Delta.

Now our government officials: I talked about them not being particularly honest, not being particularly transparent. We invited them all here, representative and the heads of the CDC, Secretary of Defense Austin, Secretary of Labor Marty Walsh... Buttigieg... Woodcock... Becerra... Fauci... Collins, together with the CEOs of Johnson & Johnson, Pfizer, Moderna, and BioNTech. None of them showed up. *None* of them showed up.

President Biden, for his part, in terms of honesty, on July 21st, just a couple of months ago, said: "If you are vaccinated, you are not going to be hospitalized, you are not going to be in an ICU unit; you are not going to die. You are not going to get COVID if you have these vaccinations." He said: "This is a pandemic of the unvaccinated."

How I wish he was right when he said these vaccines are going to be that effective! But the fact is that they haven't been.

If you take a look at what is happening in the U.K.—and again, I wish we had data in the U.S. so we could point to that data, but we don't. If they are collecting it, they are not sharing it with the American public. In the U.K., over the last seven and a half months, eighty percent of their cases have been Delta variant. Of the people who have died from COVID in the U.K. with the Delta variant, over the last seven and a half months, 63% have been fully vaccinated. Over the last four weeks in the U.K., 78% of those that have died with the Delta variant from COVID... have been fully vaccinated.

I hate to steal the thunder from one of our participants here, but in a slide, they have a very dramatic decision tree when it comes to vaccine mandates. The first decision square [asks]: "Are COVID-19 vaccines effective?"... "Yes or No?" If the vaccines are effective, then the next decision box says: *"Then mandates are pointless."* If the vaccines are effective, there is no need for mandates. If you want to get the vaccine, you got it, and you are protected, and you don't care if someone else gets vaccinated. [And then we have the] other decision line [referring to the question "Are the vaccines effective?"]... If it's no, then it also points to that exact same box. Then the mandates are pointless.

There are three realities that our federal health agencies, President Biden, and his administration are ignoring when it comes to the mandates—and, again, you have to understand the destructiveness of these mandates on our healthcare system. I have been talking to the doctors and nurses. They are the heroes of Covid, the people that had the courage and compassion to treat Covid. So many of them caught Covid. Some of them died, and most survived. Now they are treating the vaccine-injured. They will not get vaccinated. We will lose decades, decades of experience in a healthcare system that is already experiencing a significant shortage of workers. What are we doing? How insane is this?

One of the things our policymakers are ignoring is *natural immunity*. Why would we require a vaccine that is not as effective as we all hoped? Why would we force that on people with natural immunity when the science tells us those with natural immunity probably have better and more long-lasting immunity than those fully vaxxed?

Another reality that our policy makers are denying is that the vaccines are preventing transmission and preventing infection. They are not. It is obvious they are not. So, again, if you are vaccinated, and you can still get infected and still transmit, what is the rationale for the mandates? *There is no rationale.*

As that decision box said: they are *pointless*, while, at the same time being utterly destructive.

Of course, what we are really going to be discussing today, the third reality that our policymakers are denying, is the vaccine injuries.

Here Senator Johnson alludes to his first meeting with several of the participants at the prior panel he convened in Milwaukee in June 2021, and shares their motives for speaking out:

> Back then, their main message was: we just want to be seen, we want to be heard, we want to be believed. Why? Because unless the medical establishment, our doctors and our health agencies, are willing to acknowledge just the possibility of vaccine injuries.... If you are not willing to acknowledge the root cause of a condition, of an injury, of a malady, of an illness, how can you hope to cure that illness? How can you help these individuals who participated in some of the trials to benefit humanity? How can you help them recover if you are not willing to admit that vaccine injuries are real?
>
> The final slide I want to put up here is a chart that is laying out the reality of vaccine injuries. This is from the government, from the CDC and FDA's own safety early warning surveillance system, one that they touted in October. Man, they were going to pay attention to this: if they see a vaccine injury, even one that results in just the loss of a few days of work, they were going to have someone from the CDC on the phone following up on

> that vaccine injury. You are going to hear from the vaccine-injured on this panel that that is so far from the truth, so far from the reality.
>
> But if you just compare adverse events for the standard flu vaccine versus Covid, you can see that there is something happening here, something that needs to be acknowledged, something that the Walenskys, and the Faucis, and the Woodcocks, and President Biden, ought to be concerned about.
>
> So if you look over the last twenty-five and three-quarter years for the flu vaccine, on average, there have been 7,596 adverse events per year—per year. In ten months, with the Covid vaccine, we are up to 837,595.... On average, the number of deaths reported on VAERS for the flu vaccine is 78 per year. 78! The updated figures [for the Covid vaccines] today are 17,619. That is 225 times the number of deaths in just a ten-month period versus the annual figure for the flu vaccine.
>
> These vaccine injuries are real, and as the...Green Bay Packers star Ken Rutgers stated in that meeting in June, "Vaccine injuries are rare and mild until one happens to you or your loved one."[373]

Senator Johnson later added these comments, which may conclude this preface to the testimony of the Panel's chief witnesses:

> The injuries don't necessarily have to be visible to be real, to be severe, to be life-altering. It is, again, unfortunate, way more than unfortunate, it is actually outrageous that our healthcare agencies, the President of the United States, and members of his administration are completely ignoring these people and their plight.
>
> I can testify to the courage it takes to come forward. The repercussions are quite grave. The vilification, the suppression of what you are trying to say, the censorship. People who have been on this journey with me have been fired from their institutions. They have been sued. Their careers and their life as they've known it has been ended. That's why you have so very few people that are willing to come forward. Their medical licenses are threatened. The profession that they trained for decades to get good at could be taken away from them. So you understand why they are remaining silent.[374]

We can understand, which makes us all the more grateful to those—like the individuals convened at the Panel—who *are* speaking out, and telling all who will listen what most do not wish to hear.

No wonder most do not wish to hear it: the stories of the vaccine-injured, as these handful of courageous souls related, are absolutely devastating. No secondary sources can relay the power of the personal testimonies offered, all of which were stunning in their emotional eloquence. I recommend that all persons—especially the proponents of vaccine mandates—listen, firsthand, to these individuals, so their opinions may be more fully and humanely informed.

While I can here in no wise do justice to the witness borne at the hearing, a sample of that testimony can be offered. *The Highwire* spliced the words of ten vaccine-injured persons and six experts of various stripes into a montage titled "Who Will Help Us," the transcript of which I offer here in quasi-dramatic form.[375]

Who Will Help Us?

CAST:

The Vaccine-Injured:

Brianne Dressen: Injured after participating in AstraZeneca Covid vaccine clinical trial

Kyle Warner: Professional mountain bike racer, debilitated after vaccination

Suzanna Newell: Triathlete, diagnosed with an autoimmune disease, reliant on a walker following vaccination

Kellai Rodriguez: reliant on a walker following vaccination

Stephanie and Maddie de Garay: Maddie, Stephanie's daughter, is a twelve-year-old who volunteered to participate in Pfizer's clinical trials. After suffering vaccine-injury, she has been confined to a wheelchair and requires a feeding tube

Ernest Ramirez: Son died of myocarditis following Pfizer vaccination.

Cody Flint: Agricultural pilot diagnosed with perilymphatic fistual following Pfizer jab.

Shaun Barcavage: Board-certified family nurse practitioner, injured by Covid vaccine.

Doug Cameron: Permanently paralyzed following vaccination.

Dr. Joel Wallskog, MD: Orthopedic surgeon diagnosed with transverse myelitis following Moderna vaccination.

Others:

Aaron Siri, Esq.: Vaccine and civil rights attorney.

Lieutenant Colonel Theresa Long, MD, MPH, FS

Dr. Retsef Levi, PhD: MIT Sloan Faculty Co-director for Global Operations

Dr. Robert Kaplan: Stanford School of Medicine Clinical Excellence Research Center

Dr. Peter Doshi: Associate Professor of Pharmaceutical Health Services Research, University of Maryland School of Pharmacy / Editor at *The BMJ*

Kim Witczak: Consumer Representative on the FDA Psychopharmacologic Drug Advisory Committee

Scene I

Brianne: I am a wife, and a mom, and a preschool teacher.

Kyle: I'm a twenty-nine-year-old professional mountain bike racer and three-time national champion.

Suzanne: I was previously an active long distance biker and triathlete. I had no known underlying health conditions.

Kellai: I'm thirty-five years old and I spent most of the beginning of this year snowboarding and working out in the gym.

Stephanie: This is my daughter Maddie. She participated in the Pfizer Covid vaccine trial.

Brianne: I received my Covid vaccine when I gladly signed up for a clinical trial here in the United States with AstraZeneca.

Ernest: I am a father of a sixteen-year-old son. I am a single parent. I raised my boy since he was a baby. We got the Pfizer vaccine because I thought it was to protect him. I thought it was the right thing to do.

Cody: I received my first dose of the Pfizer vaccine on February first. Within thirty minutes, I developed a severe stabbing headache that became a burning sensation in the back of my neck.

Stephanie: In less than twelve hours, she developed severe abdominal pain, horrible nausea, painful electric shocks in her spine and neck. She had severe chest pain. The way she described it, it felt like her heart was being pulled out of her neck.

Shaun: I got right facial tingling, back numbness, throat tightness, tachycardia, wild fluctuating blood pressure, severe right-sided headaches and brain fog.

Suzanna: I am intermittently dizzy; my vision is blurry; my right pupil is not dilating properly; my right leg has extreme burning pain; and I also get muscle spasms and twitches.

Doug: I went to bed at ten o'clock that night. I woke up at two o'clock in the morning, paralyzed. I had a blood clot in my leg. My entire spinal chord had swollen and hemorrhaged.

Ernest: They said it was safe. Now, I go home to an empty house.

Cody: Two days after vaccination, I got in my airplane to do a job that would take only a few hours. Immediately after taking off, I knew something was not right with me. I pulled my airplane up to turn around, and felt an extreme burst of pressure in my ears. Instantly, I was nearly blacked out, dizzy, disoriented, nauseous, and shaking uncontrollably. By the grace of God, I was able to land my plane without incident, although I do not remember doing this. I've had six spinal taps over eight months to monitor my intracranial pressure, and two surgeries, eight weeks apart, to repair the fistulas. My condition continues to decline, and my doctors told me that only an adverse reaction to the vaccine or a major head trauma could have caused this much spontaneous damage.

Dr. Wallskog: I soon saw a neurologist, who diagnosed me with transverse myelitis, a rare condition that involves a demyelinated lesion of my thoracic spinal chord.

Suzanna: I see a neurologist, rheumatologist, cardiologist, gynecologist, neuro- ophthalmologist, and physical therapist, among others.

Kellai: I lost my ability to speak naturally. I have become unable to walk without a walker. I never know if or when the tremors will come or go. I can no longer cook, clean, or even pick up and hold my baby for too long before my body begins to shake uncontrollably or is thrown into excruciating amounts of pain.

Stephanie: She can't walk. She is in a wheelchair. She has a feeding tube for all of her nutrition. She has constant pain in her stomach, back, and neck. She can't feel her legs. And that's just the tip of the iceberg.

Doug: Today, I am an unemployed paraplegic who is learning an entire new lifestyle, and the only thing I did between full health and my current condition was to take a shot.

Kyle: I've been bedridden, unable to work or exercise for months. I fear that my career has officially been ended.

Cody: I don't know if I will ever be able to fly an airplane again. This vaccine has taken my career from me, and the future I have worked so hard to build.

Dr. Wallskog: My career of nineteen years that I took almost fourteen years to train for is likely over.

Stephanie: They did everything in their power to hide everything that happened to her, and that is why this is happening to all these other people and kids.

Ernest: They murdered my son. And these other people that are suffering, these kids, with all these side effects: that's child abuse, right there. I mean, why isn't something being done?

Dr. Wallskog: Assuming the FDA and the CDC would be alarmed at my diagnosis, I expected to be contacted soon after my VAERS submission. No phone call. No contact. In fact, weeks passed. I then contacted the CDC myself. They acknowledged my VAERS submission but stated my reaction was categorized as "not serious" as I had not been hospitalized and I had not died. One word describes how I felt in the months after my diagnosis: abandoned.

Brianne: We did video conferences with Peter Marks and Janet Woodcock, constant emails with Janet Woodcock and myself, directly. We have literally asked, and we have begged, repeatedly, for them to acknowledge these reactions. They declined.

Shaun: This experience has shattered my life [looks toward the others on the panel], like all of you. I know where you are. The injuries have robbed me of every moment of silence and peace. The impact on my medical career, which I love and worked so hard for, is immeasurable.

Kellai: I deserve to be heard, and treated with compassion, but instead I have been called a liar and a fake, and have even been told by the ER doctors that this is all in my head, and that there was nothing medically wrong with me.

Aaron Siri, Esq.: Among the folks that have contacted our firm are many physicians from across the country who themselves have suffered vaccine injuries. One of the things I often ask physicians who contact the firm is: will you make public the failing of our public health agencies? And that often elicits the same reaction as well. That is one of *immense* fear. The fear of retaliation from public health officials and the medical establishment.

Lt. Col. Long: After I reported to my command my concerns that, in one morning, I had to ground three out of three pilots due to vaccine injuries, the next day my patients were cancelled, my charts were pulled for review, and I was told I would not be seeing acute patients anymore.

Aaron Siri, Esq.: Everybody sitting here today—all of the physicians, the medical professionals, the PhDs who are attending today: their career is on the line to come and do this. It should not be that any physician should have to, quote unquote, "risk it all," just to advocate for their patients.

Dr. Levi: I know many mainstream scientists and medical professionals who, like me, think that the current narrative is extreme and wrong, but very few of them are willing to speak up. Any attempt to deviate from the main narrative today is faced with a wall of hostility, rejection, and even elimination from the government (including funding agencies), from public media, and, worst of all, from the scientific community itself.

Dr. Kaplan: Legitimate scientific challenges have been set aside or dismissed as quote—"misinformation"—unquote. I worry that young scientists may be worried to disclose evidence on vaccine harms. Being labeled as an "anti-vaxxer" could be a career ender.

Dr. Doshi: I am saddened that we are supersaturated as a society right now in the attitude that "everybody knows." But if hospitalizations and deaths were happening almost exclusively in the unvaccinated, why would booster shots be necessary? There's something not adding up, and we should *all* be asking: "*Is* this a pandemic of the unvaccinated?"

Kim Witczak: People should not be coerced or bribed to choose between their freedom to bodily autonomy or their livelihood and being injected. This is a human rights social justice issue.

Kellai: For everyone suffering, for everyone being pushed, guilted, and frightened into taking this thing, or not taking this thing: I see you, I hear you, I believe you, I love you, I am you.

Ernest: Once we leave here, they're going to forget about what we said here. I am going to spend Thanksgiving at the cemetery, Christmas, at that cemetery.

Shaun: I will continue to fight; I will continue to research; I will find an answer for people, or I will die trying.

Brianne: I would like to finish with a letter from a friend: "Dear Bri: I cannot take this any longer. This has taken everything away from me: my career, my family, my life. My body will not stop attacking itself, and this is beyond the worst amount of torture. They have further erased my very existence. Please accept my apologies. I must bid farewell to this world. Please tell our stories. Please make sure the world knows the cruelty imposed upon us. Goodbye, my dear friend. I will see you on the flip side. If the government won't help us, if the drug companies won't help us, *who* will help us?"

Chapter 33

THE MATRIX

Regardless of any and all other considerations, the tragic incidence of vaccine injury and death, occurring in numbers dwarfing all historic precedent, should in and of itself constitute sufficient reason to repudiate Covid vaccine mandates. No statistical number game can justify coercing a human being to risk the kind of life-altering injury or death represented by the persons on the panel, and the tens or hundreds of thousand others for whom they stand.

That truth should be self-evident.

Even so, numerous well-meaning persons —including many, such as President Biden and Governor Gavin Newsom, in positions of power—imagine mandates to be anything but unethical. On the contrary, such persons view vaccine mandates as just and righteous means of alleviating suffering and saving lives. I believe, however, that they can only maintain that position by committing the very act of violence so bitterly lamented by vaccine-injured persons themselves: namely, the act of *denying their existence altogether.*

Denial is a well-recognized psychological defense mechanism, one predicated upon a person's refusal—on account of motives largely or wholly unconscious—to acknowledge some objective reality. Because acceptance of the unwelcome truth contradicts some image or idea a person has fixed upon as integral to their very identity, that truth qualifies as psychologically intolerable. The soul cannot reconcile itself to this fact of existence, and so simply denies it, continuing to feel, think, and act in accord—not with objective reality—but the constructed universe to which it tenaciously clings.

Today, many persons have so internalized the notions that the vaccines are safe and effective and represent our best—if not our only— hope of overcoming the pandemic, that, under the guise of "misinformation" or other convenient fictions, they simply discount as illusory a whole host of objective facts that belie that position. First and foremost among these is the very existence of thousands upon thousands of human beings whose lives have been largely destroyed by the same injections the vaccine proponents invest with salvific power.

Is it rational to deny the horrific experience of so many vaccine-injured (and vaccine-killed) persons in the face of all the empirical evidence to the contrary, a small sample of which was displayed at Senator Johnson's panel? No, and any convoluted attempt to make it appear so only magnifies the patent senselessness so grotesquely on display. Maddy De Garay, in a wheelchair and dependent on a feeding tube, diagnosed with a stomach ache; Dr. Wallskog, suffering from transverse myelitis that ended his nineteen-year old professional career, told that his condition had been categorized as "not serious"; Kellai Rodriguez, whose constant tremors visibly render her unable, even, to speak normally, being told that her malady is all in her head and threatened with committal to a psychiatric ward; Brianna Dresser, volunteer in a clinical trial, discovering that, not only had the life she had known been ruined, but that her case (and so the adverse event warning that *should* figure into the trial's evaluation of the *safety* of the vaccine) had been dropped from the study results because—as she was debilitated after the first shot—she had not officially "finished" the trial.

All of this points, not to anything remotely resembling "science" or common sense, but to the sway of a tyrannical pyramid of power, some invisible matrix whose agents are among us, and that has colonized and deputized the psyche of the populace at large to imagine the illusory world it projects, its masterpiece of scientific make-believe, to be reality itself. As many of the panel witnesses so pointedly put it, people at large are *afraid* of seeing things in any other way, in part because they themselves may well be invested in that reality, and in part because they are terrified of being terminated—their own lives destroyed—if they bear witness to the truth that, for those who do not turn away, is always there in plain sight.

Another facet of this illusory reality makes the sacrifice of the vaccine-injured all the more tragic. One could, perhaps, begin to make *some* moral sense of the fate of the vaccine-injured *if* the vaccines actually worked. Yet weighty new evidence confirms what more and more persons are beginning to acknowledge: they don't, but instead just make things worse.

As Senator Johnson rightly stated, if the vaccines were truly an effective answer to the pandemic, Covid-19—after surging at the end of 2020, and naturally going into decline at the beginning of this year—would have been vanquished by the vaccine program inaugurated around the same time. Yet we all know that this is a far cry from what has actually transpired. Covid continues to plague society and degrade human life today, nor are there visible signs of its disappearance anytime soon. Indeed, quite the contrary is the case.

Despite aggressive mass vaccination campaigns, the United States, as well as other developed nations that have achieved still higher vaccination rates, saw cases surge in the summer of 2021 and reach disturbingly high plateaus: numbers comparable to or even greater than those registered before the vaccination campaign kicked into high gear. True, the U.S. has saw some tailing off again in October 2021, but, over the last several weeks that hopeful trend has begun to reverse

California, and the Bay Area in particular, can boast of one of the most aggressive vaccination campaigns in the country. Yet just yesterday, on November 10, the *San Francisco Chronicle* front-page headlines read, "State's COVID-19 Rate at 'Worrisome' Levels: Progress Stalls as Cases, Hospitalizations, Deaths Rise." The article begins:

> California's progress against the COVID-19 pandemic appears to have stalled and reversed course, as new cases, hospitalizations and deaths are once again trending upward across the state. "It's not subtle, that's for sure," said Dr. George Rutherford, an epidemiologist at the UCSF. "The numbers are increasing. Cases are up over the past three weeks."[376]

News from Europe confirms the troubling trend. In the "Around the World" section of the same issue of the *Chronicle*, you will read:

> Amid an autumn surge across much of Europe, the seven-day rolling average of daily new cases in the Netherlands has almost doubled over the past two weeks from 30.88 to 61.12 new cases per 100,000 people despite more than 80% of the adult population being fully vaccinated.[377]

Does not common sense tell us that data such as this clearly indicates that mass vaccination fails—dismally—to stop the spread of Covid, that it *cannot* serve as the lynchpin of an effective strategy to ending or even controlling the pandemic?

Today, November 11, 2021, the headline of the same section in the *Chronicle* reads: "WHO Says Cases Ebb Everywhere Except in Europe." Vaccination rates are generally relatively high in Europe, yet countries such as The Netherlands, the UK, and Germany—along with the U.S.—recorded the highest increase in Covid cases (on a percentage basis) in the world. On the other hand, the penultimate paragraph of the article reads:

> In Southeast Asia and Africa, COVID-19 deaths declined by about a third, despite the lack of vaccines in those regions.[378]

We are reading this in the *San Francisco Chronicle*, a paper so pro-vaccine that most of its Covid articles read more like pharmaceutical company propaganda than objective journalism. Yet, even so, there it is: high and climbing case rates in well-vaccinated nations, and precipitously dropping numbers in regions of the world characterized by much lower vaccination rates.

The conclusion any rational mind would draw from such information is obvious. Yet, as I have suggested, the world at large—and most especially our "health experts" and the politicians taking their cues from them—are not functioning rationally, but are caught in a rigidly controlled matrix of belief that renders minds and hearts largely impervious to fact and to reason. The same *Chronicle* article headlining the reversal of California's Covid progress ends, all too predictably, with a health expert suggesting that Californians continue to hit their collective head ever harder against the same brick wall:

> "We have three things in front of us that we can do right now," said Rutherford. "We need to get people boosted—of the things that are doable, that might be the most important. We need to get 5- to 11-year-olds vaccinated. And then we need to get people who are not vaccinated yet vaccinated."[379]

Talk about a one-track mind! Such is the reality of life in the matrix.

Of course, to the readers of this book, this recent trend should not be surprising because it is entirely in accord with the line of thinking sketched out by Dr. Geert Vanden Bossche and others aware of the hazards of mass vaccination. In fact, a paper just out from a study conducted in—tellingly—the San Francisco Bay Area region, provides (for the first time, I believe) dramatic empirical validation, *at the genomic level*, of Vanden Bossche's *theoretical* understanding of the dynamics of viral evolution.

The study, "Predominance of antibody-resistant SARS-CoV-2 variants in vaccine breakthrough cases from the San Francisco Bay Area,"[380] employed whole-genome sequencing techniques to analyze the variant profiles of 1,373 PCR-positive Covid-19 cases from San Francisco County from February 1 through June 30, 2021. This is precisely the period of the vaccine rollout, and, in those five months, the percent of the eligible population vaccinated in the county increased from two to seventy percent. Over the same period of time, the percentage of vaccine breakthrough cases in the study population increased from zero percent (primarily because almost no persons were vaccinated at the beginning of the study) to 31.8 percent—a dramatic increase reflecting not only the obvious fact that breakthrough cases appear only when a non-negligible portion of the population are vaccinees, but, as well, the dramatic upsurge in vaccine-resistant strains of Covid, especially that of Delta in June.

The findings of the study not only confirm that vaccinated individuals do contract and transmit viral infection but—more critically here—corroborate Vanden Bossche's principled insistence that *mass vaccination with a "leaky," imperfect product creates selective pressures that favor the rise of vaccine-resistant strains of Covid-19*. According to the study's abstract:

> Fully vaccinated were more likely that unvaccinated persons to be infected by variants carrying mutations associated with decreased antibody neutralization.... Differences in viral loads were non-significant between unvaccinated and fully vaccinated persons overall.... These findings suggests that vaccine breakthrough cases are preferentially caused by circulating antibody-resistant SARS-CoV-2 variants, and that symptomatic breakthrough infections may potentially transmit COVID-19 as efficiently as unvaccinated infections, regardless of the infecting lineage.[381]

The body of the paper fleshes out the crucial points:

> The proportion of antibody-resistant variants...increased from 40% to 89% while the proportion of variants with increased infectivity increased from 49% to 94%. *In unvaccinated cases, most viruses consisted of non-resistant variants* (61% and 57% based on community and UCSF testing, respectively) *in contrast to vaccinated cases, for which the proportions of non-resistant variants dropped to 34% and 20%* respectively.
>
> Overall, fully vaccinated cases were significantly more likely than unvaccinated cases to be infected by resistant variants (77.6% versus 47.7%).... Infections by the Gamma and Delta variants, which cause more pronounced decreases in Ab neutralization...were increased in fully vaccinated breakthrough infections as compared to unvaccinated infections. In contrast, variant distribution in unvaccinated cases, with alpha and epsilon predominant, was similar to estimates of prevalence locally in the community and in the state of California during the study period.[382]

What this means is that the more infectious and aggressive Delta strain gained its foothold and rose to its present dominance precisely *because* mass vaccination drove viral evolution in this direction. In the unvaccinated population, Delta did *not* surge, as it enjoyed no selective advantage over other, far more common and less infectious strains, including Alpha. The study includes a revealing graph that displays the relative prevalence of each of the variant strains (Alpha, Delta, Gamma, Iota, Epsilon, and others) in both the vaccinated and unvaccinated test subjects. Among the unvaccinated, only five percent of the test subjects were infected by Delta strains of Covid-19. Among the vaccinated breakthroughs, on the other hand, thirty-five percent of those infected carried Delta, so that *Delta appeared seven times more prevalent in the vaccinated than in the unvaccinated population.*

To my mind, this suggests that *if* the mass vaccination program had never been inaugurated, we would never have seen the surge of the more infectious, antibody-resistant Delta variant. Instead, our own immune systems, which were most likely already getting a handle on Alpha, would have naturally gained the upper hand, *especially if public health officials had promoted good health practices and effective early treatment as per the biodynamic model of Covid response.* Instead, our dysfunctional Vaccine-Distance system has made the entire situation immeasurably worse, saddling us—as the first, but surely not last, fruit of the Vaccine–Distance program—with the more difficult and dangerous Delta variant.

As Geert Vanden Bossche said right from the beginning, the whole enterprise of mass vaccination, undertaken in the midst of a pandemic, with a nonlethal vaccine, is nothing less than a "colossal blunder."

It was so in the beginning, and is so no less now, because the present policy of ever more and, inevitably, ever more imperfect vaccination, including boosters and the vaccination of children and younger populations, promises to multiply that error and its negative consequences.

More of the same from the San Francisco study:

> The predominance of immune-evading variants among breakthrough cases indicates *selective pressure for immune-resistant variants locally over time in the vaccinated population concurrent with ongoing viral circulation in the community.* In particular, the Delta variant, which is the predominant circulating lineage in the United States as of July 2021, has been shown to be *resistant to vaccine-induced immunity* as well as being more infectious than Alpha (emphasis mine).[383]

After citing additional data disclosing equivalent viral load in vaccinated and unvaccinated individuals, the study continues:

> These data suggest that symptomatic breakthrough cases are as infectious as symptomatic unvaccinated cases, and likely *contribute to ongoing SARS-CoV-2 transmission, even in a highly vaccinated community* (emphasis mine).[384]

And finally the study closes with a summary that says it all:

> In summary, our results reveal that *selection pressure in a highly vaccinated community* (>71% fully vaccinated as of early August 2021*) favors more infectious, antibody-resistant* VOCs such as the Gamma and Delta variants, and that *high-titer symptomatic post-vaccination infections may be a contributor to viral spread.* Concerns have also been raised regarding waning immunity resulting in decreased effectiveness of the vaccine in preventing symptomatic infection over time. Combined with other potential factors such as relaxation of COVID-19 restrictions and complacency due to "pandemic fatigue," these data may explain the recent steep rise in COVID-19 cases in San Francisco County and nationwide in July–August 2021. Targeted *booster vaccinations* for vulnerable populations, potentially guided by monitoring of immune correlates of vaccine efficacy, *will likely be needed in the near future to control viral spread in the community* (emphasis mine).[385]

This summary supplies a snapshot of the future awaiting us under the present Vaccine-Distance regime: 1) claims of vaccine safety and efficacy clashing with an ever-rising toll of vaccine injuries and deaths, 2) a continually waning vaccine-induced immunity that triggers calls for more and more boosters, and 3) the maintenance and intensification of contagion control methods such as masking, distancing, and lockdowns. The unending State of Emergency inevitably elicits calls for repressive vaccine mandates and other restrictions, spelling an end to anything remotely resembling a free society, especially for those who, refusing vaccination and other measures, resist what promises to become an increasingly authoritarian regime.

That is our future if we persist on our present course, a future that is, in fact, *happening now*, in of all places, France, America's own Sister-in-Revolution, the Republic born in the name of *liberté, égalité*, and *fraternité*—a nation where you will presently find these high ideals dragged in the dust, like erstwhile enemies of the Revolution, down stately boulevards in Paris or Marseille. In France, and for some months already, you must have a vaccine pass to participate at all in public life—to ride a bus, eat in a restaurant, enter a grocery store. And to what avail? Just yesterday I heard on National Public Radio that not only have such "emergency measures" been extended for *a full year*, but the French government is once again requiring children to wear masks indoors in schools, while (as is already the case with the *entire* population in Israel), those over sixty-five years of age must get a third booster shot in order to pass as "fully vaccinated" and so participate in society.

Here in America, there is still time to "hold the line" by resisting Covid-19 vaccine mandates. Such mandates are not the beginning, and will certainly not be the end, of governmental restrictions of individual rights and freedoms. Even so, they are currently the most visible and pivotal signature of that matrix that is, even as we speak, continuing to fabricate what *appears to be* and *is presented as* the objective reality of the world today, but is in fact the deception-ridden projection of a determinate network of power.

As Americans, our principal task today is to *see through* the illusions implicit in and instrumental to the program of that matrix, and so begin to reclaim the power of government in the name of We, the People. That effort, even if only partially successful, could catalyze significant political transformation. Since the foundation of such a movement need be consonant with that of America itself, and so be grounded in the dignity and sovereignty of the individual citizen, there could hardly be a better place to begin than with advocacy for *public acknowledgment of the vaccine-injured,* the effective non-existence of whom constitutes the indispensable center of the network of illusion projected by the current regime.

The lives of the vaccine-injured: Black and white, yellow and brown, red, blue, and purple...*matter*. Don't let the matrix convince you that they don't.

CHAPTER 34

FANTASY FOOTBALL: PITCHING THE NEW NORMAL

The controlling Covid narrative has a new twist. I detected its appearance by virtue of unexpected finds in two newspapers notorious (in my book, anyway) for relentlessly beating the Covid war drums. David Leonhardt's piece "Good morning. Is it time to start moving back to normalcy?" appeared in the November 12, 2021, *New York Times*.[386] Monica Gandhi's opinion piece, appearing in the November 13, 2021, issue of the *San Francisco Chronicle,* sports the title "Don't worry, COVID outbreaks are the new normal."[387]

Yes, you read that correctly. That *is* provocative, is it not? For the last twenty months, the words "Covid" and "normal" would be no more likely seen standing amicably side by side in the same sentence than would the ghosts of Adolf Hitler and Yitzhak Rabin strolling peaceably together down the streets of *Unter den Linden.*

Evidently, though, the more things stay the same, the more they change.

The respective titles of the two articles both feature the key concept that affiliates them and characterizes the new strain: *normalcy.* For the moment, let's leave the spicier Gandhi article aside and listen to what David Leonhardt, by way of a San Francisco physician, has to offer on the subject:

> Among the Covid experts I regularly talk with, Dr. Robert Wachter is one of the more cautious. He worries about "long Covid," and he believes that many people should receive booster shots. He says that he may wear a mask in supermarkets and on airplanes for the rest of his life.
>
> Yet Wachter—the chair of the medicine department at the University of California, San Francisco—also worries about the downsides of organizing our lives around Covid. In recent weeks, he has begun to think about when most of life's rhythms should start returning to normal. Increasingly, he believes the answer is: *now.*
>
> This belief stems from the fact that the virus is unlikely to go away, ever. Like most viruses, it will probably keep circulating, with cases rising sometimes and falling other times, but we have the tools—vaccines, along with an emerging group of treatments—to turn it into a manageable virus, similar to the seasonal flu.

Given this reality, Wachter, who's 64, has decided to resume more of his old activities and accept the additional risk that comes with them, much as we accept the risk of crashes when riding in vehicles.[388]

The marked lack of hysteria, the calm tone so contrary to the fear-mongering characteristic of the mainstream press for the last twenty months, represents a welcome sea change, one that clashes with a mildly alarmist *San Francisco Chronicle* headline from just two day before ("State's COVID-19 rate at 'worrisome' levels: Progress stalls as cases, hospitalizations, deaths rise"[389]). Never fear, though, brave knights and ladies of "the new normal"! Monica Ghandi, another UCSF medical expert, has an answer, of sorts. To understand it, though, we need to ignore the general cause of concern announced in that worrisome *Chronicle* headline and focus, for the moment, on the specific health crisis that elicited Ghandi's surprising Covid sally.

In California, the annual college football game between the Cal Bears (representing the University of California at Berkeley) and the Trojans (representing the University of Southern California) is a big deal. The game was originally scheduled to be played on November 13, 2021. It was, however, postponed until a more propitious date: December 4th. Why? Was it because the football players, all avid readers of that great poet Rainer Maria Rilke, wanted to celebrate the bard by doing battle on his 146th birthday?

Alas, no. Rather, in the run-up to their November 6 game against Arizona, several Cal players exhibited Covid symptoms. Ultimately, University Health Services required the whole team to undergo Covid testing not long after that game. Despite a ninety-nine percent vaccination rate in the program, no less than forty-four athletes and staff tested positive for Covid-19.

More often than not, the swift-footed Trojans thrash the Bears even when both teams enjoy full health. Can you imagine what the score might have been if all those lumbering Cal Bears were slowed down still more by Covid?

Seriously, though, a COVID outbreak is no laughing matter, even if the great majority of those who tested positive showed little or no signs of sickness. At least, in the days of old, it certainly was not anything that any socially respected medical professional shrugged off. Perhaps, though, Monica Gandhi is an avid football fan, and was unhappy to see the grand rivalry game postponed. According to her new version of the narrative, a little outbreak here or there is, after all (unlike that football game), really nothing to get too excited about. Ghandi:

> The cancellation of a highly anticipated game like this one due to COVID-19 has led to online speculation—fueled by scary headlines—about dwindling efficacy of vaccination and a return to the conditions that led to last year's deadly winter surge.
>
> But, in truth, clusters of mostly asymptomatic cases among the vaccinated, like what we're seeing at Cal, are neither cause for concern, nor unexpected with a virus that will become endemic. They are an emerging part of our new normal. And we need to start recognizing—and more important—speaking about them as such.[390]

There you have it, the punch line of this novel strain of coronavirus story: *"our new normal"*—a life, as Dr. Wachter suggests, no longer characterized by exhausting end runs to evade a Covid blitz, or continual fear of the bone-crunching tackle that might just take you out for good.

Lest there be any doubt as to what makes this more laid back, confident-in-the-pocket, "new normal" possible, Dr. Gandhi gives us the dope straight:

> Vaccines changed the game and have proven themselves to be highly effective in preventing serious illness and death from COVID-19. Because of that, what we need now is a shift in the way those in the media and in prominent public health positions think about asymptomatic or mildly symptomatic cases.[391]

Moving, now, downfield, the last para of Gandhi's piece circles back to the theme of normalcy to deliver her narrative touchdown:

> Young people have been restricted during the pandemic in the United States—despite being less at risk for severe illness—in order to protect others. We owe it to them return their lives to normal, especially when that was the promise of public health officials in the context of vaccine mandates at many colleges and universities. Football (an outside activity) was shown to be safe and lead to no transmissions in a study from last year, prior to vaccinations and in areas of high community transmission. It is too late for this Cal-USC football game, but we need to think of outbreaks differently from now on in the context of the vaccines and live our lives accordingly.[392]

I welcome the refreshing temperance exhibited by both Wachter and Ghandi, and desire a return to a kind of "normalcy" as fervently as anyone. Excessive testing and overly restrictive measures motivated more by blanket fear than objective logic certainly need be tossed from the playbook if we are to gain ground in the endeavor to reclaim more truly human lives. Even so,

I take serious issue with these op-ed writers, not because I do not think the time to reassert a kind of normalcy is, indeed, *now*, but because the premises implicit in their reclamation project do not, in my mind, jibe with either scientific truth or any code of ethics commensurate with democratic society.

Why?

Because mass and even compulsory vaccination (even while downgraded from panacea to principal tool) still figures as the indispensable center and ground of this new variant of the old controlling Covid narrative, and the imagination of what vaccination supposedly does (and what it supposedly does not do) are, in my book, steeped in that same net of illusion that should, by now, be all too familiar to all my readers. Wachter and Ghandi, far from quarterbacking the Superbowl, are rather playing Fantasy Football.

The first questionable premises pertain to the issue of vaccine efficacy. Gandhi confidently declares "Vaccines...have proven themselves to be highly effective in preventing serious illness and death." Numbers relevant to this point, as I have discussed, are hardly unequivocal. I will not dive back into the data weeds here, but, as long as we are playing gridiron games, let's go over to the NFL for some observable evidence to the contrary.

As many people know, Green Bay Packer superstar quarterback Aaron Rogers declined vaccination, and embarked upon his own (confidential) protocol of Covid "immunization," for which he was widely vilified (not to mention fined some $14,000) when he did, in fact, contract Covid and the story spilled.[393] Did Roger's game plan fail? By Gandhi's own standards, no, not really. Whatever Rogers did evidently aided his own general fitness and robust immune response, because, along with the ivermectin he reportedly took, he recovered quickly, and will be back in action after missing only a single outing.

On the other hand, it may be that only avid football fans know that Covid-19 has recently plagued one of the Packer's rivals in the NFC North: the Minnesota Vikings. The team's vigilance regarding vaccination notwithstanding, a Covid outbreak rendered at least five of its players temporarily inactive. Fully vaccinated starting center Garrett Bradbury, for instance, missed the Viking's November 7, 2021, overtime loss to the Baltimore Ravens on account of a breakthrough case, and was placed on the teams reserve/Covid-19 list, as was Harrison Smith, a defensive back. Worst of all, two days later offensive lineman Dakota Dozier was taken to the emergency room on account of Covid complications. According to Mike Zimmer, the Viking's coach, Dozier was experiencing trouble breathing. Dozier, too, was fully vaccinated.[394]

Our sample size here is, admittedly, tiny. Nonetheless, it is fair to ask: if the Covid vaccines genuinely are so highly effective at preventing hospitalization and death, why is it that it is the fully vaccinated Dakota Dozier who ends up in the ER while unvaccinated Aaron Rodgers, who followed another protocol and used ivermectin, brushes off the illness with little difficulty?

Individual differences, of course, are most likely important. In the last analysis, though, that is just one more reason why sweeping statements as to vaccine efficacy and one-size-fits all regimes can hardly be trusted. Do you think Aaron Rogers, for one, regrets punting on the vaccine? I imagine he considers $14,000 a cheap price to pay to preserve not only his best health but, as well, his own personal integrity and freedom.

So much for this aspect of vaccine (in)efficacy. Here is Gandhi's highly dubious assertion of another one: "Vaccines reduce transmission. Those who are vaccinated are less likely to get infected in the first place, and if they do, are less likely to spread the disease."[395] Gandhi does cite several studies in support of this contention which, however, contradict other evidence cited earlier in this book. Again, I do not wish to go into further data analysis here, but will merely observe that what Gandhi is speaking about—general probability of infection and transmission—is nothing other than what Geert Vanden Bossche understands as "infectious pressure."

Can we identify the ground of the difference between Gandhi's and Vanden Bossche's understanding of the situation here? Yes, readily so, as it harkens back to a fundamental point I have repeatedly stressed. The thinking underlying the controlling Covid narrative, whether this be in its older "legacy" form or this novel "new normal" variant, inclines toward the singularly myopic insofar as it disregards the complex dynamics of shifting immunological conditions and viral evolution.

On principle, it can hardly be legitimate to claim, as Gandhi does, that vaccination does such and such...*as if* conditions at one point in time remained permanently in force. Multiple studies show that vaccine efficacy fades dramatically over time, and the evolution of resistant variants, driven by mass vaccination itself, inevitably materially alter all calculations of benefit and risk. The state of the world today, with highly vaccinated countries often faring much worse than those lightly vaccinated, and indeed (as reportedly is the case in the Netherlands, Germany, and Austria) on the verge of new crises, problemizes Wachter and Gandhi's tranquilizing diagnoses.

It is thus legitimate to question whether the "new normal" pitched by these San Francisco doctors represents a reliable report on the state of the nation and the world, or will rather prove a passing figment of scientific imagination.

Its dubious veracity, however, is not all that is wrong with the "new normal" spin on the controlling Covid narrative. The core of this story—namely, "safe and effective" vaccines as the lynchpin of Covid response—remains the same, and the articles' vision of "the new normal" takes as its premise nigh universal vaccination on the one hand, and, on the other, a two-tiered society in which those who refuse to "get with the program" remain *personae non gratae:* outcasts, social exiles.

The model of "the new normal" does not only represent a kind of fantasyland, it doubles as a not-so-subtle sales pitch for mass and, finally, mandatory vaccination, a fact that comes to more or less explicit expression in Gandhi's tacit endorsement of vaccine mandates at colleges and universities and the athletic programs (like Cal football) associated with these institutions.

What is wrong with this picture? The answer, sadly, is everything, of course, that is wrong with the controlling narrative in the first place, including egregious denial of the fact of vaccine injury and death, *the incidence of which—on the gridiron as well as in other athletic arenas—already appears to be dramatically and tragically on the rise in the era of league-imposed vaccine mandates.*

This year, athletes of all ages, sports, and nations, are collapsing on the field or court. And this is happening to not one, two, or a handful, but to scores of them. In his recent piece "Elements of Refusal,"[396] Charles Eisenstein notes that "[a]thletes have been collapsing on the field and dying with astonishing frequency," and he offers a link to a compilation of headlines documenting forty-one collapses and twenty-three deaths in the last four months alone. The headlines are heartbreaking:

> "Virginia Union University football player dies after collapsing during practice"
>
> "Young footballer dies after West Bridgford match collapse"
>
> "Philadelphia Phillies prospect Daniel Brito collapses during game"
>
> "Princeton soccer player collapses on field, dies at the Hospital"
>
> "Rugby Player, 31, collapses and dies on pitch during memorial game"
>
> "15-year old girl McHi soccer player collapses during practices, later dies"[397]

This sample I have provided exhibits my English-language bias; the original list presented on the web includes many more international, non-English entries. In any event, the catastrophic inventory goes on and on and on.

A recent report on *The Highwire* puts the number of athlete collapses this year at seventy-five.[398]

Del Bigtree notes that there is no concrete proof of any causal connection between the incidents and vaccination. Even so, the numbers are unprecedented. What has materially changed that could logically account for the disturbing new phenomenon? To my mind, that question admits easy answer. It is only this year, 2021, that a great many athletic teams, at all levels, began mandating Covid-19 vaccinations.

In some nonfatal but serious instances, headlines leave little doubt as to cause. Jeremy Chardy is currently ranked as the fifty-ninth best tennis player in the world, but is presently unable to compete on account of vaccine injury ("Jeremy Chardy: I regret getting vaccinated. I have a series of problems now"[399]) while an Italian soccer play may never play again: ("Pedro Obiang, 29-Year Old Professional Footballer, Suffers Myocarditis after Covid-19 Vaccine; Possible End of Career"[400]). In some of the cases of on-field collapse, moreover, the circumstantial case for vaccine as cause appears particulary strong.

On June 29 of 2021, the whole West Indies Women's Cricket team got vaccinated. **@windies cricket** posted photos of the vaccination and tweeted:

> Over 30 West Indies Women and management staff are now fully vaccinated against Covid-19 with a few more scheduled to receive their second shots.
>
> WI vaccinated and ready to face Pakistan women! #vaccinatedontprocrastinate #vaccinesavelives[401]

On July 2, three days after the team vax, the Windies trotted out to play against the Pakistani cricketeers. Midway through the game, Chinelle Henry, one of the West Indies players, collapsed and suffered convulsions. Just a few minutes later, as Henry was loaded onto a stretcher for transport to the hospital, another player, Chedean Nation, similarly collapsed, suffered convulsions, and had to be rushed off to the ER in the wake of her teammate.[402]

No cause was given for the frightening course of events. Fortunately, in this instance, both players did recover.

A young footballer who also collapsed within days after vaccination was one of many who were not so fortunate. While mainstream media declined to make any connection, *The Covid World* (whose motto reads "Because Everyone's Story Should Be Heard"), harbored little doubt as to the probable cause of the fit, young man's out-of-nowhere demise:

> Roy Butler, Healthy 23-Year-Old Footballer Dies 4 Days After Receiving the J&J COVID-19 Vaccine.[403]

Nor did Marian Harte, Roy's aunt. She tweeted:

> My beautiful nephew Roy Butler, Waterford City Éire passed away today, after the miracle "jab"...I'm heartbroken and so so angry.[404]

Eileen Lorio, presumably another Waterford local, wrote:

> The people of Waterford are devastated to learn that a local hero, @ WaterfordFCie captain Roy Butler died on Monday of a massive brain bleed 3 days after getting the @JanssenUS J&J vax. He was a player, coach, mentor, beloved by friends and family. Media silent re vax. RIP.[405]

Monica Gandhi tells us that outbreaks of Covid test-positives are to be expected and need not cause undue concern. Insofar as her brave new world presumes nigh universal vaccination, I am afraid this "new normal" may involve not just a bunch of Cal Bears coming down with asymptomatic or mild cases of Covid, but, far more often than anyone would wish to believe possible, athletes collapsing and even dying on the field.

What can we expect when that occurs? Eileen Lorio said it all too well: *Media silent re vax. RIP.*

What else is new(s)?

CHAPTER 35

THE CRUMBLING WALL

Vaccine advocates who, like Gandhi and Wachter, advance the claim that the Covid-19 vaccines are effectively working to control (although not eradicate) Covid-19, may be able to point to data that appears to substantiate that position here, or there, for a relatively brief window of time. For the most part, however, the preponderance of evidence tips—or rather slams—the scale of truth and justice down on the dark, doomscroll-worthy side.

Stories spotlighting the inability of the Covid-19 vaccines to prevent infection and transmission of the disease are featured in any number of U.S. news outlets heading into the holiday season. "Vermont leads nation in new COVID cases and vaccination rate" reads a November 16 piece from ABCNews 10. Close to three-quarters of the Vermont population has been fully vaccinated (a percentage matched only by Rhode Island), yet *The New York Times* vaccine tracker reveals an eighty-two-percent rise in new cases over the last two weeks.[406] Colorado likewise represents one of the most highly vaccinated states in the country, with rates in excess of seventy percent. Yet Colorado, too, has recently experienced a steep rise in cases, a phenomena that has health authorities both baffled as well as distressed "What is driving Colorado's COVID surge? Not even the experts are sure" announces the November 5 issue of the *Colorado Sun*. The article states:

> Nationwide, coronavirus infections have declined from their peak earlier this fall, recently leveling out. But, in Colorado, one of the more heavily vaccinated states in the country, infections have risen. And no one is quite sure why.[407]

The piece contains a telling acknowledgment of the uncertainty that continues to shroud the world's Covid concerns:

> Even as Colorado approaches two years in the pandemic, there is still much the state's leading authorities on the virus do not know. That extends to the current surge in cases, which has defied expectations and conventional wisdom and placed hospitals in jeopardy of being overwhelmed, a risk many believed had long passed.[408]

The United States itself, although it has managed to persuade sixty percent of the adult population to vaccinate fully, lags well behind a number of other countries. Many of the most highly vaccinated nations in the world are found in Europe, the only region experiencing a dramatic "fifth wave" of Covid cases. Ireland furnishes a salient case in point. Despite vaccination rates topping ninety percent, Ireland's Covid case numbers are once more ominously on the rise. Just as telling, the current course of affairs in the Emerald Isle reveals that the phenomena of Covid-19 resurgence in locales boasting not only *high*, but the *highest* vaccination rates around is no strictly American phenomenon. A November 6th article in the Sky News ("COVID-19: Ireland's Co[unty] Waterford has one of the highest vaccination rates in the world—so why are cases surging?") begins:

> Waterford, in southeastern Ireland, epitomizes Ireland's coronavirus conundrum. Why is there a surge in COVID-19 cases in a nation where around 92% of all adults are fully vaccinated?

The article continues:

> New figures this week show that Co Waterford has both the highest vaccination rate and the highest Covid incidence rate in Ireland.[409]

Just how high is County Waterford's vaccination rate? About 99.5 percent. In other words, Waterford has largely achieved what President Biden can only dream about: complete vaccine coverage.

Yet that signal achievement has certainly *not* vanquished the virus. On the contrary, Waterford's residents currently find themselves, once more, under siege.

If your memory is short enough that you wonder why mention of Country Waterford rings a bell in your mind, recall that it is—or rather *was*—the home of Roy Butler, the young footballer who collapsed and fell down dead on the field in August, a stark reminder of the immediate risk of injury and death bedeviling any program of mass vaccination.

Gibraltar, a British colony off the coast of Spain, offers another sad Covid story. Believe it or not, Gibraltar's vaccination campaign has outstripped even County Waterford's. Essentially everybody in Gibraltar is double-jabbed, and when boosters and the vaccination of non-resident workers are accounted for, its vaccination rate comes in at an astounding 140 percent! Notwithstanding that blanket treatment, cases are recently on the rise; so much so that the authorities have felt compelled to play the Grinch. A November 17 UK *Express* headline blazes: "Gibraltar cancels Christmas celebrations amid COVID spike." The article informs us that:

> While the government has called upon the public to "exercise their own judgment," they have "strongly advised against any social events for at least the next four weeks, discouraging people from holding private Christmas events. Gibraltar has seen a steady increase in active cases of COVID-19 throughout October and November, which has gained pace over the past few days.
>
> Health Minister…Samantha Sacramento described the increase in case numbers as "drastic," encouraging people to come forward to receive their booster vaccine. The government has advised members of the public to wear masks, avoid large gatherings and maintain social distancing.[410]

Is this Wachter and Gandhi's "new normal"? No Christmas, masks, and unending "social distance"?

Even that, however, is not the worst of it. Other European nations experiencing a fifth wave have felt compelled to take yet more desperate measures. Just a few days ago, Austria announced a European first: lock down of—exclusively—unvaccinated persons.[411] No sooner, however had the order been announced, than it was revoked in favor of—once again—a total lockdown, in force for all, vaccinated and unvaccinated alike.

This is a less discriminatory measure, yet one hardly less repugnant to the population as a whole, and should serve as a kind of death blow to the fantasy that Covid-19 vaccines can be counted upon to make things right with the world. *Rather, the course of world affairs offers powerful confirmation of my analysis of the synergistic deficiencies of the Vaccine-Distance system response.* Vaccination failure drives both unchecked intensification (via vaccination of younger age groups and boosters) of the vaccine program itself *as well as* recurrent restrictive "contagion control" measures—culminating in total lock down—and vice versa. The entire strategically, tactically, and cybernetically defective system consequently results in "*persistent and often intensifying iteration of deficient response mechanisms*" that do not advance toward the goal of ending or even controlling the pandemic.

Vaccine proponents tend stubbornly to refuse to see matters in this dark light, but rather continue to find reasons to dispute such frightful conclusion. The likes of Wachter and Gandhi would undoubtedly call attention to the closing paragraphs of *The Sun's* article, which disclose that—whereas two-thirds of Coloradans are vaccinated, unvaccinated persons account for roughly that same proportion of the new Covid cases, supporting the contention that the vaccines, though indeed imperfect, do offer significant reduction in the risk of infection and thus transmission. Perhaps even more important, *The Sun* additionally states that unvaccinated Coloradans are hospitalized for Covid at four-and-a-half times the rate of the vaccinated, evidently substantiating the claim that—despite the recent surge—the Covid vaccines continue to provide potent protection against hospitalization and death.[412]

Some fighting Irishmen likewise jump on the pro-vax bandwagon, as demonstrated by the latter portions of the article on Country Waterford. The most relevant section reads:

> The current wave of infections (with daily numbers at their highest since January) differs from last winter's because of Ireland's successful vaccination rollout. Hospitalization figures, and intensive care unit admissions, are stable and decreasing slightly in recent days. It's widely accepted the "vaccine wall" has driven serious illness and death figures down.
>
> Some scientists feel that any public frustration with the high incidence rates is based on a misunderstanding of what the vaccines were supposed to achieve. "The functions of the vaccine is to stop illness and death, that's the primary goal, and the vaccines are holding up, it's great." That's the view of Professor Luke O'Neill, an immunologist at Trinity College Dublin, and one of the country's best-known scientific figures during the pandemic.[413]

Professor O'Neill's assertion represents a willful twisting of the truth. Traditionally, the function of a proper vaccine is to prevent infection and disease, not merely ameliorate symptoms, and the Covid mass vaccination program was originally aggressively promoted as a means to that definitive end. O'Neill's stance offers just one of numerous examples of the way unhappy developments have compelled proponents of the controlling narrative continually to "move the goalposts" to sustain their story.

Leading figures on both sides of the issue today acknowledge that whatever protection the vaccines do offer wanes—and dramatically so—over time, often plummeting toward zero in a matter of months. The protection referred to here applies not merely to incidence of disease but, as well, to incidence of serious illness and death. Evidence of that decay and its disastrous consequences has already been documented in Israel as well as other places around the world.

Recent news out of Belgium, for instance, must be disturbing for those pinning their hopes on any sort of "vaccine wall." On November 7, a Belgian news organ out of Antwerp reported that (as translated into English) "Anyone who thinks that the ICU is full of unvaccinated patients is no longer right." The report cited Dr. Kristian Deckers of the Hoofdarts-GZA (a Belgian health center) to this effect:

> Anyone who thinks that the ICU is full of unvaccinated patients is no longer right. Right now, here, we see that a majority of patients have breakthrough infections. Very different from a few weeks ago, when the majority in the ICU was still unvaccinated but right now that is not true anymore. The patients in the ICU of our hospitals in GZA, I checked it yesterday, are all vaccinated.[414]

Tangible evidence of vaccine failure, and indeed broad recognition of such, surfaces, too, in the cry for boosters sounding with increasing urgency all around the world. Gibraltar, proud bearer of the world's universal vaccination standard, cancelled Christmas in part to smooth the way for the rollout of its booster program. Just a few days ago, Boris Johnson announced the more or less inevitable. In order to be considered "fully vaccinated" in England, one will now need to secure a pass verifying that you have received not two, but three shots.[415]

United States health agencies have—in marked contrast to President Biden himself—showed rather more reluctance to embrace boosters wholeheartedly. But the continuing crisis around the nation has precipitated an increasing push for boosters, one that, again, amounts to a tacit admission of vaccine failure. On November 12, Tony Fauci, in an interview for *The New York Times Daily* podcast, signaled the likely denouement of the government's persistent adherence to the present system of response: namely, following Israel and Britain's lead, and requiring all those who wish the privileges accorded to "the fully vaccinated" to obtain boosters. Dr Fauci:

> We're starting to see waning immunity against infection, and waning immunity, in the beginning aspect, against hospitalization. And if you look at Israel, which has always been a month to a month-and-a-half ahead of us in the dynamics of the outbreak, in their vaccine response, and in every other element of the outbreak, they are seeing a waning of immunity, not only against infection, but against hospitalizations, and to some extent, death, which is starting now to involve all age groups. It isn't just the elderly. So if one looks back at this, one can say: "You know, it isn't as if

a booster is a bonus. A booster may actually be an essential part of the primary regimen that people should have.[416]

I mentioned that, not so very long ago, the FDA had shown itself to be, at best, lukewarm about recommending boosters to the general population, and indeed voted decisively (14 to 2) against doing so.. The policy that remains—nominally—in force today, though five states (Arkansas, California, Colorado, New Mexico, and West Virginia) have already willfully cast it aside.[417]

Why did the FDA show such reticence? Claims that the original regimen provide sufficient protection are fast falling by the wayside. Other notable reasons which may well have played a role in the FDA's reluctance (and certainly *should* have done so) reflect the darker side of any ambitious booster program. *More shots administered, means, inevitably, more adverse events; more vaccine-injuries and deaths.* Moreover, experience teaches that boosting always comes at an immunological cost, and—like repeated doses of any antibiotic—tends to promote increasing tolerance, or resistance, on the part of the target entity; here, Sars-CoV-2.

Now, as Covid cases spike, boosters may be all the rage, but two short months ago immunologists were less shy about spelling out the reasons why boosting—especially when repeated—may well be a very, very bad idea. Here are relevant passages from a September 15 *New York Times* piece:

> What the Israeli data show is that a booster can enhance protection for a few weeks in older adults—a result that is unsurprising, experts said, and does not indicate long-term benefit.
>
> "What I would predict will happen is that the immune response to that booster will go up, and then it will contract again," said Marion Pepper, an immunologist at the University of Washington in Seattle. "But is that three-to four-month window what we're trying to accomplish?"
>
> In younger people, officials must balance the limited benefit of a third dose with the risk of side effects like blood clots or heart problems.... And repeatedly stimulating the body's defenses can also lead to a phenomenon called "immune exhaustion," Dr. Pepper said. "There's obviously some risk in continuously trying to ramp up an immune response...If we get into this cycle of boosting every six months, it's possible that this could work against us.[418]

Boosters promise no sure way out of the dysfunction inherent in the Vaccine and Distance system of response. On the contrary, they play right into the intrinsic deficiency of the system.

It is time *now,* before this runaway train speeds further down the track, to clear our minds, flex our political muscles, and—Democrats and Republicans alike—demand that our government turn toward ways and means that can promise to bring an end to Covid pandemonium, and not stubbornly and stupidly persist in policies that promise more of the same, while violating essential human freedoms.

Even so, the power to make this change does not begin, or end, with the government, but with We, the People. Yet much of the populace still seems effectively inoculated against hearing anything other than what "health experts" have to say, declining to shoulder the obligation of independent, critically informed thought that civic responsibility demands. Vanden Bossche and others have been crying from the rooftops for months. Barely a whisper of that warning voice has penetrated the stone wall built by the matrix of powers that be.

Of late, though, winds have begun to change. Could it be that this imposing edifice—like that of the "wall" of protection afforded by the Covid-19 vaccines—may soon crumble before our eyes?

Chapter 36

THE REAL ANTHONY FAUCI

Shortly before Thanksgiving in November 2021, Robert F. Kennedy Jr.'s book *The Real Anthony Fauci* appeared. It is an impressive work supported by exhaustive research. The number of footnotes in its first, hundred-page-long chapter exceed by two hundred or so all of those so far appended to the book you are currently reading. Either Kennedy has been working on his text far longer than I have on mine, or any number of research assistants have aided and abetted his efforts, or he is superman.

In any event, the book itself should—if it is given the attention it merits—figure as a kind of milestone in the fight against the reigning Covid cabal. Here are some of Kennedy's own choice words on the topic:

> Lamentably, Dr. Fauci's failure to achieve public health goals during the COVID pandemic are not anomalous errors, but consistent with a recurrent pattern of sacrificing public health and safety on the altar of pharmaceutical profits and self-interest.... In exalting patented medicine Dr. Fauci has, throughout his long career, routinely falsified science, deceived the public and physicians, and lied about safety and efficacy....
>
> All his strategies during COVID—falsifying science to bring dangerous and ineffective drugs to market, suppressing and sabotaging competitive products that have lower profit margins even if the cost is prolonging pandemics, and losing thousands of lives—all of these share a common purpose: the myopic devotion to Pharma.... Tony Fauci does not do public health; he is a businessman, who has used his office to enrich his pharmaceutical partners and expand the reach of influence that has made him the most powerful—and despotic—doctor in human history.[419]

This is clearly a most damning allegation, and not one to which, five months before the time of this writing, I myself would have been able to respond "yea" or "nay" with any degree of real knowledge or conviction. I say "five months" because today is, indeed, five months to the day since I first sat down to write a letter to President Joe Cambray in a vain effort to head off the imposition of vaccine mandates at Pacifica, the institution under whose aegis I am currently, via Zoom, teaching my course on Rilke and American psychologist James Hillman, "The Poetic Basis of Mind," for what may be the last time.

As evidenced by my inclination to write that letter, I had already formed certain definite opinions about Covid in general, and the Covid vaccines in particular. I owed the drift of those opinions, at that time, in no small measure, to both the spiritual intuition and investigative pursuits of Monika, my wife, who began looking more deeply into the whole Covid matter long before I. Nonetheless, five months before today my knowledge on the topic was still rudimentary. I'd done only minimal research of my own, and had little real sense of the full complexity of the Covid issue. If I had read the cited sentences from Kennedy (and much else in his book) in late June 2021, I may have been inclined to credit the veracity of his statements, but I would have had little real basis for informed, independent judgment. In short, whether I may have agreed or disagreed, I could not have professed to have truly *known* what Kennedy was talking about.

Now, some hundred and fifty days later and thirty-five chapters into a book I never intended to write, I like to imagine that has changed somewhat. I have done a good deal more of my own investigation, and pursued my own critical inquiry into various facets of the Covid controversy. That effort, and the writing it has engendered, has enabled me to arrive at my own conclusions, with which—if you have acted the part of a faithful reader—you will by now yourself be well-acquainted.

How do those conclusions jibe with the tale told in *The Real Anthony Fauci*?

Reading Kennedy's opus (and especially his first, Covid-centric chapter), I find very little that is strange, and much that is all too familiar, even as he elaborates certain crucial topics in much more depth than I have. As far as the essential lineaments of the whole Covid phenomena—the organizing plot, central characters, and chief motifs proper to a *counternarrative* that contests the controlling Covid story—I find we are very much on the same page.

How does this story end? In its *official* version, it does *not* conclude with the end of the pandemic. Now, especially with the emergence of yet another "variant of concern" (Omicron) that is nowhere in sight. Nor is this end necessarily even *desired* by the matrix of powers that be, because an indefinite extension of pandemic conditions and its accompanying social psychology best serves the aims of financial enrichment and social control. Indeed, the last chapter of *this* version of the story does not culminate in the end of the pandemic, but rather with the end of democracy; with, that is, what Covid World has so vividly exhibited: an apocalyptic extinction any political and moral order premised on the principles of freedom and love.

In reflecting upon these matters in the light of Kennedy's new book, I have come to realize that the mainstream response to the Covid crisis represents nothing less than a coordinated siege on the human body, soul, and spirit, one that effectively works to undermine not one or two of the foundational stones of free society, but many of them. Below, I note six of the chief fronts of this new world war. They are: (1) the war on science; (2) the war on nature; (3) the war on medicine; (4) the war on the body and public health; (5) the war on democracy (on our democratic system of governance); and (6) the war on society. Below, I touch upon each of these in turn, not so much to rehearse the arguments already presented in the body of this book as to supplement and amplify those with choice material from *The Real Anthony Fauci*:

1. The War on Science

This features as one of the chief themes of my own book. Kennedy, too, alleges that the worldwide Covid response has systematically prostituted science, perhaps most obviously in its mishandling of the facts of the matter:

> If the COVID-19 pandemic has revealed anything, it is that public health officials have based their many calamitous directives for managing COVID-19 on vacillating and science-free beliefs about masks, lockdowns, infection and fatality rates, asymptomatic transmission, and vaccine safety and efficacy, which took every direction and sowed confusion, division and polarization among the public and media experts…
>
> Dr. Fauci's libertine approach to facts may have contributed to what, for me, was the most troubling and infuriating feature of all the public health responses to COVID. The blatant and relentless manipulation of data to serve the vaccine agenda became the apogee of a year of stunning regulatory malpractice.
>
> The shockingly low quality of virtually all relevant data pertinent to COVID-19, and the quackery, the obfuscation, the cherry-picking and blatant perversion would have scandalized , offended and humiliated every prior generation of American public health officials…The "mistakes" were always in the same direction—inflating the risks of coronavirus and the safety and efficacy of vaccines in order to stoke public fear of COVID and provoke mass compliance.[420]

2. The War on Nature

I have repeatedly emphasized that the concerted effort to entirely discredit the organic basis of health in general as well as the very idea of natural immunity in particular (so that the role of the latter may be usurped by vaccination) functions as the theoretical as well as practical core of the Vaccine-Distance system. Here is one of Kennedy's long riffs on this theme:

> I was struck, during COVID-19's early months, that America's Doctor [Anthony Fauci], apparently preoccupied with his single vaccine solution, did little in the way of telling Americans how to bolster their immune response. He never took time during his daily White House briefings from March to May 2020 to instruct Americans to avoid tobacco (smoking and e-cigarettes/vaping double death rates from COVID); to get plenty of sunlight and to maintain adequate vitamin D levels ("Nearly 60 percent of patients with COVID-19 were vitamin D deficient upon hospitalization, with men in the advanced stages of COVID-19 pneumonia showing the greatest deficit"); or to diet, exercise and lose weight (78 percent of Americans hospitalized for COVID-19 were overweight or obese). Quite the contrary, Dr. Fauci's lockdowns caused Americans to gain an average of two pounds per month and to reduce their daily steps by 27 percent. He didn't recommend avoiding sugar and soft drinks, processed foods, and chemical residues, all of which amplify inflammation, compromise immune response, and disrupt the gut biome which governs the immune system. During the centuries that science has fruitlessly sought remedies against coronavirus (aka the common cold), only zinc has repeatedly proven its efficacy in peer-reviewed studies. Zinc impedes viral replication, prophylaxing against colds and abbreviating their duration... Yet Anthony Fauci never advised Americans to increase zinc uptake following exposure to infection.
>
> Dr. Fauci's neglect of natural immune response was consistent with the pervasive hostility toward any non-vaccine intervention that characterized the federal regulatory gestalt. On April 30, 2021, Canadian Ontario College of Physicians and Surgeons threatened to delicense any doctor who prescribed non-vaccine health strategies including Vitamin D. "*They are trying to erase any notion of natural immunity,*" says Canadian vaccine researcher Dr. Jessica Rose, Ph.D., MSc, BSc (emphasis mine). "Pretty soon the incessant lies and propaganda will have successfully instilled in the masses that the only hope for staying alive is via injection, pill-popping, so in sum, no natural immunity." In a podcast interview on On October 1, 2021, *Washington Post* reporter Ashley Fetters Maloy pretended to expose "misinformation" about COVID-19 by broadcasting misinformation:

> There's a pervasive idea that your body and your immune system can be healthy enough to ward off COVID-19, which, of course, we know it's a novel coronavirus. No one's body can. No one's body is healthy enough to recognize and just totally ward this off without a vaccine.

Clearly, this is false information. Through 2020, before vaccines were available, some 99.9 percent of people's natural immune systems protected their owners from severe illness and death.[421]

3. The War on Medicine

This represents another red thread in my argument, the treatment of which culminates in the presentation and discussion of The Physician's Declaration in Part IV of this volume. Yet the Rome summit convened in September of 2021, whereas the most recent chapter of the War on Medicine commenced in earnest as soon as Covid-19 appeared in America, at which time (in part on account of Trump's endorsement of hydroxychloroquine [HCQ]) it quickly became embroiled in partisan politics. I alluded only in passing to the nefarious means by which HCQ was suppressed; Kennedy devotes an eighteen-page chapter to the sordid story. He offers like treatment of ivermectin and as well as Fauci's disastrous and indefensible promotion of the toxic pharmaceutical remdesivir.

Most important, though, remains an overview of the medically as well as morally catastrophic direction of the Vaccine-Distance program as a whole. Kennedy states:

> [Fauci's] critics argue that Dr. Fauci's "slow the spread, flatten the curve, wait for the jab" strategy—all in support of a long-term bet on unproven vaccines—represented a profound and unprecedented departure from accepted public health practice. But *most troubling were Dr. Fauci's policies of ignoring and outright suppressing the early treatment of infected patients* who were often terrified. "The Best Practices for defeating an infectious disease epidemic," says Yale epidemiologist Harvey Risch, "dictate that you quarantine and treat the sick, protect the most vulnerable, and aggressively develop repurposed therapeutic drugs, and use early treatment protocols to avoid hospitalizations."
>
> Risch is one of the leading global authorities in clinical treatment protocols.
>
> Risch points out a hard truth that should have informed our COVID control strategy: "Unless you are an island nation prepared to shut out the world, you can't stop a global viral pandemic, but you can make it less

> deadly. Our objective should have been to devise treatments that would reduce hospitalization and death. We could have easily defanged COVID-19 so that it was less lethal than a seasonal flu. We could have done that very quickly. We could have saved hundreds of thousands of lives."
>
> Dr. Peter McCullough concurs: "Using repurposed drugs, *we could have ended this pandemic by May 2020* and saved 500,000 American lives, *but for Dr. Fauci's hard-headed, tunnel vision on new vaccines and remdesivir* (all emphasis mine)."[422]

In addition to challenging Fauci's paradigm of treatment, Kennedy cites numerous distinguished doctors who pointedly object to the authority he wields, deriding what amounts to a bureaucratic takeover of the practice of medicine by practically inexperienced "health experts" who were simply not qualified to prescribe or proscribe medical practice:

> Risch, McCullough, and Kory are also among the hundreds of scientists and physicians who express shock that Dr. Fauci made no effort to identify repurposed medicines. Says Kory: "I find it appalling that there was no consultation process with treating physicians. Medicine is about consultation. You had Birx, Fauci, and Redfield doing press conferences every day and handing down these arbitrary diktats and not one of them ever treated a COVID patient or worked in an emergency room or ICU. They knew nothing."[423]

Kennedy's book, too, via the words of knowledgeable doctors, sets forth in very concrete terms how the pandemic *should* have been handled:

> Dr. McCullough argues that, as COVID czar, Dr. Fauci should have created an international communications network linking the world's 11 million frontline doctors to gather real-time tips, innovative safety protocols, and to develop the best prophylactic and early treatment practices. "He should have created hotlines and dedicated websites for medical professionals to call in with treatment questions and to consult, collect, catalogue, and propagate the latest innovations for prophylaxing vulnerable and exposed individuals, and treating early infections, so as to avert hospitalizations." Dr. Kory agrees: "The outcome we should have been trying to prevent is hospitalization. You don't just sit around and wait for an infected patient to become ill. Dr. Fauci's treatment strategies all began once all these under-medicated patients were hospitalized. By that time, it was too late for many of them. It was insane. It was perverse, It was unethical."[424]

The outrage sounded here by Dr. Kory finds resonant echo in other choice quotations that cap off a searing critique of the immorality inherent in Dr. Fauci's regime:

> Dr. Fauci's choice to deny infected Americans early treatment was not just bad public health strategy; it was, McCullough avows, "Cruelty at a population level." Says McCullough: "Never in history have doctors deliberately treated patients with this kind of barbarism."[425]

The power of that regime extends far beyond the halls of government and hospital corridors, impinging upon the very neural network of medical research and science itself. I close here with Kennedy quoting McCoullough:

> [Dr. McCullough:] "'America's Doctor' has never, to date, published anything on how to treat a COVID patient. It shocks the conscience that there is still no official protocol. Anyone who tries to publish a new treatment protocol will find themselves airtight blocked by the journals that are all under Fauci's control."[426]

4. The War on the Body and Public Health

The largely science-free, no-holds barred mass vaccination campaign that features as the centerpiece of the Fauci-led system of Covid response constitutes what may well be considered a War on the Body and Public Health, representing, as it does, a policy that recklessly endangers the health and wellbeing of countless individuals as well as the population as a whole.

I have relied on Geert Vanden Bossche's ideas pertaining to viral evolution to explain the danger mass vaccination poses at the population level. Kennedy's book makes clear, meanwhile, that Dr. Vanden Bossche was not the only one warning about the hazards of a mass vaccination program undertaken with "leaky" vaccines.

From the outset of the pandemic, the long pre-pandemic history of failure with coronavirus vaccines (remember that SARS-CoV-2 represents a novel strain of a *class* of viruses that have been around forever) inclined many vaccinologists to be skeptical of the attempt to invent a Covid-19 vaccine that might confer sterilizing immunity and thus exert "lethal pressure" on the disease. At a certain juncture, it indeed became quite clear that *none* of the candidate Covid-19 vaccines would clear that hurdle. Kennedy recalls Dr. Fauci's noteworthy response to that discouraging news:

> Instead of declaring defeat and retreating to the drawing board, Dr. Fauci cheerfully announced that none of the first generation COVID vaccines was likely to prevent transmission. The news should have cratered the entire project. Leading virologist, including Nobel Laureate Luc Montagnier, pointed out that a non-sterilizing, or "leaky," vaccine could not arrest transmission and would therefore fail to stop the pandemic. Even worse, vaccinated individuals, he warned, would become asymptomatic carriers and "mutant factories" blasting out vaccine-resistant versions of the disease that were likely to lengthen and intensify rather than abbreviate the pandemic...[And] Dr. Peter McCullough warned that mass vaccination with a leaky vaccine during a pandemic "would put the world on a never-ending booster treadmill."[427]

The Real Anthony Fauci additionally provides a lucid exposition of one of the chief hazards haunting any mass vaccination program, namely antibody-dependent enhancement. There exists, in fact, a variety of means by which vaccination can seriously compromise (rather than enhance) our immunological defenses. I have tended to foreground the manner in which vaccination can suppress the versatility and efficacy of our immune response by training the body to depend upon what—on account of viral mutation—become ill-matched and thus ineffective antigenic responses. Yet antibody-dependent enhancement includes a distinct, and in many ways still more destructive mechanism, that Kennedy (following accepted scientific terminology) calls "pathogenetic priming."

In antibody-dependent enhancement, vaccination, by "priming" the immune system (even as one may "prime" a lawn mower before pulling the starter cord), induces conditions that lead the immune system to *overreact* if it subsequently encounters the wild virus. That overreaction can in and of itself be so extreme as to cause serious injury or death, and did indeed do so in *all* of the early animal experiments with coronavirus vaccines. Many researchers accordingly expressed deep concern about the possibility of Covid-19 vaccines inducing antibody-dependent enhancement. As Kennedy observes, Anthony Fauci himself tacitly recognized the danger in a March 26, 2020, White House briefing:

> The issue of safety is something I want to make sure the American public understands: does the vaccine make you worse? And there are diseases, in which you vaccinate someone, they get infected with what you're trying to protect them with [sic] and you actually enhance the infection. That's

the worse possible thing you could do—is vaccinate somebody to prevent infection and actually make them worse.[428]

ADE (antibody-dependent enhancement) represents just one means by which vaccination may cause serious injury and death. Like other vaccine-related dangers, it may manifest in the short or long term, as its deleterious action can kick in whenever the vaccinated host encounters the virus. Its prevalence in the context of the Covid-19 vaccines remains unclear, largely because—as Kennedy highlights—Dr. Fauci and the network of power he commands have mounted a concerted, multipronged effort to suppress evidence of vaccine injury and death, including evidence of that potentially caused by antibody-dependent enhancement.

I have amply documented some of the principal means of that campaign, including: (1) Maintenance of a dysfunctional reporting system (VAERS) and, more generally, the wholesale failure of regulatory bodies to monitor vaccine safety in any meaningful manner whatsoever, and; (2) The systematic censorship of any material bearing witness to vaccine injury or death in mainstream and social media outlets. Kennedy notes a number of additional methods of suppression. Allowing the CDC to discourage autopsies in deaths following vaccination (the fourth of six specific means enumerated by Kennedy) falls under the aegis of #1 above, but Kennedy's own first-mentioned means of suppression merits special notice:

> Dr. Fauci's first approach was to abort the three-year clinical trials at six months and then vaccinate the controls—a preemption that would prevent detection of long-term injuries, including pathogenic priming. Regulators initially intended the Pfizer vaccine trial to continue for three full years, until May 2, 2023. Because the FDA allowed Pfizer to unblind and terminate its study after six months—and to offer the vaccine to individuals in the placebo group—*we will never know whether vaccinated individuals in the trial suffered long-term injuries* (emphasis mine), including pathogenic priming, that cancelled out short-term benefits. Science and experience tell us that many vaccines can cause injuries like cancers, autoimmune diseases, allergies, fertility problems, and neurological illnesses with long-term diagnostic horizons or long incubation periods. A six-month study will hide these harms.[429]

We should note that (as per Kennedy's sixth point) so too will *vaccinating the entire population,* which end, if largely attained, can serve to hide vaccine injuries over the long haul. The tale Kennedy tells in this connection is all too familiar:

> Dr. Fauci presided over a progression of increasingly draconian forms of coercion to compel vaccination of the entire population. With his open encouragement, universities, schools, businesses, hospitals, public employers, and a litany of other societal power centers simultaneously launched numbing waves of strong-arm tactics to compel unwilling Americans to submit to vaccination, including threats of discrimination, job loss, exclusion from schools, parks, sports and entertainment venues, bars restaurants, military service, public employment, travel and healthcare....
>
> Whether intentional or not, the effect of this escalation was, increasingly, to eliminate the control group—which, coincidentally, would permanently hide the evidence of vaccine injuries. This motivation...explains Dr. Fauci's reckless and ferocious drive to vaccinate every last American, even those who have natural immunity and nothing to gain from vaccination, Americans below fifty, even kindergarten-age children with zero risk from COVID, and pregnant women, despite a nearly complete lack of information about the jab's impact on the fetus.[430]

As per its status as the central pillar of the Vaccine-Distance model, "Dr. Fauci continued to insist that fully vaccinating the entire population was the only path to ending the pandemic," ignoring the fact that "COVID vaccines prevent neither transmission nor infection, nor reduction in viral loads,"[431] and so are entirely unsuited to that end. Consequently, in Kennedy's words:

> Physicians and scientists complained that Dr. Fauci's vaccine promotions constituted a vast, unprecedented population-wide experiment, with shady record- keeping and no control group. Meanwhile, the actual data suggested that the COVID vaccines were causing far more deaths than they were averting.[432]

This last statement, of course, directly contradicts the mainstream narrative. Kennedy, like myself, records the revision of the party line forced after general recognition of the vaccine's limitations, and, as well, the illusory premises grounding the new spin on the story:

> By August, 2021, Dr. Fauci, the CDC, and White House officials were reluctantly conceding that vaccination would neither stop illness nor transmission, but nevertheless, he told Americans that the jab would, in any case, protect them against severe forms of the disease or death...
>
> Real-world data from nations with high COVID jab rates show the complete converse of this narrative; the resumption of infections in all those countries accompanied an explosion of hospitalizations, severe cases and death among the vaccinated! Mortalities across the globe, in

> fact, have tracked Pfizer's deadly clinical trial results, with the vaccinated dying in higher numbers than the non-vaccinated. These data cemented suspicions that the feared phenomenon of pathogenic priming has arrived, and is now wreaking havoc.[433]

The Real Anthony Fauci backs up these momentous assertions with hard data from Gibraltar, England, Wales, Scotland, Israel, Vermont, and Cape Cod—all highly vaccinated areas. I will not rehearse the telling results, but recommend that you confirm the facts (by way of Kennedy's book and other relevant sources) yourself, and draw your own conclusions.

Correlatively, *The Real Anthony Fauci* also exhibits graphs based on data collated by The Johns Hopkins University Coronavirus Center (a dedicated *proponent* of mainstream medicine and the vaccine agenda) that displays dramatic spikes in deaths in the period immediately following the rollout of a mass vaccination program in twenty-four countries spread widely across the globe. Kennedy notes: "Critics suggest that the shocking and predictable rise in COVID deaths following vaccination is evidence of long-feared pathogenic priming." While acknowledging that this qualifies as a fear rather than a proven fact, he likewise observes: "Officials have offered no other compelling explanation as to why the vaccine consistently precipitates disproportionate injuries and deaths among the jabbed."[434]

Until "health experts" do offer *persuasive, fact-based* evidence to the contrary, critics of the mass vaccine program appear to me to be more than justified in regarding that offensive not as humanity's salvation or best line of defense against Covid-19, but unfriendly fire that, whatever the intentions of its proponents, amounts to a clandestine war against humanity.

5. The War on Democracy

Kennedy's fifth point, which concerns means employed by Dr. Fauci to suppress consequential regard of vaccine injury, offers a ready transition to my fifth war front. Kennedy noted:

> Dr. Fauci populated the key FDA and CDC committees with NIAID, NIH, and Gates Foundation grantees and loyalists to insure rubber-stamp approvals for his mRNA vaccines, without any long-term injury studies. More than half of FDA's VRBPAC (Vaccine and Related Biological Products Advisory Committee), which approved EUA's for Moderna, Johnson & Johnson, and Pfizer, and granted final licensure to the Pfizer vaccine,

were grant recipients from NIH, NIAID, BMGF, and pharmaceutical companies. More than half of the CDC's ACIP committee participants were similarly compromised.[435]

This is just one instance of the systemic corruption that compromises the administration of public health in this country. Taxpayers pour billions of dollars into federal agencies that, rather than operating independently of industry influence, are largely subject to it. Kennedy:

> From the moment of my reluctant entrance into the vaccine debate in 2005, I was astonished to realize that the pervasive web of deep financial entanglements between Pharma and the government health agencies had put regulatory capture on steroids. The CDC, for example, owns 57 vaccine patents and spends $4.9 of its $12.0 billion-dollar annual budget (as of 2019) buying and distributing vaccines. NIH owns hundreds of vaccine patents and often profits from the sale of products it supposedly regulates. High level officials, including Dr. Fauci, receive yearly emoluments of up to $150,000 in royalty payments on products that they help develop and then usher through the approval process. The FDA receives 45 percent of its budget from the pharmaceutical industry, through what are euphemistically called "user fees." When I learned that extraordinary fact, the disastrous health of the American people was no longer a mystery; I wondered what the environment would look like if the EPA received 45 percent of its budget from the coal industry![436]

This is hardly governance "of, by, and for the People." When these captured agencies presume to exercise autocratic control over the practice of medicine and violate the sanctity of the doctor-patient relationship, we are surely justified in regarding such as constituting an intolerable infringement of the American people's natural right to health freedom.

This corruption of government agency represents one prominent feature of a sociopolitical landscape strewn with landmines that are threatening to blow up and maim or kill democracy. Both Kennedy's book and this present volume document myriad ways by which Covid-19 has served as an excuse for systematic violation of the human rights that constitute the foundation of democracy. Chief among these is freedom of speech, yet Kennedy (and here I cite from Kennedy's forward to Mercola and Cummins' *The Truth about Covid-19*) writes:

> The very Internet companies that snookered us all with the promise of democratizing communications have created a world where it has become

> impermissible to speak ill of official pronouncements, and practically a crime to criticize pharmaceutical products.... Tech/Data and Telecom robber barons...are rapidly transforming America's once proud democracy into a censorship and surveillance police state....
>
> The imposition of censorship has masked this systematic demolition of our Constitution including attacks on our freedoms of assembly (through social distancing and lockdown rules), on freedom of worship (including abolishing religious exemptions and closing churches, while liquor stores remain open as "essential service"), private property (the right to operate a business), due process (including the imposition of far reaching restrictions against freedom of movement, education, and association without rule making, public hearings, or economic and environmental impact statements), the Seventh Amendment right to jury trials (in cases of vaccine injuries caused by corporate negligence), our right to privacy and against illegal searches and seizures (warrantless tracking and tracing), and our right to have governments that don't spy on us or retain our information for mischievous purposes.[437]

6. The War on Society

It's critical to acknowledge that, objectively speaking, the U.S. Covid Response, under the command of Dr. Anthony Fauci, has been a disaster from beginning to end. Kennedy notes that the U.S. represents only four percent of the world's population but accounted for 14.5 percent of COVID deaths over the course of the first year of the pandemic. As of September 30, 2021, the 2,107 deaths per million registered in the United States translates into a mortality rate over twenty-five percent higher than that of much-vilified Sweden, almost twice that of currently hard-hit Germany, more than four times that of Denmark, six and a half times that of India (remember when India's Covid catastrophe headlined the news almost daily?), more than twenty times that of Kenya's ninety-seven deaths per million, and more than two thousand times that of Tanzania (which logs in at 0.86).[438]

These partial statistics advertise a general truth that cannot be frequently enough reiterated: that for the most part, across the globe today, high vaccination rate generally correlates not with lower, but rather higher, mortality rate. Of all the major continents, Africa has by far the lowest vaccination rate: only ten percent or less of the population there has been fully vaccinated. The vaccination rates of North America and Europe (the highest in the world) are *six times that* (roughly sixty percent).[439] Yet, as these cited statistics suggest, Africa has suffered proportionally much less mortality than North American or Europe.

The reasons for this are unclear, but could involve the phenomena of antibody-dependent enhancement in highly vaccinated nations, and/or wider use, in Africa, of treatments such as HCQ that have been banned or discouraged in Europe and North America.

The figures cited are relevant to the whole course of the pandemic, including developments during the current year (2021) after vaccine rollouts. Yet the policies instituted in the United States at the outset of the pandemic bear their fair share of the blame for the giant "F" (for failure) Kennedy sees written all over Dr. Anthony's Fauci Covid-19 report card. Kennedy notes:

> Dr. Fauci's strategy for managing the COVID-19 pandemic was to suppress viral spread by mandatory masking, social distancing, quarantining the healthy (also known as lockdowns), while instructing COVID patients to return home and do nothing—receive no treatment whatsoever—until difficulties breathing sent them back to the hospital to submit to intravenous remdesivir and ventilation. This approach to ending an infectious disease contagion had no public health precedent...Predictably, it was grossly ineffective; America racked up the world's highest body counts.[440]

We are speaking, here, of the ubiquitous "Distance" aspect of the Vaccine-Distance system, the scientific rationale for which is not one whit better than that of the "Vaccine" part. Kennedy continues:

> Peer-reviewed science offered anemic if any support for masking, quarantines, and social distancing, and Dr. Fauci offered no citations or justifications to support his diktats. Both common sense and the weight of scientific evidence suggest that all these strategies, and unquestionably shutting down the global economy, caused far more injuries and deaths than they averted.[441]

I referenced the destructive consequences of masking, quarantining, and social distancing any number of times in this book, but did not delve into the relevant issues—which deserve concerted attention—in any depth. Kennedy does, at least more so than I, and I encourage my reader to acquaint herself with the deeply consequential reckoning offered in *The Real Anthony Fauci* and other relevant sources.

Critically informed consideration of these matters is all the more important because the game plan associated with the Vaccine-Distance system remains in force, unchanged. Much of the populace appears to accept that masking, distancing, and even lockdowns represent rational, effective (even if imperfect), and indeed indispensable means of curtailing the pandemic, constituting—along with vaccination—a first and last line of defense against Covid chaos. Yet the physical, economic, and sociopsychological consequences of these measures can hardly be overestimated, even if not always subject to ready measurement.

Kennedy offers these remarks regarding lockdowns:

> Anthony Fauci seems to have not considered that his unprecedented quarantine of the healthy would kill far, far more people than COVID, obliterate the global economy, plunge millions into poverty and bankruptcy, and grievously would constitutional democracy globally. We have no way of knowing how many people died from isolation, unemployment, deferred medical care, depression, mental illness, obesity, stress, overdoses, suicide, addiction, alcoholism, and the accidents that so often accompany despair.[442]

The benefit that accrued from the policy initiative?

> Studies have strongly suggested that lockdowns had no impact in reducing infection rates. There is no convincing difference in COVID infections and deaths between laissez-faire jurisdictions and those that enforced rigid lockdowns and masks.[443]

As far this last mentioned topic is concerned, Kennedy cites a number of sources contesting the efficacy of masking. One straightforwardly asserts:

> "Regional analysis in the United States does not show that [mask] mandates had any effect on case rates, despite 93 percent compliance. Moreover, according to CDC data, 85 percent of people who contracted COVID-19 reported wearing a mask."[444]

Nor has science ever substantiated the efficacy of social distancing measures: for instance, the famous—and largely arbitrary—six-foot rule.

Yet let's go back to the volatile subject of masks for a moment. Not only, Kennedy claims, has science failed to establish benefit for masking, numerous studies highlight a wide range of real harms associated with it. I will leave it to my readers, once again, to acquaint themselves, via Kennedy's *The Real Anthony Fauci* and other sources, with the extensive and varied medical arguments against masking, but I cannot bypass Kennedy's cogent evocation of the sociopsychological damage inflicted by this presently all-too-common practice:

> Dr. Fauci observed in March 2020 that a mask's only real efficacy may be in "making people feel a little better." Perhaps he recognized that what masking lacked in efficacy against contagion, it compensated for with powerful psychological effects. These symbolic powers demonstrated strategic benefits for the larger enterprise of encouraging public compliance with draconian medical mandates. Dr. Fauci's switch to endorsing masks after first recommending against them came at a time of increasing political polarization, and masks quickly became important tribal badges—signals of rectitude for those who embraced Dr. Fauci, and the stigmata of blind obedience to undeserving authority among those who balked. Moreover, masking, by amplifying everyone's fear, helped inoculate the public against critical thinking. By serving as persistent reminders that each of our fellow citizens was a potentially dangerous and germ-infected threat to us, masks increased social isolation and fostered divisions and fractionalization—thereby impeding organized political resistance.[445]

That little piece of cloth, pulled over mouth and nose: what a powerful tool of disconnection and disaffection; what a potent weapon in the War against Society, one more critical front of that undeclared war, raging in America and much of the world, for the last twenty-odd months.

Kennedy offers these comments regarding the quasi-military strategy informing Dr. Fauci's policy:

> All of Dr. Fauci's prescriptions and communications seemed intended to maximize stress and trauma: enforced isolation, mandated masking, business closures, evictions and bankruptcies, lockdowns, and separating children from parents and parents from grandparents. We now know that fear, stress, and trauma wreak havoc on our immune systems.[446]

These wreak havoc on the human immune system, yes, but also, perhaps still more fatally, on the web on interconnections that comprise the fabric of society itself.

~

Before embarking upon these delineations of six "fronts of war," I alluded to the contrast between two competing Covid narratives; the mainstream story or controlling narrative, and the counter-narrative that informs both this book and *The Real Anthony Fauci*. The two stories—like two roads at a crossing—head in different directions, and one cannot travel both. It is consequently incumbent upon each and every individual to decide which path to follow: whether to believe it right and good and just to stay the course prescribed by the official Covid narrative—to believe its premises, and to condone the measures (including mandates) that represent its sociopolitical consequences, or whether, on the other hand, to affirm the contrary. This course represents holding that the world currently presented to us as reality is a projected image bred of falsehood, greed, the unbridled will to power, ignorance, and illusion—a nefarious enchantment which, however, *can be broken* by a courageous exercise of free will, discerning intellect, and the feeling heart that abhors the prospect of bondage, isolation, division, servility, inequity, and fear that are the signposts of the officially prescribed Right Way.

Although we no longer live in the era of kings, each and every individual, by virtue of their own power of conscious choice, acts the role of kingmaker, and so must decide which sovereign spirit they wish to serve: whether they wish to kneel before the image of America's Doctor and the chaos he brings in train, or to step back from the present pandemonium and pay homage to the king of kings, the *logos* that abides in quiet splendor in the innermost recesses of each and every human soul, in the temple of the mind, in the throne room of the sacred heart.

PART VI

POSTSCRIPT I

COVID WORLD, AUGUST 2023

In a December 4, 2021, substack piece titled "The Human Family," writer Charles Eisenstein imagines how Covid World might end.[447] As the threat posed by SARS-CoV-2 finally recedes, people will lapse into complacent disinterest as to exactly *why* it may have done so (efficacious vaccines? natural diminution of viral virulence?). As life returns more or less to normal, the whole Covid moment will be chalked up as a blip on the map of history; one most sane people would sooner forget than remember. Who doesn't want to leave a nightmare behind with the break of day?

I begin *Covid and the Apocalypse of the Modern Mind* (the sequel to *Two Roads*) by taking issue with Eisenstein's augury. Even so, today (late July 2023), it may appear that he was mostly right. The controversy swirling around all things Covid has largely calmed down.[448] People can see each other smile again, and most bustle about business as usual, concerned more about the war in Ukraine or continued inflation than masks or vaccine mandates.

Or so it may seem—at least, to the casual observer.

Yet open those lazy eyes just a bit, and it is not hard to see the Covid-sparked firestorm raging on, and even gaining force.

I began writing this first volume of *Reset or Renaissance* (*Two Roads: An American Scholar's Covid Chronicle*) in late June 2021, and finished it before the end of that year. Since that time, I have been working principally on the more historically and philosophically oriented volume 2 (*Covid and the Apocalypse of the Modern Mind*), but the contemporary stream of current Covid-related affairs naturally ran (and continues to run) on.

In the present book (*Two Roads*), I document developments that contest the mainstream Covid narrative on multiple fronts, including (1) the origin of SARS-CoV-2 virus; (2) the availability of safe and effective protocols of early treatment for Covid-19; (3) the efficacy of the "distance" aspect of the official vaccine-distance system of response, including lockdowns and masks; (4) the safety and efficacy of the Covid-19 vaccines; (5) the propriety or legality of steps taken (by government, industry, mainstream and social media, medical boards, academic journals, and other branches of the matrix) to police conduct and control the flow of Covid information; and (6) the prospect (and indeed present reality) of centralized systems of corporate-influenced power, on the domestic as well as on the international front, exercising social and political control in a manner incommensurate with the conditions of impartial scientific inquiry, the sanctity of the physician-patient relationship and democratic society.

Throughout the last year and a half, news on these fronts has continued to crackle; over the last few weeks, it has positively ignited. This is not surprising. From the outset, it was clear that the issues raised by Covid and the official response to it were not passing matters, but involved concerns central to human life and culture.

It is not remotely possible to supply anything like a comprehensive update on all the relevant issues. Data from new studies of a variety of Covid-sensitive matters has come in; pharmaceutical companies as well as government officials have been compelled, by force of law, to disclose previously hidden sources of information; Elon Musk's acquisition of Twitter led to the disclosures contained in the so-called Twitter Files; a plethora of lawsuits challenging the propriety of mandates, the FDA's directives on ivermectin and other aspects of government, professional, and academic policy have been filed and argued; Republican-led House committees have led investigations and interrogated high-profile witnesses pertaining to many if not all the aforementioned areas of concern.

While no exhaustive coverage can be proffered,[449] I can, with an eye toward a fit postscript to my account of Covid affairs, review some of the most significant recent developments, well aware that the tide of events will continually outrun any coverage I provide.

This much, at any rate, can be confidently affirmed: On every front,[450] history has validated—rather than cancelled or ameliorated—the deep concerns expressed in *Two Roads: An American Scholar's Covid Chronicle*.

1. Origin of the SARS-CoV-2 Virus

The lab-leak hypothesis, once branded and vilified as "conspiracy theory" has by now been widely, if not universally, accepted. Those in favor include the FBI and its director, Christopher Wray. "The FBI has for quite some time now assessed that the origins of the pandemic are most likely a potential lab incident" Wray told Fox news at the end of February 2023.[451] Roughly a week later, the House Select Subcommittee on the Coronavirus Pandemic held a hearing titled "Investigating the Origin of COVID-19." On March 8, the Committee published a press release headed: "COVID Origins Hearing Wrap Up: Facts, Science, Evidence Point to a Wuhan Lab Leak."[452] The "Key Hearing Takeaways" draw upon testimonies by Dr. Robert Redfield, former director of the CDC; Nicholas Wade, former science and health editor at that (dependably conservative news outlet) *The New York Times*, and Jamie Metzl, a former Clinton administration official and geopolitical commentator with knowledge of Chinese affairs.

The trio provided testimony pertaining to: the biological grounds favoring the lab leak over the natural zoonotic transmission hypothesis (Redfield); extensive efforts by China to preclude discovery of the origin of the virus (Metzl); how Drs. Fauci and (Francis) Collins "used unverified data to dismiss the lab-leak theory in favor of natural transmission"[453] (Wade); how "scientists kept in line with the natural origin camp led by Drs. Fauci and Collins because of their dependence on governments grants"[454] as well as the media's failure to challenge a questionable narrative (Wade).

I tell the gist of this story—at least the most damning part, implicating Fauci, Collins, Jeremy Farrar, and others in a conspiracy to quash the lab-leak theory—already in *Two Roads*.

Two very recent footnotes to the rather sordid affair are especially notable.

Remember Senator Rand Paul's most explosive exchange with Dr. Tony Fauci? In a July 20, 2021, Senate hearing, Paul effectively accuses Fauci of perjury on account of the latter's testimony that NIH did *not* fund gain-of-function research in Wuhan. In response, Fauci, waving the paper representing offending research, asserts that "the paper that you are referring to was judged by qualified staff up and down the ladder as NOT being gain-of-function." When an incredulous Senator responds that facilitating an animal virus's capacity to infect humans clearly constitutes gain-of-function, Fauci angrily and emphatically declares: "Senator Paul, you do *not* know what you are talking about, frankly. And I want to say that officially. You do not know *what* you are talking about."[455]

Recent disclosures, however, reveal that not only did Senator Paul know very well what he was talking about but so (naturally) did Fauci.

The relevant material dates from the fateful day of February 1, 2021; the day when Fauci sounded the alarm and engaged in complex machinations to kill the lab-leak hypothesis in the bud. Central to that effort was a call to Jeremy Farrar of the Wellcome Trust. An internal Fauci email to other relevant personnel (including Dr. Collins), sent 5:58 p.m. on February 1, details the contents of that discussions. When first made public, the *entire email* after

Fauci's introduction ("Folks: The call with Jeremy Farrar, Wellcome...") was *redacted;* the whole of what should be publicly vital information on a topic of preeminent importance to public health was blotted out. As a consequence, however, of ongoing work on the part of the House Select Committee on the Coronavirus that email has finally been *unredacted*, enabling the public to see, in this instance, the quality and character of the public service purchased with its tax dollars.

Predictably, the whole of it cries cover-up. In the context of Fauci's charged exchange with Senator Paul, however (one in which, remember, he is defending himself against an unofficial charge of perjury), one sentence toward the middle of the email stands out.

Wuhan University is right down the block from the Virology Lab. Fauci wrote:

> The suspicion was heightened by the fact that scientists in Wuhan University are known to have been working on gain-of-function experiments to determine the molecular mechanisms associated with bat viruses adapting to human infection, and the outbreak originated in Wuhan.[456]

On August 8, 2023, Senator Rand Paul sent ***a letter of criminal referral*** to Matthew Graves, the U.S. attorney for the District of Columbia. The letter begins:

> Dear Mr. Graves:
>
> I write to request your office open an investigation into the testimony made to the United States Senate Committee on Health, Education, Labor and Pensions on May 11, 2021, by Dr. Anthony Fauci, former Director of the National Institute of Allergy and Infectious Diseases (NIAID).
>
> In response to my questioning at the May 11, 2021, hearing, Dr. Fauci testified that the NIH has not ever and does not now fund gain-of-function reserach in the Wuhan Institute of Virology. In a subsequent hearing, I warned Dr. Fauci of the criminal implication of lying to Congress and offered him the opportunity to recant his previous statements. In response Dr. Fauci stated that he had "never lied before the Congress" and "did not retract that statement." Dr. Fauci's testimony is inconsistent with facts that have since come to light.[457]

Senator Paul goes on to cite the (now unredacted) text of the February 1 email and identifies additional instances of gain-of-function research at Wuhan funded by the NIH. His letter concludes:

> Before Congress, Dr. Fauci denied funding gain-of-function research, to the press he claims to have a dispassionate view on the lab-leak hypothesis

> and in private he acknowledges gain-of-function research.... A congressional hearing, however, is not the place for a public servant to play political games—especially when the health and wellbeing of American citizens is on the line.
>
> For this reason, I request that you investigate whether Dr. Fauci's statements to Congress on May 11, 2021, violated 18 USC # 1001 or any other statute.
>
> Sincerely, Rand Paul MD
> United States Senator

In a subsequent interview with Fox News, Paul states: "I don't think there's ever been a clearer case of perjury in the history of government testimony, and I don't say that lightly....He's caught dead to rights here."[458]

The breaking news does not, however, stop there. Enter Robert Kadlec, the godfather of the biosecurity state (see Volume II) and (more recently) former assistant secretary of the Office for Response Preparedness Response at HHS. As detailed in a *Fox & Friends* spot with Ainsley Earhardt, Australian investigative journalist Sharri Markson interviewed Kadlec in connection with her work on an article recently published in *The Australian* newspaper "Wuhan Cover-up: Wuhan, Lab Leak Suspicions, Anthony Fauci and How the Science Was Silenced":

> There were two things that really were quite shocking. The first is that he [Kadlec] directly said that Anthony Fauci decided to protect his own reputation and the reputation of his Institute which was funding the risky coronavirus gain-of-function research at the Wuhan Institute of Virology, and that's why Anthony Fauci was motivated to downplay any suggestion of a lab leak....The second part to this that was so fascinating was that Robert Kadlec said that their investigations indicate that it was vaccine research by the Chinese military in conjuction with the Wuhan Institute of Virology that they think led to the creation and outbreak of Covid-19.[459]

So much for the first footnote to the Wuhan story. If you want to know all the gory details, I am sure you will be able to find them in Robert F. Kennedy Jr's forthcoming book, *The Wuhan Cover-Up: How US Health Officials Conspired with the Chinese Military to Hide the Origins of COVID-19.*[460]

Meanwhile, on July 18, Bloomberg ran a story based on information obtained from a (July 16) HHS memo: "US Stops Funding to Chinese Lab at the Center of Covid Controversy."[461] The first sentence reads, "The Biden Administration formally halted the Wuhan Institute of Virology's access to US funding, citing unanswered safety and security questions for the facility at the center of the Covid lab leak theory."[462] Undoubtedly, this is good news, and a fit denouement to the Wuhan debacle. Yet was there ever a more catastrophically glaring instance of the adage "too little too late"?

(Late-breaking news: Tony Fauci is not the only one at legal risk on account of the gain-of-function research and its cover-up. According to the August 14 installment of *The Defender:*

> The families of four people who died from COVID-19 and one person injured by the virus are suing EcoHealth Alliance…and a cohort of government and elected officials, hospitals, military, personnel and others. According to the complaint filed Aug. 2 in the Supreme Court of the State of New York, the defendants exposed the plaintiffs to "undue risk and actual harm"—"whether accidental or intentional"—by helping to fund and conduct gain-of-function research, create and release COVID-19, and conspire "to cover up" these actions.[463]

So the Covid saga continues, as the scene shifts, more and more, to the courts…)

2. Early Treatment Options and the Practice of Medicine

I just mentioned a forthcoming book on the Wuhan cover-up. In fact, by this time, a sizable library of Covid-related books has materialized, including a number of titles authored (or coauthored) by the "rebel" physicians featured in these pages. Anyone wishing to flesh out their knowledge of the *other* side of the Covid story (the side exposed in these pages), can avail themselves of the firsthand accounts available in such books as Robert Malone's *Lies My Gov't Told Me: And the Better Future Coming*; Scott Atlas's *A Plague upon Our House: My Fight at the Trump White House to Stop COVID from Destroying America;* Peter McCullough's *The Courage to Treat Covid-19: Preventing Hospitalization and Death while Battling the Bio-pharmaceutical Complex*; and Pierre Kory's *War on Ivermectin: The Medicine That Saved Millions and Could Have Ended the Pandemic*. McCullough and Kory's books in particular document their authors' tireless efforts to counter the greed-driven obsession with vaccines and other patent-worthy drugs with ***real*** medicine; *medicine that does not dismiss safe and effective treatments simply because saving lives may mean losing corporate dollars.*

Despite the failing credibility of all aspects of the controlling Covid narrative—including its pretense of authentic medical expertise—the attack upon those physicians who dare to contest the reign of "the bio-pharmaceutical complex" continues unabated. As recently as last week (August 4, 2023), the American Bureau of Internal Medicine instituted formal proceedings against doctors Pierre Kory and Paul Marik. Kory and Marik's FLCCC reported the development in these terms:

> The ABIM Credentials and Certification Committee has recommended that FLCCC co-founders, Paul Marik, MD and Pierre Kory, MD, MPA should have their ABIM certifications revoked for spreading what the committee considers "false or inaccurate medical information." The committee concluded that the published peer-reviewed clinical, and observational data that create the foundation of the FLCCC protocols, educational materials and public statements are not "consensus driven scientific evidence." In reaching their recommendation, the committee cites NIH and CDC guidelines as well as several studies that have been largely disproved or questioned for their glaring flaws, conflicts of interest or poor design. Additionally, the committee cites a National Public Radio story that was later corrected for falsely reporting that overdosing of ivermectin was causing a surge in emergency room admittance.[464]

The practical action however, is by no means flowing in one direction only. In August 2022, Marik and two other physicians sued HHS and the FDA in a U.S. District Court in Southern Texas,[465] alleging "that the FDA have illegally interfered with the practice of medicine." While Marik, Bowden, and Apter "acknowledge the FDA's authority to regulate drugs," they claim that the FDA has no authority to "prohibit, direct, or advise against off-label uses of drugs approved for human uses." [466] By way of evidence substantiating their claims of personal and professional harm (which harm includes loss or threatened loss of licensure for prescribing ivermectin) effected by illegal FDA speech, the plaintiffs point to six FDA publications that, in the strongest possible terms, warn against use of ivermectin to prevent or treat Covid-19.

Although the district court judge granted the defendant's motion to dismiss, the consequent appeal landed the case in the Fifth Circuit U.S. Court of Appeals, where oral argument commenced on August 9, 2023. Because the motion to dismiss was granted largely on the basis of the (supposedly) nonbinding character of the information offered by the FDA, the argument naturally revolved around the issue of the effective force borne (or not) by the language employed by the FDA in its ivermectin-related tweets, posts, and publications.

Fifth District Judge Jennifer Walker, one of three-judge panel hearing the appeal, put FDA attorney Ashley Honold on the defensive from the get-go. Referring to the notorious FDA tweet featuring a split image photo of a vet and a horse on one side and a (masked) doctor and patient on the other and bearing the caption "You are not a horse. You are not a cow. Seriously, Y'all. Stop It," the judge pressed Honold on the imperative character of the FDA's language.

> **AH:** Good morning, and may it please the Court, Ashley Honold for the United States. This case is about informational statements made by the United Staes Food and Drug Administration to warn consumers about the dangers of using certain drugs. FDA made these statements in response to multiple reports of consumers being hospitalized after self-medicating with ivermectin intended for horses available for purchase over the counter without the need for a prescription. FDA did not purport to require anyone to do anything, or to prohibit anyone from doing anything....
>
> **JW:** What about where it said: "No, stop It." Why isn't that a command? That seems to me a command. If you were in English class, they would say that was a command. "Stop it!" That is different from: "We're providing helpful information."
>
> **AH:** Your honor, the language that the FDA used in these tweets were merely quips. I don't think these quips changed the substance of FDA statements.
>
> **JW:** Is that a command? "Stop It!"?
>
> **AH:** The tweets about the horse ivermectin were intended to warn consumers that they should not use ivermectin intended for animals, and that this could be unsafe.
>
> **JW:** I'm sorry, can you answer the question, please? Is that a command: "Stop it!"?
>
> **AH:** Your honor, in some contexts those words could be construed as a command, but...[467]

To understand the force of the plaintiff's complaint in this context, one need know that that FDA communication slid seamlessly between warnings not to take horse medicine and statements discouraging the use of *any and all* sorts of ivermectin—including that long official approved for human use—for treatment of Covid-19. For instance, below the split image mentioned above, the FDA tweet reads:

> Why You Should Not Use Ivermectin to Treat or Prevent COVID-19.
>
> Using the Drug Ivermectin to treat COVID-19 can be dangerous and even lethal.
>
> The FDA has not approved the drug for that purpose.[468]

The FDA here makes no distinction between types of ivermectin, implying that use of any form of the drug for Covid treatment "can be dangerous and even lethal." This, morever, counts as only one of six similar instances of FDA speech cited by the plaintiffs as (unlawfully) dissuading use of ivermectin for use or prevention of Covid-19.

As a practical matter, many recognize that, in point of fact, government policy *did* render ivermectin unavailable to many doctors and patients. Pharmacies refused to fill prescriptions; doctors who sought to prescribe the drug (like the plaintiffs in the case) were condemned and often sanctioned. Against this background, Honold's claim that the "FDA was not regulating the off-label use of drugs.... The FDA explicitly recognizes that doctors do have the authority to prescribe ivermectin to treat COVID"[469] rings peculiarly hollow.[470] The latter sentence, in particular, constitutes hypocritical backtracking aimed at covering the FDA's legal behind, *even while amounting to a tacit concession that the FDA's aggressive anti-ivermectin campaign lacked sound scientific basis.*[471] The war on ivermectin, after all, was never really about horse paste, and the whole horse-hooplah was *created* largely by the government's own refusal to support or even tolerate exploration of regular (non-veterinary) grade ivermectin as a treatment for Covid-19.

Yet to return to the legal argument: One could naturally claim, as Honold did, that the FDA possesses and must retain its right to provide information pertaining to drug safety. Honold, in fact, claimed that the agency possessed "sovereign immunity" in this respect; that its speech was fully protected so long as it performed the function of providing medical information.

Judge Jennifer Walker, however, was not necessarily buying it.

> AH: If the FDA is merely making information statements, they do have sovereign immunity...
>
> JW: Is the FDA *ever* responsible for making these public statements? If they make statements that are false, or grossly misleading, or wrong, can they

> ever be held responsible, or are they allowed to make...whatever statements they want without any oversight?[472]

A good—a very good—question. We await the judges' answer to it in the form of the verdict in the case.

Meanwhile, too few persons remain aware of, or have ready access to, safe and effective protocols of Covid prevention and (still more critically) early treatment. Meanwhile, Pfizer has added to its coffers by virtue of sale of its antiviral Paxlovid, an expensive drug of questionable efficacy and safety. Meanwhile, the overt or covert war on ivermectin (cf. the ABIM's action against Marik, Kory, and the FLCCC), and indeed upon most all health and medical measures that threaten pharmaceutical company profits, goes on, costing lives as well as piles and piles and piles of the people's dollars.

3. D-Day: Lockdowns and Masks

I think it's fair to say that the question of lockdowns is by now, a settled one. Anyone, anywhere who still thinks they were a good idea (let alone a legal one) is living (like too many of the rich and powerful) in another world. We hear from one source after another of the incalculable generational damage done, especially to minority communities and to children. The counterveiling benefit? A January 2022 meta-analysis out of Johns Hopkins (yes, Johns Hopkins; as readers of *Two Roads* will know, hardly a hotbed of Covid policy dissidents) focusing upon the reduction in mortality achieved through lockdowns, tells it like it is in language admirably frank for a scientific publication:

> Our study finds that lockdowns had little to no effect in reducing COVID-19 mortality.... However, lockdowns during the initial phase of the COVID-19 pandemic have had devastating effects. They have contributed to reducing economic activity, raising unemployment, reducing schooling, causing political unrest, contributing to domestic violence, loss of life quality, and the undermining of liberal democracy. These costs to society must be compared to the benefits of lockdowns which our meta-analysis has shown are little to none. Until future research based on credible empirical evidence can prove that lockdowns have large and significant reductions in mortality, lockdowns should be rejected out of hand as a pandemic policy instrument.[473]

Another influential meta-analysis published not so long ago addresses the efficacy of another chief feature of the Distance dimension of the vaccine-distance system of response: masks. Cochrane Library Reviews represent the gold standard in scientific meta-analyses. Any paper issuing from Cochrane generally possesses unusual authority. In January 2023, Cochrane published a paper titled "Physical Interventions to Interrupt or Reduce the Spread of Respiratory Viruses," an update of research concerning this question that dates back well over a decade, but includes a number of new Covid-relevant studies. What was the chief conclusion regarding masks? The key "Main Results" sentences read:

> We, included 12 trials (10 cluster-RCTs) comparing medical/surgical masks versus no masks to prevent the spread of viral respiratory illness (two trials with healthcare workers and 10 in the community). Wearing masks in the community probably makes little or no difference to the outcome of influenza-like illness (ILI)/COVID-19 like illness compared to not wearing masks...confidence interval (CI) 0.84 to 1.09; 9 trials, 276,917 participants; moderate-certainty evidence.[474]

In light of the intense controversy surrounding mask use, these are certainly noteworthy conclusions. Perhaps equally so was the response the paper evoked from the proponents of the mainstream narrative. Even though the moderate-certainty level evidence is comparable to that characteristic of many if not most Cochrane Review studies,[475] statements diluting or denying the outcome sprang up as spontaneously as Spartan soldiers from soil strewn with dragon teeth.[476]

Bowing to the pressure, Cochrane editor-in-chief Karla Soares-Weiser took the unprecedented step of publishing a clarificatory statement "on behalf of Cochrane." I cite the beginning and a clause near the end of the statement:

> Many commentators have claimed that a recently updated Cochrane Review shows that "masks don't work," which is an inaccurate and misleading interpretation.... We are engaging with the review authors with the aim of updating the Plain Language Summary and abstract.[477]

Just as Rand Paul was clear (Fauci's fulminations notwithstanding) that gain-of-function means gain-of-function, the language of the original Cochrane study is plain enough. The inexpert layman may be excused for imagining that if an intervention "makes little or no difference," that means it doesn't work. Nor is it difficult to surmise the hidden import of the phrase "*We are engaging with the review authors with the aim of...*" While it's not clear to whom this royal "We" refers, what is evident is that the researchers themselves, including lead author Tom Jefferson (author of almost twenty Cochrane Library Reviews over the span of roughly two decades and involved in this particular subject since 2006), did not sanction Soares-Weiser's unauthorized amendment of their conclusion.[478] After the publication of Soares-Weiser's "clarification," Tom Jefferson reiterated, "There is just no evidence that they [masks] make any difference. Full stop."[479]

Another, still more egregious instance of political interference in the science of masks revolves around the quality of the data and data analysis the CDC relies upon to make policy determinations. A preprint appearing just a little over a week ago (July 11, 2023), "An Analysis of Studies Pertaining to Masks in Morbidity and Mortality Weekly Report: Characteristics and Quality of All Studies from 1978 to 2023," casts the reliability of CDC "science" in serious doubt.

In case you are not familiar with the *Morbidity and Mortality Weekly Report* (*MMWR*), the paper's authors inform its readers of the nature and importance of the report.

> *MMWR* is a weekly scientific journal without external peer review overseen by the CDC to publish data on nationally notifiable infectious diseases, which can then be used for program planning, evaluation, and policy development. It is considered their primary avenue for disseminating scientific information and is often referred to as "the voice of CDC."[480]

Insofar as "Mask policies during Covid is one topic that has been highly influenced by data published in the *MMWR*," the paper's authors set out to study, in detail, "the scientific process in the journal" and so "describe and evaluate the nature and methodology of the reports and appropriateness of conclusions in *MMWR* pertaining to masks."[481]

The results were disturbing; at least for those who presume that "the voice of CDC" speaks with *real* scientific authority. Here are relevant conclusions:

> *MMWR* publications pertaining to masks drew positive conclusions about mask effectiveness over 75% of the time despite only 30% testing masks and <15% having statistically significant results. No studies were randomized, yet over half drew causal conclusions. The level of evidence generated was low and the conclusions drawn were most often unsupported by the data....
>
> With regard to the topic of mask effectiveness, our findings highlight the journal's lack of reliance on high quality data and a tendency to make strong but unsupported causal conclusions about mask effectiveness.[482]

In case you missed upshot of all this, the authors spell it out in no uncertain terms:

> Our findings raise concern about the reliability of the journal for informing health policy[483]

The policy import of these results, as well as those others reported in this section, are consequential enough, but of greater moment is the general point, made over and over in *An American Scholar's Covid Chronicle,* that the enmeshment of science and politics today breeds the corruption of both. Within the various branch offices of our ruling technocracy, dishonesty and deception spread like a quickly metastasizing cancer, infecting the vital scientific as well as political organs of American life.[484]

As a matter of fact (as indicated by the more than a decade-and-a-half of research included in the Cochrane meta-analysis), the truth that masks do not work has long been known—at least, among those experts most qualified to judge. Perhaps the most decisive public testimony on the subject has been furnished by a professional whose job description, *unlike* that of a physician or public health administrator, centers squarely on the task of protecting the public (most especially, workers) from toxic agents on the loose.

One iteration of that testimony, delivered before the New Hampshire State Senate in early April 2022, kicks off as follows:

> My name is Stephen Petty. I am a certified Industrial Hygienist, a certified safety professional and engineer. I have been working 45 years in the field of health and safety. I have spent my entire life trying to protect workers, and the public, from toxins.[485]

The SARS-CoV-2 virus may not be a toxin of quite the same ilk as, for instance, asbestos; nonetheless, the same principles of effective (or ineffective) protection apply.

In his testimony, Petty confirms what we just learned from Hoeg, Aslam, and Prasad's review of CDC research: namely, that it is fatally flawed. The mask studies cited by the CDC in defense of their policy recommendations fail on at least two counts: they lack a control group comprised of *unmasked* individuals *and* fail to account for serious confounding factors (such as differences in the quality of ventilation in cohort environments). Petty believes these deficiencies render any conclusions from the CDC studies scientifically useless. In line with the Cochrane Review results, he cites other, more valid studies that *do* compare rates of Covid infection in masked and unmasked control cohorts and do *not* find statistically significant differences between the two groups.[486]

Yet it is not the (necessarily very imperfect) epidemiological analyses that most persuasively substantiate Petty's view that masks don't work. His own rock-solid conviction stems from knowledge long established and universally accepted in his field. Petty:

> We have in Industrial Hygiene what we call the hierarchy of controls. The most effective is...engineering control; the least effective is PPE [personal protective equipment]. PPE for respiratory protection is respirators....The interesting thing is that masks don't even fit in the hierarchy; they're below it. They're not even part of it.

This means industrial hygienists have long regarded masks as a defective means of personal protection, so much so that they have no place in the industrial hygiene practitioner's professional toolbox.

Respirators, however, do—even if it's a lowly place. What is the difference between a respirator and a mask? Petty: "You cannot seal a mask, by definition. A mask that seals is a respirator."[487]

Given that inability to *seal* a mask, anyone can readily understand why elementary physics dictates that masks will not work—*especially* when it comes to protecting against the SARS-CoV-2 virus. Petty:

> A Covid particle is one-thousand times smaller than the cross section of a human hair. I ask everybody the simple question: "When you wear your mask, can you slip a human hair by the side of your mask?" Of course you can, especially below the eyes. It's a super-freeway for the virus to come and go. The source control argument is bogus. Source control means the person wearing the mask...somehow, those viruses can't escape the mask. That's just nonsense. If you have this super-highway, the virus doesn't care where it's coming in or going out.[488]

What then is the real, practicable solution to the threat posed by the SARS-CoV-2 virus—at least from the industrial hygiene angle? As Petty emphasizes repeatedly in his testimony, his profession has long recognized that it is *engineering* changes—ventilation and circulation mechanisms that dilute, disperse, and even destroy contaminants or toxic particles—that can create a safe (or at least much safer) ambient environment. It is precisely that kind of engineering that has long ensured that you can safely fly in an airplane *without* that worse-than-useless piece of cloth or swath of plastic, disfiguring your face.

I will not rehearse here all manifold reasons why masks not only do not work *but are positively harmful to physical and mental health*—especially, of course, if you are a child.[489] Let me instead move toward a conclusion by citing one more pointed remark from Stephen Petty:

> You can imagine that for somebody who has spent his whole life defending workers...how infuriating it is to see people propose solutions that cannot and do not work.[490]

Petty's pleas have not always fallen on deaf ears. In the aftermath of his testimony in Kentucky, that state *reversed* its statewide mask mandate. Federal officials, however, are another story. Even if they hear Petty loud and clear,[491] they do not—for their own reasons— choose to listen.

4. V-Day: Vaccine Safety and Efficacy

Unfortunately, but predictably, the story with regard to vaccine safety and efficacy is more of the same. An April 2023 article by Dr. Yaakov Ophir (one referencing publication of a study he conducted with two colleagues) begins by acknowledging what he regards, at this point in time, as common knowledge:

> Two key bricks seem to have fallen from the COVID-19 vaccine's narrative—the one about their fantastic efficacy against infections and the one about their superb safety.

...before turning to the last resort of "the safe and effective" mantra:

> However, one stubborn narrative brick seems to stand still, leading many people to believe that the booster doses of the vaccine are capable of providing long-term protection against severe illness and deaths (despite their failure to protect against infections).

...and putting this, too, in question:

> But is this brick really that strong? Does the existing scientific literature really support the notion that the two types of protection are independent of each other—that the protection against severe illness and deaths somehow remained high while the protection against infections disappeared?[492]

You can probably guess the author's conclusion.

It has always seemed strange to me that a vaccine that does not protect against infection—which, after all, I believe, has (in accord with the aim of herd immunity) always been the *ostensible* purpose of vaccines—could nonetheless prove truly effective in the prevention of serious illness and death. Evidently, I was not wrong to wonder at this logic. Ophir and his colleagues clarify that actually *demonstrating* (as opposed to imagining) that it does indeed do so, depends upon a concept called "conditional probability," one too often neglected or misapplied.

Examining three classes of evidence, including data from Israel referenced by U.S. health authorities, the authors found that (just as in the above-cited review of MMWR-based mask "science") conclusions drawn as to efficacy of prevention of serious illness or death—conclusions relied upon in order to direct public health policy—*lack any sound scientific basis*. In the author's words:

> The widely accepted medical narrative today, as if the booster doses of the mRNA vaccines prevent severe illness and deaths despite their failure to protect against infections, lacks scientific support. It is more likely that this proclaimed efficacy against severe illness and deaths is merely a wishful myth, which has no empirically grounded evidence.[493]

Of course, proponents of the mainstream narrative typically dismiss counter-claims as "misinformation." The problem with this is that the purveyors of "misinformation" appear to be the ones in command of the facts and employing sound scientific reasoning in drawing conclusions; the ones, in short, trafficking in something approaching REAL science as opposed to myth and propaganda.

After all, from the very beginning of Covid World, proponents of the controlling narrative systematically depended upon—not dialogue and debate—but suppression of dissenting views. What conclusion would a rational person draw from this fact?

I do not, however, wish to spend another moment on the matter of vaccine efficacy. *In my view, the whole question should be dismissed as moot.* Why? Because it makes neither scientific nor ethical sense *even to debate* vaccine efficacy if the vaccines are revealed to be not safe but dangerous and all too frequently cause significant injury or death.

Ophir evidently believes that most people—despite the contrary official platform—no longer regard the Covid vaccines as "safe." *Two Roads* made an impassioned case as to why there is every reason—not to believe, but to *know*—that this is in fact the case, and indeed emphatically and tragically so.

The news over the last eighteen months or so (I mean the *real* news, which of course you will not find in your mainstream paper) has only served to put exclamation point after exclamation point to this opinion. To anyone willing not to look away, but to stare the facts in the face, the evidence of widespread harm—grievous, tragic harm—is devastating.

For starters, all one need to do (if, that is, you do not yourself know any vaccine-injured persons) to get a feel for subject, is to log onto canwetalkaboutit.org (subhead: "Let's Break the Silence about COVID-19 Vaccine Injury and Death") or React19.org (the organization founded by Brianna Dressen) and read some of the countless stories posted there by the vaccine-injured. React 19 posts a directory of different kinds of injuries, so an interested person can find the particular class of calamity he or she may wish to learn more about. The directory includes: Brain fog, clotting, death, dermatologic fatigue, food allergies, GI issues, head pain, heart issues, inflammation, limb weakness, MCAS, muscle or joint pain, neuropathy, paraesthesias, POTS, psychiatric, sleep issues, tinnitus, tremors, and twitching.

These, remember, are not hypotheticals. You will find many stories under each and every heading, and many persons suffer from multiple severe issues.

The worst part is, however, that the list of injuries or illnesses connected to the vaccine keeps growing.[494] It is, moreover, not merely the Covid dissident community that is making the relevant connections. For instance, just a few weeks ago, in early July, *Science* magazine published an article linking the Covid vaccines to autoimmune disorders, including small fiber neuropathy and POTS.[495]

The wall of silence surrounding vaccine injury and death is (slowly, perhaps, but surely) crumbling. After all, the number of people inside keeps growing, and the prisoners are ever more determinedly hacking at that wall.

Just how common is vaccine-induced injury in the case of the Covid-19 vaccines? There is relatively recent and terribly telling evidence on that score, too. After a protracted legal battle that should not have been necessary, public defenders finally forced the CDC to release data from the V-safe system the CDC itself had set up to monitor the success of the Covid-19 vaccines. How did this system—originally touted as a far more reliable vaccine-safety monitoring system than VAERS—operate?

V-safe consists of a cell-phone app one could sign up for (voluntarily) upon receiving vaccination. The vaccinated were encouraged to do so, because once registered in the V-safe system users could not only report adverse events (not necessarily a draw for those enthusiastically embracing the vaccine program) but also receive updates as to the appropriate time to secure your second dose and other information designed to maximize the success of the vaccination campaign. Available as early as December 2020, when the very first Covid vaccines were administered, just over ten million people registered for V-safe, the vast majority of those doing so from December 2020 through May 2021. As access to the vaccines remained limited during that period, the pool of those who registered for V-safe probably represents persons generally enthusiastic about the vaccine program (the early birds!) and so likely *not* particularly looking for a means of reporting vaccine injury. On the contrary, these were most likely individuals hoping and expecting to be in the vanguard of those bearing witness to the fervently desired success of the novel vaccines.

The actual results from the V-safe system, however, revealed all too clearly why the CDC was so loathe to make those results available to the public. Far from demonstrating the safety of the Covid-19 vaccines, V-safe data confirms what one might well expect from the VAERS data. The V-safe system reveals the Covid-19 vaccine program—when evaluated from the point of view of its safety—to be nothing short of a catastrophe.

We often hear that vaccine adverse events do transpire, but are rare—*very* rare; on the order, perhaps, of one in a million. In other words, such events are nothing that anyone need really be concerned about, because you, or your loved one, are as likely to be struck by lightning as to be seriously harmed by a vaccine. The V-safe data, however, gives the lie to this fantasy—at least in the case of the Covid vaccines. The data reveals that of the ten million V-safe registrants, almost *800,000 were so adversely affected by the vaccine that they were compelled to seek medical help.*[496] In case you are not so fast with your math, that's not one in a million, or one in every 100,000, or 10,000, or 1,000, or even one in a hundred, but rather roughly *one in every thirteen persons* (7.7 percent). Moreover, not only did the majority of the adverse event reports register very soon after vaccination, but of the 7.7 percent that sought medical care, most were compelled to do so not once, or twice, but (on average) *three times,* a fact that suggests the serious nature of the adverse consequences.

The bad news does not stop there. In addition to the aforementioned pool, roughly 2,500,000—*another twenty-five percent of the pool of 10,000,000—were adversely affected enough that they were either forced to miss work or school or could not perform other normal functions.*[497] This means that—while about one in thirteen participants were compelled to see their doctor, or visit urgent care or the hospital, and usually multiple times— roughly *one in every three* participants suffered *some* kind of non-trivial health event in the wake of vaccination.

No wonder it took 463 days and two lawsuits (brought by ICAN) to force CDC to release the V-safe data[498]: data that could, and should have been made public in the first part of 2021, *before* the vast majority of persons were vaccinated. If the data had been made available, and duly publicized, it may well have seriously dampened the avid enthusiasm that accompanied the vaccine roll out. Evidently, the last thing the CDC wanted to do was to drop a wet rag on the vaccine fever just heating up. That, however, does not in the least excuse the sore betrayal of public trust.

There is much more that might be said about the V-safe data; the interested reader can explore the data for him/herself on the convenient interactive dashboard made available by ICAN.[499] One last point, however, may be worthy of special note. The V-safe data showed infants or young children in the newborn to three-year-old age class to be susceptible to serious adverse events (incidents that require medical care) at roughly the same rate as older persons. Of the approximately 13,000 zero to three-year-olds registered in the system, just over one thousand, or 7.2 percent, were so adversely affected (and again, most reports registered within days after vaccination) as to require medical attention.

On the *Highwire* episode spilling the V-safe beans,[500] ICAN's Aaron Siri makes the point that *if over seven percent of infants and preschoolers who contracted Covid were so affected as to need medical care, the public health alarm bells would be ringing at a deafening volume* as experts announced the acute danger posed by the disease to this dear and vulnerable class of persons. Yet, despite having the bulk of the V-safe data available to them by May 2021, and knowing that zero to three-year-olds *were at virtually no risk of serious harm from Covid-19 itself*, the relevant authorities nonetheless forged ahead with approval of the vaccines for infants and preschoolers in June of that year.

Even as I leave any further examination of the V-safe data to my reader, we unfortunately do not need to look far to discover further distressing instances of heartless disregard for the health and welfare of the most vulnerable among us—not only infants but also pregnant women and the unborn. This time, the data comes from Switzerland and Germany, but there is every reason to assume the results are generally applicable, at least in the United States and other European nations.

Addressing the group Doctors for Covid Ethics in Zurich this summer (2023), Dr. Konstantin Beck—a statistician, former adviser to the German minister of health, and currently a professor at the University of Lucerne—presented research revealing *a direct link between Covid-19 vaccination and a disturbing increase in miscarriages and stillbirths.* Speaking in competent if imperfect English, Beck opened his presentation ("Women and Children First: Baby Gap and Young People's Excess Mortality in Switzerland") with these words:

> It is an honor for me to be invited, but, on the other hand, the topic is so awful. I must say, I was never researching on such a . . . bad . . . story. I think it's a very important topic, and we shouldn't keep silent about it, because there aren't many people talking about it, and it's important that the message is distributed.

He continued:

> "Women and Children First"—That's my motto. . . . Given this emergency, you are to protect the most vulnerable first; the children, the pregnant, the unborn, those who have their lives still ahead. During Covid, we did not follow this ethical code of conduct. We exposed the most vulnerable unnecessarily to new risks that outweighed by far the original pandemic risk.[501]

What is the data that supports Beck's contentions? Beck and fellow researcher Raimund Hagemann were spurred to undertake their analysis by what they call the "baby gap," a dramatic drop in live births in Switzerland in 2022. Each and every month of that year saw a historically low number of births, contributing to an overall 8.5 percent reduction in live births. In Zurich, the drop was almost twice that at 16.5 percent. The last roughly comparable (thirteen percent) such drop occurred in 1914, when young Swiss men went off to fight in World War II.

Beck and Haigemann were hardly the only ones aware of the baby gap, and various hypotheses have been put forward in explanation. Beck identified objective reasons for rejecting all of these. The notion that Covid-19 infection reduced fertility rates, for instance, simply does not comport with data revealing a 2021 *spike* in birth rate following the first wave of infection near the beginning of the year and, too, data disclosing *a relatively constant rate of pregnancy and so no evidence of any reduction in fertility during the relevant time period.*

What Beck did find, however, was *a tight correlation between vaccination rate and the drop in births.* Adjusting time lines to account for ninth months of pregnancy, Beck displayed a graph showing *the drop in birth rate closely mirroring increasing rates of vaccination.* Given data indicative of *a relatively constant rate of pregnancy,* one may surmise that the historic lows were the effect of an increase in the percentage of pregnancies that did not reach term on account of miscarriages and stillbirths. Both German and Swiss health insurance data are consistent with this supposition insofar as that information base reveals "clear and significant increase in the number of pregnancy complications treated" beginning in the last quarter of 2021, as well as a dramatic (20%) rise in stillbirths in Germany during that period.[502]

Beck concluded that—while correlation does not *prove* causation—the consistent close linkage between dropping birth rates and rising rates of vaccination makes spontaneous abortion triggered by the latter the most likely explanation for Switzerland's historic baby gap. It is so all the more, Beck contends, *because what is known—and what is* not *known—about the vaccine's effect on pregnancy offers no good reason to reject this theory; on the contrary.*

According to Beck, "Anyone who had read a leaflet from the manufacturer" could easily learn that *there had been little or no consequential testing of the effects of the leading Covid vaccines on pregnant mothers, at the same time that ground for concern did exist as to the adverse effect of the vaccine on infants.* Beck, however, by no means believes it is or was chiefly the responsibility of the Swiss or German citizenry to notice and register this truth; rather, it was the relevant authorities who could and should have anticipated the very real possibility of serious adverse effects of the Covid vaccines on developing embryos, and should *never* have recommended its use by pregnant mothers.

As disturbing as all this is, Konstantin Beck had still more bad news to share—news focusing not so much on the entry into life as the exit from it. Upon careful analysis of relevant data—the same data used by the Swiss Federal Office of Statistics (FOS)—Beck arrived at a very different conclusion than the office—namely, while the FOS claimed no significant increase in *excess mortality* in 2021 and 2022, Beck did find such, an increase most marked among children (birth to nineteen) and, especially, young adults in the twenty-to-thirty-nine-year age group. With respect to the latter age group, Beck found a fourteen percent increase in excess mortality, a figure all the more notable when considered against the background of a consistent trend of (slightly) decreasing mortality rates over the course of prior years.

So who is right, Beck or the FOS? In yet another instructive instance of how it is all too easy for government officials to bank upon the presumption of superior authority even while pursuing inferior (and, in too many instances, fraudulent) methods of research design or statistical analysis, Beck demonstrates how both (a) an unwarranted expectation of an artificially high mortality rate for 2021 to 2022, and (b) aggregation of all age groups effectively *concealed* the excess mortality exposed by his more scrupulous and discriminating methodology. If you build into your model an expectation of a sudden jump in mortality (perhaps ostensibly on account of Covid-19, but that assumption cannot be legitimately posited in calculations of *excess* mortality, or mortality above a historic norm), your definition of "excess" will naturally be tainted, and any significant change artificially absorbed by your excessive "expectation." It is also not difficult to understand how age group aggregation can disguise real effects. If the great majority of deaths transpire in older age groups, but the analysis is not age-stratified, statistically significant difference peculiar to lower age groups will be masked by aggregation.

Beck, moreover, points out that the FOS *did* register a worrisome decrease in the overall health of the young Swiss population as measured by a frightening (almost 600 percent) increase in the incidence of strokes, heart attacks, and other debilitating adverse events. Given this disturbing data, "we should not wonder," Beck notes, "why we have an ongoing excess mortality in this age group." Beck concludes with words that leave little doubt as to his own opinion as to what may be the cause of the decrease in health and increase in mortality among younger age groups:

> To sum up: We see relevant health problems in the data for 2021/2022.
>
> We started vaccination in the year 2021 and 2022. We did *not* see the same relevant health problems in the year 2020 when we had a population that was not protected by vaccination and had to cope with a more aggressive virus.[503] That's the baseline. [504]

Beck is not alone in his findings. In fact, his statistical research echoes and supports the more spectacular results relevant to the U.S. population arrived at by financial analyst Edward Dowd, author of the 2022 book *Cause Unknown*.[505] Dowd draws his numbers from the CDC's own data. Like Beck, he finds significant *excess mortality*[506] in all age groups, but focuses special attention on young(er) adults—millennials between the ages of twenty-five and forty-four. His most telling results are jaw-dropping:

> From February 2021 to March 2022, millennials experienced the equivalence of a Vietnam war, with more than 60,000 excess deaths. The Vietnam war took 12 years to kill the same number of healthy young people we've just seen die in 12 months.[507]

Dowd, like Beck, does not shy from sharing his view as to the cause of what he terms a virtual "democide"—death by government.

> Those deaths occurred the same time as vaccine mandates were announced, and boosters approved. This younger population is not particularly at risk for Covid,[508] and the size and timing of this spike in fall 2021, raises clear questions about the potential contribution from the vaccines and boosters.[509]

Dowd notes, too, that a great many millennials, who comprise the core of the work force, had no choice but to vaccinate on account of mandates and employer requirements—no choice, that is, if they wanted to keep their jobs. It is also true that younger persons, while less susceptible to serious harm from Covid, are *more* susceptible to certain serious adverse effects, such as myocarditis-induced cardiac arrest.

Mandates and myocarditis: Dowd's data suggests this may be a killing combination.

What of data for 2022? It is still bad, very bad, though not as bad as 2021. You can read about it in Dowd's (December 2022) book, or on an associated website.[510]

I just mentioned myocarditis, and while *cardiac issues comprise the largest class of potentially fatal vaccine adverse events,* it is far from the only major cause of such. A recent (July 28, 2023) article in *The Epoch Times* reports on another deeply disturbing development. The first paragraphs of the piece ("mRNA Covid Vaccines May Be Triggering 'Turbo Cancers' in Young People") reports:

> Experts are seeing a puzzling rise in cancer in people under 50 that appears biologically different from late-onset cancers. While some claim cancer rates have been rising for decades and attribute the increase to sugary drinks, life-style, and sleep disruptions, others say mRNA COVID-19 vaccines have caused an emergence of "turbo cancers."
>
> Although there is no official medical definition for what doctors are calling "turbo cancers," the term is commonly used to define aggressive, rapid-onset cancers resistant to treatment—primarily in young healthy individuals following COVID-19 vaccination. These cases often present in a late stage with metastasis and quickly turn fatal.[511]

If such "turbo cancers" are a real thing, they could obviously contribute significantly to the excess mortality among young adults identified by Beck and Dowd.

Pathologist Dr. Ryan Cole, for one, bears witness to the actuality of the tragic phenomena, one my reader will recognize as *consistent with the wide range of atypical medical phenomena, including unexpected virulent cancers, PA Deb Conrad observed on her watch,* "terrifying" her to the degree that she would sooner lose her treasured job than risk the Russian roulette of Covid-19 vaccination. Dr. Cole:

> Physicians are seeing multiple types of cancers in their day-to-day practices—and in young patient cohorts where you typically don't see cancer. Although the increase in cancer has been blamed on missed screening, you know it isn't due to missed screenings because young people don't typically get screened.... What's happening is these cancers we're used to seeing, their growth patterns and their behavior are completely out of character.... So "turbo cancer" is something that wasn't there, and all of a sudden it's everywhere.[512]

One of the worst features of these "turbo cancers" is that they exhibit atypical cell behavior and do not respond to traditional cancer treatment. This, combined with their aggressive speed, means that diagnosis is all too often a death sentence: something no doctor wants to deliver and no patient wants to hear.

Is there any knowledge as to what may be causing these cancers? Researchers are making incremental progress on this score. Two days after injecting fourteen mice with a Pfizer Covid-19 booster shot, one of them died of malignant lymphoma, exhibiting abnormally enlarged organs and cancerous lymphoma in the heart, kidney, liver, spleen, and lungs. This represents the *first* documented case of malignant lymphoma in mice. If subsequent experiment confirms causality, Pfizer can add this novel result to its list of accomplishments.

Yet triggering cancerous lymphoma is just one of multiple and diverse mechanisms of harm associated with the mRNA Covid vaccine platform. Much more research is required in this area; oncologist, cancer researcher, and nuclear radiologist Dr. William Makis has suggested no less than nine possible mechanisms by which mRNA vaccines might cause turbo cancers. The first five (in an abbreviated rendition) are as follows:

1. The current COVID-19 mRNA vaccines contain pseudouridine-modified mRNA, which attenuates and alters the activity of key proteins in the innate immune system, impairing cancer surveillance;
2. Vaccination alters T-cell signaling that induces profound impairment in type 1 interferon and cancer surveillance;

3. The shift of the antibody IgG4 caused by repeated mRNA vaccination could create a tolerance for spike protein and impair the production of the antibodies IgG1 and IgG3 and cancer surveillance;
4. The spike protein produced by the body after COVID-19 mRNA vaccination may interfere with important tumor suppressor proteins—P53, BRCA1, and two tumor suppressor genes.
5. The spike protein may interfere with DNA repair mechanisms…[513]

I will leave it to the interested reader to investigate the remaining mechanisms, if one is so inclined. If the reader wishes further edification as to the recognized dangers of mRNA platform "vaccines," one may wish to read the free (downloadable) booklet provided by Doctors for Covid Ethics, "mRNA Vaccine Toxicity."[514] On its website, the group introduces the text as follows:

> Readers of our website will be aware that the mRNA vaccines that have been used against COVID-19 have caused injury and death on a scale unprecedented in the history of medicine. This book argues that these harms had to be expected from the first principles of immunology. Furthermore, they are not limited to the COVID vaccines alone; instead, they are inherent in the mRNA technology as such. We must therefore expect that future mRNA vaccines against other viruses or bacteria will be similarly toxic. mRNA technology will never be safe to use for vaccination against any infectious agent.[515]

The last sentences here refer to the well-known fact that, owing to diverse practical and economical advantages afforded by the novel mRNA technology, the biopharmaceutical complex is very likely planning to employ this platform for a wide array of future products. The Doctors for Covid Ethics statement represents an urgent warning against public compliance with this course of action, an admonition that should be heeded in light of our collective experience with the Covid-19 vaccines.

Perhaps, though, my reader remains skeptical: *I do not see my family, friends, and colleagues dropping like flies; virtually all of the people I know who were vaccinated did not suffer much, if any, harm. Besides, I do not see any real causality proven in any of these statistical analyses. Has anyone actually demonstrated a concrete, causal link between Covid-19 vaccination and death, or are these alarms all based on mere statistical analysis, plausible but unproven mechanisms of harm, and other less than definitive methods of argument?*

As for the *first* objection above, two responses may be ventured. First, it should be realized that, given the sheer quantity of persons vaccinated, the frightening number of casualties suggested by the various studies cited may be *somewhat* masked by the magnitude of the populations in question here; those affected, even if tragically numerous, are "spread out" in a still wider sea of people. Secondly, I expect more and more persons *do* know of more and more people who have suffered injury or death that *may in fact have been caused by the vaccine, whether or not this was consciously recognized.* Of course, the controlling narrative ("vaccines are safe and effective") steers us deliberately and even derisively away from considering vaccination as the cause of ailment, injury or death, except in the most obvious cases—and usually, even then.

Still—as Ed Dowd would undoubtedly argue—how, except by way of mass inoculation with an experimental product, is one plausibly to explain recent *spectacular* rises in all-cause mortality, droves of young vibrant athletes suddenly collapsing and dying,[516] or perfectly healthy teens dying in their sleep? If you need visual aids, or a reality a check on this score, get Dowd's book. It has many pictures you'll *not* want to see and the headlines of many—too many—stories you'll not want to read.

Speaking of mortality, let's turn to the second objection articulated above. As a matter of fact, in early July of this year (2023), the preprint of a paper employing autopsy analysis in order to establish (or disprove) a causal relationship between death and vaccination appeared in *The Lancet.* The abstract of the study, authored by Risch, McCullough and six others (including those with specific expertise in autopsy analysis), supplies relevant context:

> Background: The rapid development and widespread deployment of COVID-19 vaccines, combined with a high number of adverse event reports, have led to concerns over possible mechanisms of injury, including systemic lipid nanoparticle and mRNA distribution, spike-protein-associated tissue damage, thrombogenicity, immune system dysfunction and carcinogenicity. The aim of this systematic review is to investigate possible causal links between COVID-19 vaccine administration and death using autopsies and post-mortem analysis.

...clarifies the methods applied:

> Methods: We searched all published autopsy and necropsy reports relating to COVID-19 vaccination up until May 18, 2023...After screening...[we] included 44 papers that contained 325 autopsy and one necropsy case.

> Three physicians independently reviewed all deaths and determined whether COVID-19 vaccination was the direct cause or contributed significantly to death.

...and shares the relevant results:

> Findings: The most implicated organ system in COVID-19 vaccine associated death was the cardiovascular system (53%).... The mean time from vaccination to death was 14.3 days. Most deaths occurrred within a week from last vaccine administration. *A total of 240 deaths (73.9%) were independently adjudicated as directly due to or significantly contributed to by COVID-19 vaccination.* [517]

The authors proceed to put the gist of the matter in a nutshell, even while calling (urgently) for further research to corroborate (or challenge) their findings:

> Interpretation: The consistency seen among cases in this review with known COVID-19 vaccine adverse events, their mechanisms, and related excess death, coupled with autopsy confirmation and physician-led death adjudication, suggests there is *a high likelihood of a causal link between COVID-19 vaccines and death in most cases.* Further urgent investigation is required for the purpose of clarifying our findings. [518]

The paper naturally contains rich information pertaining to potential mechanisms of harm, which I cannot detail here. Noteworthy, too, is the reference to excess death (or mortality). The study elaborates this theme in a manner that corroborates and amplifies what I have shared from Beck and Dowd, and a lengthy passage near the end of the paper serves to cap this entire discussion of Covid-19 vaccine safety:

> The large number of COVID-19 vaccine-induced deaths evaluated in the review is consistent with multiple papers that report excess mortality after vaccination. Pantazatos and Seligmann found that all-cause mortality increase 0–5 weeks past injection in most age groups resulting in 146,000–187,000 vaccine-associated deaths in the United Staes between February and August of 2021. With similar findings, Skidmore estimated that 278,000 people may have died from the COVID-19 vaccine in the United States by December 2021.... Aarstad and Kvitastein...found that among 31 countries in Europe, a higher population COVID-19 vaccine uptake in 2021 was positively correlated with increased all-cause mortality[519] in the first nine months of 2022 after controlling for alternative explanations. Furthermore, excess mortality for non-COVID-19 causes has been detected in many countries since the mass vaccination program

> began. [Here the authors cite six separate studies]. Pantazatos estimated that VAERS deaths are underreported by a factor of 20. If we apply the underreporting factors to the May 5th, 2023, VAERS death report of 35,324, the number of deaths in the United States becomes 706, 480. If this extrapolated number of deaths were to be confirmed, the COVID-19 vaccines would represent the largest medical failure in human history.[520]

Finally, the paper authors explore—as is both fit and necessary—the wide-ranging ramification of their findings, should they be confirmed:

> If a large number of deaths are indeed causally linked to COVID-19 vaccination, the implications could be immense, including: the complete withdrawal of all COVID-19 vaccines from the global market, suspension of all remaining COVID-19 vaccine mandates and passports, loss of public trust in government and medical institutions, investigations and inquiries into the censorship, silencing and persecution of doctors and scientists who raised these concerns, and compensation for those who were harmed as a result of the administration of COVID-19 vaccines.[521]

The penultimate sentence here is rich with irony. I read the preprint not on *The Lancet* but on *The Daily Sceptic.* Why? Because within twenty-four hours of its publication, it was *removed* by the journal. *The Lancet* provided its own nebulous reasons for its action, but I think my reader will, by this time, be well-attuned to the deeper, thoroughly *un*scientific reasons why the Risch-McCullough paper's life span on *The Lancet* was no longer than that of a fly in May.

In sum, what exactly suggests that Covid-19 vaccines are *not* safe, but poorly tested, extremely dangerous toxic agents that no sane person who treasures life and health should admit into their body? *Nothing, but* the tortured witness of numberless vaccine-injured persons whose tragic plight is confirmed by unprecedented numbers of VAERS reports, damning V-safe data, and an ever-growing inventory of debilitating side effects (from POTS to turbo cancers); the corroborative testimony of PAs, nurses, and conscientious doctors who should know; lack of adequate testing combined with *numerous* recognized or suspected mechanisms of serious and indeed lethal harm; preliminary confirmation of the same by autopsy analysis and dead laboratory mice; disturbing increases in spontaneous abortion linked to the jab; skyrocketing rates of excess mortality reported from around the world correlated, temporally *and* quantitatively, with increased rates of mass vaccination; young, fit athletes regularly collapsing and dying before our eyes; healthy sons and daughters dying inexplicably in sleep; and, finally, the continued censorship and brutal silencing of those who dare to try to tell this side of the story.

What, on the other hand, speaks *for* the safety of the Covid-19 vaccines? *Nothing, but:* shoddy "science," bought officials, and mainstream media that robotically toes the party line; ideological indoctrination of physicians and the public at large; the "hag of superstition"[522] and the mindless mantra that far too many drink like Jonestown Kool-Aid: *"Safe and effective, safe and effective, safe and effective,"* a phrase that echoes endlessly down the long halls of hell.

5. Civil Rights and Liberties

The civil liberty issues raised by Covid-related policies are so multiple and significant, and so much has happened (usually involving lawsuits) and continues to happen on so many fronts that even a satisfactory abstract would far exceed the limits of this brief postscript. Some of the chief areas of contestation include the legality of vaccine mandates at colleges and universities; the reinstatement and compensation of employees wrongfully fired for refusing vaccination; undue infringement upon the rights of religious liberty in the form of blanket rejection (or simple preclusion) of religious exemptions; discrimination and disciplinary action against physicians who question "consensus science" by medical boards and universities; and collusion of government, social media platforms, mainstream media, and other major players (e.g. TNI) in the systematic censorship and suppression of free speech, especially on those social media platforms that today play such a central role in the exchange of ideas and opinions essential to democracy.

To provide a rough sketch of the contours of this vast, complex, and ever-changing landscape, I begin with brief mention of some of the most recent developments.

Today, the 15th, finds us in mid-August 2023. Within the last few minutes, a story on the academic front appeared in my email inbox: "Rutgers Set to Kick Out Students Today unless They Comply with COVID Vaccine Mandate." The article opens thus:

> As of today, Rutgers remains one of fewer than 100 universities out of 2,679 four-year colleges and universities that refuse to let go of COVID-19 vaccine mandates and, according to anonymous sources, Rutgers is planning to dis-enroll noncompliant students beginning today.[523]

It includes an editor's note, that reads:

> Children's Health Defense in August 2021 sued Rutgers University, claiming its COVID-19 vaccine mandate violates the right to informed consent and the right to refuse unwanted medical treatments. The case, still pending, is likely headed to the U.S. Supreme Court.[524]

In fact, the district court initially decided the case in Rutger's favor. It has since been appealed to the United States Court of Appeals for the Third Circuit. The verdict reached by that body, however, may well be a way station en route to the highest court in the land. Such is the preeminent importance of diverse legal questions raised by Covid policies that have transformed the American political, social, and legal landscape.

As far as Rutger's historical record is concerned, the cited article notes that on January 8, 2021, at the very beginning of the Covid-19 vaccine rollout, Rutgers had announced, "With our stance of human liberties and our history of protecting that, the vaccine is not mandatory." The story continues to document the retraction of that pledge, ending with an ominous assertion, the general pertinence of which reaches far beyond its narrower purview: "The pandemic is nowhere near over at Rutgers, not by a long shot."[525]

Yesterday's (August 14) inbox included a story detailing developments in yet another of the plethora of cases countrywide seeking legal redress for harm suffered because of (allegedly discriminatory) vaccine mandates. Here, teachers employed by New York State and its Department of Education have sued on account of what they contend were ill-considered automatic rejections of applications for religious exemptions. The most pertinent portion of the story reads:

> State Supreme Court Judge Ralph J. Porizo today heard arguments from both sides in the case of DiCapua v. City of New York, filed in February by Teachers for Choice and other fired NYC DOE employees…Nearly 300 people gathered outside the courthouse today [8/14] to support the plaintiffs who in April filed a motion for class certification, citing that all members of the class were affected by the same errors of law and that "the auto-generated, vague, and conclusory denials" of religious exemptions were all "arbitrary and capricious."…
>
> In addition to deciding whether to certify the class, Judge Porzio will render a decision on the question of Article 78—whether to overturn the DOE's determination on the religious exemptions and offer relief to plaintiffs. If the plaintiffs win class status and win relief, all members of the

class would be reinstated...with full seniority and no break in service and back pay and attorney fees.[526]

The topic of religious exemption is a hot one of late, with lawsuits seeking to protect the right to such exemption proceeding in several states. One such effort was recently crowned with a rare, perhaps pivotal success. On April 18, 2023, a federal judge ordered that Mississippi reinstate the religious exemption option last available in 1979. The April 20 edition of *The Mississippi Free Press* reports:

> A federal judge struck down the State's long-standing childhood vaccine requirements for public or private school attendance, saying the State must allow religious exemptions like most others already do. Mississippi is one of just six states that only permits childhood vaccine [exceptions] for medical reasons, with no religious exemptions.
>
> The Texas-based Informed Consent Action Network funded the lawsuit, filed in September 2022, arguing that the lack of religious exemptions for vaccines violates the First Amendment's guarantee of the free exercise of religion. On Tuesday...Judge Sul Ozerden agreed with ICAN's argument.... The Mississippi State Department of Health "will be enjoined from enforcing (Mississippi's compulsory vaccination law) unless they provide an option for individuals to request a religious exemption from the vaccine requirement." The State could still appeal the ruling, however.[527]

The State, however, did not. The beginning of an official July 17 news release reads as follows:

> JACKSON—the Mississippi State Department of Health (MSDH) will begin offering religious exemptions Monday, July 17, 2023, in addition to the existing medical exemption process in compliance with the federal court order entered in April 2023. Detailed information is now available on our website along with the proper forms to be completed and a statement from the Board of Health.[528]

Not that the Board is happy about it! The news release continues:

> "MSDH stands with the Board of Health in support of the current School Vaccination Law which has protected our children for over 40 years," said State Health Officer, Dr. Daniel Edney.[529]

Dr. Edney may stand where he will. The fact is, the "current" school vaccination law—which has *not* included religious exemptions for forty years—now does so. It is true that the state may require (as the release informs us) interested parents not only to fill out the appropriate form but to come in for a personal appointment and watch "a vaccine education video." I do not, however, think these slight burdens will put off the sizable party of parents who have been agitating for the return of Mississippi's religious exemption for many, many years, yet—despite substantial support—were unable to achieve a legislative breakthrough.

The hope that the legal precedent set by the Mississippi might help the like cause in other states was somewhat dampened when the Connecticut U.S. Appellate Court for the Second Circuit recently agreed with a district court ruling upholding the state's 2021 law rescinding religious exemptions for vaccination. The August 4 ruling issued by a three-judge panel was not, however, unanimous, but rather included a forceful dissent.

It is not difficult to grasp at least one leading feature of Judge Joseph Bianco's contention that the *factual basis* of the majority opinion was insufficiently established:

> Although Connecticut asserts that this differing treatment between religious and secular exemptions[530] was prompted by a substantial increase over recent years in the number of religious exemptions, and an acute risk of an outbreak of disease, Connecticut fails to explain how 44 states and the District of Columbia have maintained a religious exemption for mandatory state vaccination without jeopardizing public health and safety.[531]

Another crucial clause of Judge Bianco's dissent reveals the extent to which concerns emerging from Covid World are gradually redefining general perceptions pertaining to vaccines and public health policy. Judge Bianco:

> Not only is the majority opinion's holding incorrect at this stage given the factual allegations in this case, but its analysis also has troubling implication for the future of the Free Exercise Clause as it related to all types of vaccination requirements for students and other members of the public, including COVID-19. In other words, under the majority opinion's analysis, *a state or other government entity could expand mandatory vaccination requirements and simultaneously eliminate religious exemptions (while maintaining broad medical exemptions) and easily satisfy the low constitutional bar of rational basis review by invoking generalized concerns about public health and safety.* (emphasis mine)[532]

This is exactly what happened in many contexts, including (as the story previously cited indicates) that of the New York State Department of Education's employment policies.

No doubt encouraged by Judge Bianco's dissent, the chief plaintiffs in the case (which include three Connecticut parents) vowed to appeal the decision to the Supreme Court.

> [We] respectfully disagree with the court's conclusion that the removal of the religious exemption in Connecticut does not infringe upon the free exercise of religion under the First Amendment, or the Fourteenth Amendment's guarantee of equal protection under the law.... We fully intend to seek review of this decision in the U.S. Supreme Court to obtain equal justice for all children—not only in Connecticut but in every state in the nation.[533]

Whether or not we will in fact see a religious exemption case argued before the Supreme Court remains to be seen. I do believe, though, that such is very likely in the long if not the short run and is so largely because consciousness of the issue has been raised and, indeed (for many, at least), transformed by the coercive policies implemented and enforced during the pandemic.

Freedom of speech represents another essential civil liberty put at risk and indeed systematically violated by a wide variety of Covid World measures. The freedom of physicians to express the scientific judgments that contradict or contest the mainstream "consensus" comprises a particular, and peculiarly critical, class of free speech concerns.

One would naturally hope that the domains of science and medicine would be immune to the practice of *policing* opinion and silencing dissent, actions suited to the exercise of hegemonic power but *not* the pursuit of truth. We have, however, seen how—on the contrary— institutionalized forms of authority in scientific and medical circles have consistently been deployed to enforce an artificial "consensus" and maintain dogmatic positions, which (like the catechisms of some fundamentalist theocracy) can often be challenged only at the cost of violent retribution. The case of Dr. Renata Moon represents an exemplary and profoundly disturbing case in point.

Dr. Renata Moon boasts a distinguished twenty-five-year career as a board-certified pediatrician—one unmarked by any allegations of professional misdemeanor or malpractice—as well as a six-year tenure teaching at Washington State University (WSU). Dr. Moon, however, entertains serious reservations about the safety of mRNA vaccines and has resisted endorsing its use for children (as a pediatrician, her special clientele). Consequently, Senator Ron Johnson invited Dr. Moon to offer testimony at the official roundtable discussion sponsored by the senator on December 7, 2022. After fulfilling formal university requirements that might enable her to attend without compromising her academic obligations, Dr. Moon did testify, *not* —as she made amply clear—as a representative of WSU but as a private individual and practicing physician.

Dr. Moon was aware of the potential repercussions of her actions; she knew of no few colleagues whose refusal to toe the party line on vaccines had resulted in loss of licensure or threats thereof. The subsequent actions of her academic employer nonetheless took her by surprise. In the aftermath of her testimony, she received a threatening memo from WSU noting that WSU felt obligated to "report" her doings to the Washington Medical Commission (WMC). If her testimony had not itself been public, one might say the university "ratted" on her. Furthermore, as the language of the memo itself adumbrates,[534] WSU ultimately judged Dr. Moon's testimony *sufficient grounds to allow her long-standing contract to expire.* To put the matter bluntly, she was fired.

Dr. Renata Moon received notice of the non-renewal of her contract on June 29, 2023, two years to the day after I began writing the letter to Pacifica Graduate Institute (the school at which I myself no longer teach because of Covid strictures) that inaugurated the writing of this book.

The organization Informed Choice Washington rightly opines that, on account of Dr. Moon's historic contributions to WSU's Floyd College of Medicine—she in fact helped *found* the school—her termination must be regarded as "far from routine."[535] Dr. Moon herself certainly considered that to be the case; so much so, that she inaugurated proceedings to seek legal redress, not only for the personal damage suffered but, more broadly, for the gross violation of essential civil liberties represented by the joint actions of WSU and WMC.

I will let relevant clauses from the declaratory complaint that Dr. Moon filed as part of the lawsuit to tell the gist of the story:

> On December 7, 2022, at the invitation of United States Senator Ron Johnson, I appeared before a hearing in the Kennedy Caucus Room in Washington, D.C. entitled "COVID-19 Vaccines: What They Are, How They Work, and Possible Causes of Injuries." I spoke as a private citizen on personal time regarding concerns about the dangers of COVID-mRNA vaccines. At the hearing, I testified that I have direct knowledge of a significant rise in myocarditis; showed a blank informational package insert personally taken from a sealed box of mRNA vaccine, which makes it impossible to have informed consent discussions with patient's parents; and stated that other reputable countries have stopped giving these vaccines to children.

I also state that physicians speaking out about the dangers of the experimental COVID-19 mRNA vaccine have had their licenses threatened.

Though the information stated was perfectly factual and occurred during a proceeding organized by a United States Senator for the sake of fact-finding, on March 3, 2023, my employer, Washington State University (Elson S. Floyd College of Medicine) informed me of the following:

> "...Physician Professionalism...The Washington Medical Commission (WMC) supports the position taken by the Federation of State Medical Boards (FSMB) regarding COVID-19 vaccine misinformation, "Spreading inaccurate COVID-19 vaccine information contradicts that responsibility, threatens to further erode public trust in the medical profession and puts all patients at risk." The WMC has asked the public and practitioners to report possible spread of misinformation. There were components of your presentation that could be interpreted as a possible spread, as such we are ethically obligated to make a report to the WMC to investigate possible breach of this expectation."

Washington State University's Elson S. Floyd College of Medicine has not alleged that I committed malpractice as my testimony in Washington D.C. had nothing to do with patient care. They allege that they are following edicts set by the WMC when they threaten my medical license for simply speaking words and having "unauthorized" opinions. My "unauthorized" opinions were based on personal experiences and scientific data. This is a chilling threat to the Constitutional right to free speech, the very foundation upon which our Constitutional Republic is built.

I was born in the United States of America as a first generation proud American. My parents fled political persecution from behind the Iron Curtain of communism to legally immigrate to the USA. My parents and millions of other immigrants left everything behind and moved from the hell that their countries had become for one simple reason: FREEDOM. Our constitutional rights, which protect our freedom of speech and civil liberties, are precious beyond measure. Please stop this blatant trampling of our Constitutional rights.[536]

The pandemic *over?* Talk of *amnesty* when hostile forces have never relinquished their advanced positions, or stopped firing big guns? Perhaps the fear of the coronavirus itself has receded, but the plague of authoritarianism left in its wake continues largely unabated.

Remember the tangible agony expressed by doctors Byram Bridle and Donald Welsh in view of the *officially sanctionel* yet *violent and thoroughly unscientific* persecution of dissent in academic and medical circles in Canada in

2021? Evidently, it remains every bit as bad, or worse, here in the United States, two or three years later. Evidently, powerful parties and institutions within the U.S. are not at all appalled by the methods once employed to control the flow of information behind the Iron Curtain. "*The WMC has asked the public and practitioners to report…the possible spread of misinformation.… We are ethically obligated to make a report.*" Chilling words, indeed!

Moreover (as Matt Taibbi suspected long ago), the most prominent of the many of such parties is none other than the executive branch of the U.S. government. That, however, is another story. If you are not familiar with it already, I'll say this much up front: it's a whopper.

Long, long ago—I mean in July 2021—in the chapter "Dissing Democracy: Power and Misinformation," I noted journalist Matt Taibbi's observation that the U.S. government appeared to be colluding with major social media platforms as those platforms—under the cover of "content moderation"—systematically censored disfavored Covid-related speech. Taibbi noted that, if this were indeed the case, such practice constitutes a grave violation of the Constitution. The relevant passage from chapter 7 of *Two Roads* reads:

> Taibbi advances the cogent argument that if YouTube is consulting with federal agencies such as the CDC, FDA, and NIH as it develops its moderation guidelines with respect to health-related mis- and disinformation, then persons such as the Weinsteins are in fact suffering from what is not only *de facto* but indeed *de jure* state censorship in direct violation of the First Amendment. Such a practice creates a situation in which government agencies are not only making public health policy, but are also controlling the parameters for private and public debate of the relevant issues.

Two years down the road (that same, *too* well-traveled road), novel developments have confirmed Taibbi's suspicions to a nightmarish degree, and indeed to an extent that he himself could hardly have imagined. Two such development are of outstanding importance. Let's begin with the first dramatic episode, one in which Matt Taibbi himself plays a leading role.

After a notoriously conflicted process, Elon Musk's much-publicized purchase of Twitter was formalized in late October 2022. The iconoclastic Musk, a self-professed champion of free speech, decided to provide a few select journalists and authors access to internal Twitter files (emails, screenshots, and chatlogs), in part, to shed light on how the company's often-controversial "content moderation" decisions may have been reached. Matt Taibbi and Michael Shellenberger were two of the six writers given access to the files, and who (as per prior agreement with Musk) eventually made accounts of their findings available on Twitter. Taibbi himself posted the first lengthy "Twitter Files" entry on December 2, 2022. Over the course of the next several months, many more followed, until a disagreement between Musk and key writers scuttled the project in March.

Covid-related speech, though hardly the only controversial topic involved (the Hunter Biden laptop story as well as Donald Trump's Twitter ban were two other high-profile topics) certainly counted as one of the chief areas of concern for those reporting on the Twitter Files. Twitter had long functioned as one of several major social media platforms that consistently censored disfavored Covid-related speech, and the release of the Twitter Files shed light upon the extent to which that practice reflected not merely *collusion* but also active *coercion* on the part of many departments of the U.S. government, as well as an impressive galley of ancillary academic and private organizations.

As a consequence of their reporting of the Twitter Files, Taibbi and Shellenberger testified at the March 9, 2023, House Select Committee hearing on the weaponization of the federal government chaired by Congressman Jim Jordan. The following excerpts from the opening statements of each of the two writers provide a telling glimpse of the frightening reality Shellenberger and Taibbi encountered upon examination of the infamous Twitter Files.

Shellenberger testified first and began by citing one of the most famous, important, and prescient speeches in American history. Shellenberger:

> In his 1961 farewell address, President Dwight Eisenhower warned of "the acquisition of unwarranted influence…by the military-industrial complex." Eisenhower feared that the size and power of the "complex," or cluster, of government contractors and the Department of Defense would "endanger our liberties or democratic processes." How? Through "domination of the nation's scholars by Federal employment, project allocations, and the power of money." He feared public policy would "become the captive of a scientific-technological elite."

The author of *An American Scholar's Covid Chronicle* cannot help but make special note of President Eisenhower's reference to the nation's scholars, and his keen concern that the undue influence of a technological elite might preclude them from fulfilling the mission of their high office. Shellenberger proceeds to disclose the disturbing gist of his findings:

> Eisenhower's fears were well-founded. Today, *American taxpayers are unwittingly financing the growth and power of a censorship-industrial*

> *complex run by America's scientific and technological elite, which endangers our liberties and democracy.* I am grateful for the opportunity to offer this testimony and sound the alarm over the shocking and disturbing emergence of state-sponsored censorship in the United States of America....

...before fleshing out the relevant facts...

> The Twitter Files, state attorneys general lawsuits, and investigative reporters have revealed a large and growing network of government agencies, academic institutions, and nongovernmental organizations that are actively censoring American citizens, often without their knowledge, on a range of issues, including on the origins of COVID, COVID vaccines...and many other issues.

...and identifying critical mechanisms of coercive control:

> Government officials have been caught repeatedly pushing social media platforms to censor disfavored users and content. Often, these acts of censorship threaten the legal protection social media companies need to exist, Section 230.[537]

Matt Taibbi followed Shellenberger to the stand, and his testimony amplified and concretized Shellenberger's statements. After briefly recounting how he came to work on the Twitter Files, Taibbi proceeds to the heart of the civil rights matter:

> The original promise of the Internet was that it might democratize the exchange of information globally. A free internet would overwhelm all attempts to control information flow, its very existence a threat to antidemocratic forms of government everywhere.
>
> What we found in the Files was a sweeping effort to reverse that promise and use machine learning and other tools to turn the internet into an instrument of censorship and social control. Unfortunately, our own government appears to be playing a lead role.

Taibbi delves into some of the specifics of the parties, governmental and nongovernmental, involved:

> We learned Twitter, Facebook, Google, and other companies developed a formal system for taking in moderation "requests" from every corner of government: the FBI, DHS, HHS, DOD, the Global Engagement Center at State, even the CIA. For every government agency scanning Twitter, there were perhaps 20 quasi-private entities doing the same, including

> Stanford's Election Integrity Project, Newsguard, the Global Disinformation Index, and others, many taxpayer-funded.

And, like Renata Moon in her statement, charges the relevant parties of behavior one might find behind the Iron Curtain or, alternatively, as one of America's own historic versions of the same:

> A focus of this growing network is making lists of people whose opinions, beliefs, associations, or sympathies are deemed to be misinformation, disinformation, or malinformation. The latter term is just a euphemism for "true but inconvenient." Plain and simple, the making of such lists is a form of digital McCarthyism.

Taibbi also makes very clear that we are dealing with actions that pose multiple very serious and practical dangers for the affected persons:

> Ordinary Americans are not just being reported to Twitter for "deamplification" or de-platforming, but to firms like PayPal, digital advertisers like Xandr, and crowdfunding sites like GoFundMe. These companies can and do refuse service to law-abiding people and businesses whose only crime is falling afoul of a faceless, unaccountable, algorithmic judge.
>
> As someone who grew up a traditional ACLU liberal, this sinister mechanism for punishment without due process is horrifying.

Horrifying indeed; nor can the people turn to their historic ally, the press, for critical aid, because (to its undying shame) the mainstream press itself has gone turncoat:

> Another troubling aspect is the role of the press, which should be the people's last line of defense in such cases.
>
> But instead of investigating these groups, journalists partnered with them. If Twitter declined to remove an account right away, government agencies and NGOs would call reporters for *The New York Times, Washington Post,* and other outlets, who in turn would call Twitter demanding to know why action had not been taken.
>
> Wittingly or not, news media became an arm of a state-sponsored thought- policing system. [538]

The "censorship industrial complex" exposed by Shellenberger, Taibbi, and others' reporting on the Twitter Files is nothing short of terrifying to any defender of democracy, as it reveals the U.S. government and a host of powerful accomplices engaged in a naked Orwellian plot to control the minds, hearts, and pocketbooks of the people. Yet, as sensational as the Twitter File episode may have been, the relatively short-lived release of files soon assumed the character of an opener to another, far more consequential headliner show: *Missouri v. Biden* (*Murthy v. Missouri* as of October 2023).

Missouri Attorney General Eric Schmitt and Louisiana Attorney Jeff Landry filed suit against the federal government in May 2022 alleging that President Biden and his administration were "working with social media giants such as Meta, Twitter, and Youtube to censor and suppress free speech, including truthful information, related to COVID-19, election integrity, and other topics, under the guise of combating 'misinformation.'"[539] Subsequently, several other notable parties joined the case as plaintiffs, including Jay Battacharya and Martin Kuldorff, coauthors of The Great Barrington [Massachusetts] Declaration, and Dr. Aaron Kheriaty, former professor of psychiatry and director of the medical ethics program at the University of California Irvine (UCI). He was fired for refusing to comply with UCI's vaccine mandate. In July 2023, during a later phase of the case, Robert F. Kennedy Jr.'s kindred class action suit on behalf of individuals suffering alleged White House-sponsored censorship was consolidated with *Missouri v. Biden.*

Because chief plaintiffs in *Missouri v. Biden* included State Attorneys General (not merely private individuals or citizen organizations), the plaintiffs won significant powers of legal discovery, enabling them to pursue previously unavailable avenues of accumulating evidence. In late fall, 2022, attorneys for the plaintiffs issued subpoenas for a number of prominent White House officials, and were able to secure deposition of (among others) Dr. Anthony Fauci. The value of Fauci's lengthy testimony, was, however, somewhat impaired by the aging doctor's evidently fast-deteriorating powers of memory. Repeated grilled about contacts with various relevant parties, Fauci used the phrase "I don't recall" 174 times in the course of his deposition.

Then came the Twitter Files. Not only did the files open new troves of evidence the plaintiff's attorneys in *Missouri v. Biden* could put to very good use, the publicity surrounding Musk and the Twitter Files cast a bright spotlight on the issue of government-sponsored censorship in Covid World. When Judge Terry A. Doughty of the U.S. district court (Western Louisiana, Monroe Division) handed down a verdict on the plaintiffs' request for preliminary injunction on July 4, 2023 (a date the judge obviously chose for its potent symbolic resonance), the story made front-page headlines all over the country, including *The New York Times* and *Washington Post.*

The judgment, however—though a ringing victory for free speech in America, and one consequential response to the profound concerns voiced by Taibbi and Shellenberger—was not one those so-called liberal newspapers applauded. Judge Doughty granted the plaintiff's request for preliminary injunction, prohibiting the government (including the DOJ, DHH, State Dept., CDC, and FBI) from contacting diverse social media companies "for the purpose of urging, encouraging, pressuring, or inducing in any manner the removal, deletion, suppression, or reduction of content containing protected free speech."[540] The order also enjoined the government from substantive contact with academic programs based at Stanford and the University of Washington that materially aided and abetted government censorship (e.g., the Election Integrity Partnership, the Virality Project, and the Stanford Internet Observatory).

While, technically, the ruling granted only a preliminary injunction, such a ruling, especially when supported by a lengthy (155 page), forceful, and unequivocal opinion, clearly indicates how the judge intends to rule on the case. As Judge Doughty himself writes:

> The Plaintiffs are likely to succeed on the merits in establishing that the Government has used its power to silence the opposition. Opposition to COVID-19 vaccines; opposition to COVID-19 masking and lockdowns; opposition to the lab-leak theory of COVID-19; opposition to the validity of the 2020 election; opposition to President Biden's policies; statements that the Hunter Biden laptop story was true; and opposition to policies of the government officials in power. All were suppressed.[541]

The date of issuance was not the only signature of Judge Doughty's intent to mark the historic importance of his decision; the character and substance of his opening remarks[542] evidently do so as well. Those remarks make multiple reference to leading figures of the Enlightenment, or Age of Reason, including several of America's own founding fathers.

Judge Doughty:

> *I may disapprove of what you say, but I will defend to the death your right to say it.* —Evelyn Beatrice Hill, *Friends of Voltaire, 1906*
>
> This case is about the Free Speech Clause in the First Amendment to the United States Constitution. The explosion of social-media platforms has resulted in unique free speech issues— this is especially true in light of the COVID-19 pandemic. If the allegations made by Plaintiffs are true, the present case arguably involves **the most massive attack against free speech in United States' history.** In their attempts to suppress alleged

disinformation, the Federal Government, and particularly the Defendants named here, are alleged to have blatantly ignored the First Amendment's right to free speech.

Although the censorship alleged in this case almost exclusively targeted conservative speech, the issues raised herein go beyond party lines. The right to free speech is not a member of any political party and does not hold any political ideology. It is the purpose of the Free Speech Clause of the First Amendment to preserve an uninhibited marketplace of ideas in which truth will ultimately prevail, rather than to countenance monopolization of the market, whether it be by government itself or private licensee.

Plaintiffs allege that Defendants, through public pressure campaigns, private meetings, and other forms of direct communication, regarding what Defendants described as "disinformation," "misinformation," and "malinformation," have colluded with and/or coerced social-media platforms to suppress disfavored speakers, viewpoints, and content on social-media platforms. Plaintiffs also allege that the suppression constitutes government action, and that it is a violation of Plaintiffs' freedom of speech under the First Amendment to the United States Constitution.

The First Amendment states:

Congress shall make no law respecting an establishment of religion or prohibiting the free exercise thereof: ***or abridging the freedom of speech,*** *or of the press; or the right of the people peaceably to assemble, and to petition the Government for a redress of grievances—First Amendment, U.S. Const. amend. I (emphasis added).*

The principal function of free speech under the United States' system of government is to invite dispute; it may indeed best serve its high purpose when it induces a condition of unrest, creates dissatisfaction with conditions as they are, or even stirs people to anger . . . Freedom of speech and press is the indispensable condition of nearly every other form of freedom.

The following quotes reveal the Founding Fathers' thoughts on freedom of speech:

For if men are to be precluded from offering their sentiments on a matter, which may involve the most serious and alarming consequences, that can invite the consideration of mankind, reason is of no use to us; the freedom of speech may be taken away, and dumb and silent we may be led, like sheep, to the slaughter. —George Washington, March 15, 1783.

Whoever would overthrow the liberty of a nation must begin by subduing the free acts of speech. —Benjamin Franklin, Letters of Silence Dogwood

Reason and free inquiry are the only effectual agents against error. —Thomas Jefferson

Thus spoke (or wrote) Judge Doughty. Did the Biden administration hang its head in shame, admit grave error, and pledge to honor the spirit of the fathers and the letter of the law? Hardly. Even though Judge Doughty's order provided a list of exceptions ensuring that the government would be free to act so as appropriately to counter criminal activity or national threats, the government claimed that "irreparable harm" would be suffered if the injunction were enforced. The Biden administration accordingly immediately filed an appeal to the Court of Appeals for the Fifth District, and requested a stay of the injunction. On July 14, the Fifth Circuit granted an administrative stay, putting enforcement of the injunction on hold until the Fifth Court could rule on the merits of the case.

Proceeding on an expedited schedule as befit the weight of the proceedings, a three-judge panel of the Fifth Circuit (justices Jennifer Walker Elrod, Don Willet, and Edith Brown Clement) heard oral arguments on the case on August 10. While the verdict, still outstanding, will likely be rendered soon, chief counsel for the plaintiffs, John Sauer, was audibly on fire, memorably comparing government social media censorship to an extended book-burning campaign. The government's legal counsel Daniel Tenney's defense, on the other hand, limped along rather miserably. The judges, for their part, did little to disguise their discomfort with Tenney's attempt to deny coercion on the part of the government. Mimicking the kind of veiled threats employed by federal agents to coerce media platforms, one judge wryly insinuated: "That's a really nice social media company you've got there. It would be a shame if something happened to it!" Another parroted the government saying "Jump!" and a company exec responding "How high"?[543]

So, all signs point to the likelihood (though not, of course, the certitude) that the Fifth Circuit will reinstate Judge Doughty's injunction, either in its original or in some modified form.

That decision, however, will almost certainly not be the end of the legal road for *Missouri vs. Biden.* All pundits agree that, whichever way the judges rule, the case is very likely heading for the Supreme Court. It is there that the highest court in the land may have a chance to address "the most massive attack on free speech in United States history," and perhaps prescribe some legal remedy for the unprecedented "censorship industrial complex" that constitutes an existential threat to democracy in America.[544]

6. Systems of Control

In the course of discussing the previous topics, we have per force already touched upon diverse systems of social control, many of which are today functioning in a way incommensurate with both impartial science and free society. In the wake of 9/11, one would often hear talk of so-called terrorist cells. It should be evident from what has already been shared that medical boards and like professional medical organizations (the Washington Medical Commission [WMC], for instance, or the American Bureau of Internal Medicine) are today violently enforcing a rigid orthodoxy and so operating as cells of tyranny, contributing to what one writer has called "the biomedical security state."[545] It would be destructive enough if the influence of such organizations did not extend beyond the purview of medicine itself, but the brand of authoritarianism they exercise both reflects and spills out into the larger body politic, entering into an unholy alliance with industry, government agency, media, and other organs in the mutually-reinforcing system of social oppression I call (after the film by that name) the matrix.

I delve more systematically into this complex but enormously important subject in *Covid and the Apocalypse of the Modern Mind,* devoting the better part of the whole first section of that book ("The Great Reset and the Dialectic of Enlightenment") to the topic. Even so, I wish to conclude this postscript, this late update of my *Covid Chronicle,* by noting two important recent developments pertinent to the subject.

I have just alluded to the manner in which medical orthodoxy, rigidly enforced by dictatorial licensing boards and other official bodies, can all too easily infect society at large with kindred forms of intolerance and coercive control. Yet mechanisms of ideological and social persuasion do not always function by way of the kind of naked display of power exhibited by licensing boards or universities that fire respected teachers for voicing "unauthorized" views.

In fact, the contrary is often the case. Some of the actions that most effectively expand the reach of a given system of belief (and, coordinately, the forms of social praxis that support that system) may not appear at all coercive or authoritarian. Instead, these may often appear under the auspices of laudable enterprises designed only to serve the public good. The recent burgeoning of health centers in public schools represents one textbook case in point.

On the face of it, the idea of school-based health centers (SBHCs) sounds unobjectionable and in many respects may, indeed, function as a convenient and effective means of providing more children (especially those in underserved communities with inferior access to medical services) more and better healthcare. It is also an idea that has been around for over two decades. Numerous SBHCs have been in operation for years. Even so, the recent maverick-size wave of monetary and organizational support channeled into SBHCs on the federal as well as state level is unprecedented.

In May 2022, the U.S. Department of Health and Human Services (HHS) granted $25 million to 125 SBHCs to strengthen and expand healthcare services. Still more significantly, a month or so later, in June 2022, the federal government passed the Bipartisan Safer Communities Act. The act empowered HHS to disburse $50 million in grants to states "for the purpose of implementing, enhancing, or expanding the provision" of healthcare in SBHCs in coordination with Medicaid or the Children's Health Insurance Program (CHIP). The Center for Medicare and Medicaid Services (CMS) was charged with administrative oversight of the program. Nor are state officials lagging in the effort to boost SBHCs. In fall 2022, for instance, the governor of Georgia announced an allotment of $125 million to expand the SBHC program in that state.[546]

What is the rub here? Organizations such as the Georgia Coalition for Vaccine Choice[547] fear that mechanisms put in place for the administration of healthcare in the newly enhanced and empowered SBHCs can all too easily enable health and school officials to perform an end run around parental choice—a special concern, naturally, when controversial health measures may be in question.

According to CMS, SBHC services include efforts "to prevent disease, disability, and other health conditions or their progression" by means of immunizations and well childcare.[548] At the same time, the parental consent forms distributed by SBHCs legally authorizing them to provide services may be unclear—and even deliberately ambiguous—as to exactly what services a parent sanctions by signing a general consent form. The first half-page of such a form from one Georgia school[549] appears as follows:

~

Georgia Highlands Medical Services
Cummings Elementary School Based Healthcare
CONSENT FORM

____________ ____________ ____________

Student Grade Home Room Teacher Student Last Name

In order for your child to receive services with Georgia Highlands Medical Center at Cummings Elementary School, this consent form must be completed.

I hereby voluntarily give my consent for ____________ to receive health services with Georgia Highland Medical Services at Cummings Elementary School. I further authorize any healthcare provider and professional staff working for the clinic to provide such medical tests, diagnoses, procedures and treatments as are reasonably necessary and advisable for the medical evaluation and management of my child's healthcare.

I understand that my signing this consent allows the healthcare provider and professional clinic staff of Georgia Highlands Medical Services at Cummings Elementary Schools to provide comprehensive health services which includes physical and behavioral health services.

~

"In order for your child to receive..." What elementary school parent does not want to authorize knowledgeable school-based staff to help their child if he or she suffers injury or a sudden ailment at school? Yet child advocate attorney Justine Tanguay writes:

> This year, many schools will be sending home blanket consent-to-treat forms for parents to sign. Parents need to be aware that these forms are not the traditional authorizations requests to the school nurse to give first-aid or treat minor illness.[550]

Regarding the form itself, reporter Suzanne Burdick notes:

> The form says nothing about parents being notified before, during, or after treatment...The form does not clarify who determines what services are "reasonably necessary or advisable" and does not explain how parents will be involved in that process.... The form does not clarify what specifically falls into the category of "physical and behavioral health services" or how parents will be involved in the determination for what services their child may need.[551]

Parental concern may well be heightened upon discovery that the School Based Health Alliance—a group that works to support SBHCs—receives funding from both HHS and Merck, even as HHS allocated nearly $5 million to research led by a Merck consultant to explore so-called Announcement Approach Training.[552] Merck is the company that markets the highly controversial HPV vaccine (Gardasil), the target population for which are young, predominantly school age persons, especially preteens and adolescents. What constitutes Announcement Approach Training? One can guess well enough from the title. The approach involves health providers *simply "announcing" that the HPV vaccination will be part of a routine examination, instead of prefacing any discussion of the topic by first reaching out to the child's family.*

Regrettably, the kind of overly "comprehensive" health consent form scripted for Cummings Elementary seems tailor-made for the Announcement Approach, which (while clearly designed to maximize uptake of the HPV vaccine) could otherwise conceivably run afoul of informed choice or parental consent laws. Those restrictions notwithstanding, it seems to me that the so-called Announcement Approach has been much in vogue since the advent of Covid, not only in SBHCs but in society at large—as if the authorities believed it best to treat Americans as if we were a nation of school children.

SBHCs could perform a great service—*if* health centers were administered in such a way as to accord due respect to informed consent and parental choice. Yet the behavior of pharmaceutical companies, medical boards, and compliant government agencies hardly inspires faith on that score. As Georgia attorney and co-director of the Georgia Coalition for Vaccine Choice puts it, "It's unfortunate that we have to approach this [SBHCs] with the thought: How could this be abused? But that's where we are." [553]

Corporate industry, medical boards, universities, social media companies, even SBHCs, and (of course) the U.S. government itself—all of which participate in the complex of power I call "the matrix." Yet, as *Missouri v. Biden* (currently *Murthy v. Missouri*) shows, even the behemoth of the U.S. government may potentially be reined in by concerted citizen action. The government, after all, is technically and ethically answerable to its employers—we, the people—and legally beholden to each and every clause of the Constitution, the body of law that represents the moral charter of the nation.

Yet, is there some scenario in which the mechanisms of social control gets so out of hand that the people, and even the U.S. Constitution, would officially be made subject to some *superior* institutional authority? *Unthinkable,* you might say. *Despite all the craziness that went down in Covid World, this is still the United States of America.* And yet, the current administration, whether in deliberate collusion with the technocratic elites of the world or not, is leading us in just that direction, one that Americans, jealous of their national sovereignty as well as personal freedoms, must abhor.

Imagine all the very *worst* aspects of Covid World—the fearmongering and exaggerated hyping of a deadly pandemic; the peremptory imposition of a host of indiscriminate and dictatorial measures; the greed-driven obsession with experimental vaccines and deliberate marginalizing of genuinely safe and effective health measures; compulsory mandates and harsh punitive measures for those who refuse the jab; vaccine passports and digital IDs (such as the Europe Unions's Green Pass) and the systematic suppression of science and free speech in mainstream and social media under the guise of combating misinformation…in short, all that engendered Covid World. Imagine all of this neatly wrapped up, packaged and delivered for reuse to VIPs who *still* think that all of the foregoing represents *enlightened* leadership and an apt model for future success. On top of that, imagine granting—not any state or national government—but some *international* organization with the unilateral authority to engender and implement something like Covid World again, and—by force of a legally binding "treaty" that supersedes the sovereignty of nations—compel the people of the world to comply with its edicts.

Imagine all this, and—*voilà!*—you hold in the palm of your hand the two lengthy and detailed documents known as the zero draft of the WHO Pandemic Treaty and the newly amended version of the *International Health Regulations* (IHR), promulgated by the WHO.[554] Imagine all this, and you have nothing less than a made-to-order dystopia on your doorstep, a quasi- (or not so quasi-) totalitarian takeover of world government under the aegis of public health (or, in the current parlance of the WHO, their "One Health" initiative).

This nightmarish scenario is no dream but threatens to become an all-too concrete reality within the span of mere months. The WHO has been working steadily on this grand scheme for a while, and moving forward on it with deliberate speed. In the works for WHO knows how long, the zero draft of the Pandemic Treaty was first made public on February 1, 2022; a revised version was published on June 2, 2023. Amendments to the IHR were proposed in mid-December 2022, and a revised version of the proposed amendments published on February 6, 2023. The whole package is scheduled for approval in May 2024, when adoption of the proposals requires nothing more than a simple majority of the 194 countries presently belonging to the WHO.[555]

In the case of successful passage, all member countries would be legally bound by the edicts of the WHO as spelled out in the approved documents. In order for the WHO orders to acquire the force of law in the U.S., the President need not even sign nor the Congress debate and confirm because, technically speaking, the proposals do not represent "new" initiatives (even if they clearly do), but merely revisions of agreements previously approved and already in force.

If you are an American, you may well be saying to yourself: This cannot be. It cannot possibly be true that my government has the power to surrender the sovereign rights guaranteed by the Constitution, the supreme Law of the Land, which the government itself, in our republican form of rule (our constitutional democracy), is forever bound to observe and obey, and which can only be amended by the due process the Constitution itself prescribes. It is not conceivable that measures and regulations promulgated by some conglomerate international body, whose administrators are in no wise elected by or otherwise representative of the people of the United States, can bind American citizens so as to restrict lawful prerogative within this country, or abrogate the sovereign rights guaranteed by the Constitution. No WHO One Health measure—let us say, a mandate prescribing compulsory vaccination by some new mRNA platform drug, or an edict prescribing universal masking or new lockdowns, or a requirement that I carry a digital health ID in order to travel, or the banning of disfavored speech by the Czars of Public Communication at the WHO—none of these or any similar WHO-sponsored orders could legally bind my action, my medical choices, my right to travel, or my liberty to voice my opinion on matters of the moment owing to my standing as a constitutionally protected citizen of a sovereign nation.

So one might think. Yet some say that any assurance on that score would be ill-founded. On account of legalities related to the binding force of other international agreements and war treaties, approval of the Pandemic Treaty and IHR documents could effectively make me a loyal subject of—no God, sovereign nation, or even king of kings—but the Almighty WHO, which, by the wave of the magic IHR/Pandemic Treaty wand, might suddenly accede to a position very like supreme ruler of the globe.

That is a consummation devoutly to be… STOPPED!

If you as yet do not understand in detail why, James Roguski, the nerve center of #StopTheTreaty, #StopTheAmendments, and #ExitTheWHO initiatives, gives 10 compelling reasons why—for anyone who values liberty and human dignity—the so-called Pandemic Treaty represents something not so very far from the quintessence of evil. He then proceeds to list 10 more why the same can be said, with still greater conviction and practical urgency, of the proposed amendments to the IHR regulations.[556]

Roguski has been working on the matter for some time, and—to keep pace with revisions of the relevant WHO documents—his top-ten list has morphed somewhat, but here's my rendition of one version of his list for the Pandemic Treaty:

1. As I suggested in introducing this whole delightful subject, if you thought Covid and the official response to it was your idea of a good time and suitable governance, we can look forward to indefinite repetition/extension of the same or like joy-rides. The so-called Pandemic Treaty would "dramatically expand the role of WHO . . . providing a legally binding framework convention that would hand over enormous additional legally binding authority to WHO" recognizing "the central role of WHO in the prevention, preparedness, response and recovery from future pandemics."[557]

2 & 3. Naturally, this would require a new tremendously elaborate bureaucracy. Don't think "WHO" is a Brechtian enough moniker for the doings of this noble international organization? Never fear, now you and your country will be ruled by the new executive body called *The Conference of Parties,* conveniently (see #4) abbreviated COP. The establishment, maintenance, and operation of the organization run by this politburo would siphon many *billions* of dollars off from member countries, as the yearly budget of this bureaucracy would be many times the current budget of the entire WHO.

4. No need to worry about petty U.S. lawsuits like Missouri vs. Biden. The treaty would empower WHO to take the business of censorship into its own hands, AND throw in unprecedented surveillance capacities for good measure. Approval of the WHO documents would thus, in one fell swoop, virtually ensure the meteoric rise of what Dr. Aaron Kheriaty, in a new must-read book, calls the "Biomedical Security State"—except that it would be no nation state in charge, but the WHO COP.[558]

5. If Operation Warp-speed weren't speedy or recklessly risky enough for you, the treaty would license still more accelerated production, approval, and distribution of novel experimental drugs and injections (including, presumably, future mRNA vaccines).

6. Concerned about GOF (gain-of-function) research? Well, lay those concerns aside, because there will be nothing you or anyone else can do about it. The Pandemic Treaty would remove all restrictions on GOF worldwide, more or less ensuring a steady stream of man-made pandemic disasters for the WHO to prepare for and "respond" to.

7. Ever heard of Event 201, Dark Winter and the other War Game-like simulations that incubated Covid World? If not, please plunge into volume 2 of *Reset or Renaissance* and learn about how the technocrats of the world regularly train to take such good care of the rest of us. The WHO treaty, by the way, would fund many more such war-games to the tune of billions and billions *more* dollars. After all, practice makes perfect!

8. If you thought the official powers-that-be did such a wonderful job aiding the *human* world's response to COVID, and that your beloved cat, dog, horse, or favorite coyote deserve a piece of the action, now WHO's new "One Health" aegis will extend WHO skill and wisdom over the face of the entire globe, including the animal world (pet, wildlife, and agricultural management) and indeed all natural eco-systems, under the umbrella of public health administration.

9. Passing reference to furry friends, however, should not for a moment divert attention from the fact the WHO's primary aim is to infiltrate every aspect of human life. Thus it's new and newly hegemonic "One Health" concept is matched by a kindred "Whole of Government —Whole of Society" approach. On the health front, all of this of course means Centralization Deluxe, so that you can forget about anything like the old-fashioned doctor-patient relationship or recognition of the importance of individual difference in medicine or any other domain. Mindless, faceless totalizing UNI/CONFORMITY, here we come!

10. Just in case the supreme Police Power of WHO in its new guise as world COP wasn't clear enough, the latter would have its executive and enforcement capacities lodged in a formal "Global Review System," empowering it systematically to review the compliance of member nations with all its dictates, and to take suitable remedial/punitive (including financially based) measures in case of non-compliance.

Can all this conceivably be true? I am afraid one cannot make this stuff up (unless perhaps, one's name is Orwell, or Huxley, or—perhaps...Stalin?) If the above were not terrifying enough, Roguski tells us that (believe it or not), the Pandemic Treaty is not even the worst of it; that the amended IHR comprise a still more immediate and practical threat to human life and liberty.

For your edification and mine, I will give just the headlines of one version of Roguski's top ten for the IHR.

1. CHANGE FROM ADVISORY TO MANDATORY
2. POTENTIAL RATHER THAN ACTUAL EMERGENCIES
4. ALLOCATION PLAN (WHO director gets control over production/ distribution of health products and MCMs[559] such as vaccines)
5. MANDATORY MEDICAL TREATMENTS
6. GLOBAL HEALTH CERTIFICATES
7. LOSS OF SOVEREIGNTY
8. UNSPECIFIED ENORMOUS COSTS
9. CENSORSHIP
10. OBLIGATIONS OF DUTY TO COOPERATE

While the last four items overlap with the Pandemic Treaty top ten, the higher ranked ones convey a sense of why Roguski views the IHR amendments as of still greater immediacy and practical moment. They make concrete and practicable wholesale transfer of enormous power to the WHO and speak of concrete measure (such as global health certificates and mandatory medical treatments) that could fundamentally alter the reality of our world virtually overnight.

The combination of the first and second listed items possesses especially sinister implications. The first nakedly hands unprecedented power to the WHO, while the second suggests that no actual health emergency even need transpire to trigger whatever measures the WHO wishes to take, as the mere potential of a health threat (determined, of course, by WHO itself) suffices. Practically speaking, that means the world would be subject to WHO edicts most any time, most anywhere.

My attentive reader may be disturbed by an omission. I've listed only nine reasons above. What happened to number 3? In fact, I deliberately left it for a last, special mention because (in my mind, at least) number 3 virtually says it all. In Roguski's list it reads:

3. DISREGARD FOR DIGNITY, HUMAN RIGHTS AND FREEDOMS

Is Roguski here assessing the broader implications of the IHR amendments after a fashion not explicit in the language of the proposed changes? No, on the contrary, Article 3 of the existing, *unamended* language of the IHR enjoins the WHO and member nations ever and always to act in such a manner that shows *"respect for dignity, human rights and fundamental freedoms of people."*[560] The amended version of the IHR does not revise or modify this clause; it simply removes—deletes it!—altogether. The WHO today clearly believes that the phrase "respect for dignity, human rights, and fundamental freedoms of people" articulate aims no longer commensurate with its ideological or practical mission; but instead represent inconvenient or untenable ideals that can only get in the way of its work.

As far as Covid World is concerned—as well as the current character of the WHO and its pet project—this deliberate omission, the deafening sound of that intentional silence, does, I think, say it all.

PART VII

POSTSCRIPT II

THE KENNEDY CANDIDACY AND THE ANATOMY OF PRO-VAX PREJUDICE

Thanksgiving 2023

I originally hoped to publish *Two Roads* early in 2022 when the pandemic was still in full swing. Once I realized I was writing a book rather than a (very long) letter, I donned my seven-league boots, intending to wade midstream into public debate on ivermectin, vaccine mandates, and other controversial issues. I will not enter here into why the book did not appear sooner.[561] From the perspective of the present, however, I can see how the delay yields gain as well as loss, novel opportunity no less than missed chances. We are still just beginning to come to terms with—not the (largely resolved) day-to-day Covid crises—but with the legacy of Covid World, the deeper meaning of the relevant events. What are we are to make of everything that transpired in the course of the pandemic and everything that—despite the lifting of the public health emergency—is still going on?

To speak of one concrete boon: the delay in getting this book to press opened the door for me to write the August 2023 postscript, expanding the temporal reach of this book and carrying many of its arguments to more emphatic conclusion. While the saga of Covid-19 is very far from complete, "Covid World, August 2023" brought *An American Scholar's Covid Chronicle* to some kind of satisfactory end—not the end of the road, to be sure, but to a well-earned layover nonetheless; a place where I could, in good conscience, pull off my boots and count a good day's work said and done.

Or so I thought. Now, three months later, I am no longer confident this first volume is indeed completed. As I work over the copyedited draft of the text, I find that quarter-year turn has once more triggered the itch of the pen and that the "angel of the book" is urging me not to let time gone by go to waste, but somehow, someway, to make good use of it again.

The current moment—shortly before Thanksgiving 2023—is one ripe with significance for the story I have told (or at least *began* to tell) in *Two Roads*. It is now exactly two years since Robert F. Kennedy Jr's *The Real Anthony Fauci* appeared. It is roughly two years, as well, since I finished the chapter in *Two Roads* devoted to that tome and so brought the main body of *Two Roads* itself to a close. So much for "a backward glance o'er travel'd roads," but what of the way ahead? If it is now two years since Kennedy's *Fauci* appeared, it is also one year (or just under) until America elects a new president in November 2024.

An American presidential election is always a historic affair. Yet 2024 is of uniquely powerful relevance to the world opened and explored in *Two Roads*. It is so, of course, because RFK Jr. himself is running. Not only is he running, but as of early October of this year, RFK Jr.—having suffered crucifixion by the Democratic Party to which his father and uncle and he himself once belonged—is doing so as an Independent. In the much-publicized Quinnipiac Poll published November 1, Kennedy was polling twenty-two percent in a head-to-head contest between Biden and Trump, and out-polling them both with two constituencies that typically augur which way the political tide is flowing: Independents, and younger voters (in this poll, those eighteen to thirty-four years of age).[562]

Not bad for a Covid dissident scorned as an "anti-vaxxer," even if his name *is* Kennedy.

I do not, however, want to use this additional bit of text to talk to you about RFK Jr.—at least not directly, or exclusively. I do, however, want to talk about his "brand"—or rather, the way he and others of like mind are branded "*anti-vaxxers*" and the peculiarly insidious type of prejudice associated with that label.

The topic is of signal importance. The whole landscape of Covid World was decisively shaped by the vaccine-centric agenda and policies of mass vaccination continue to function as a lynchpin of public health policy. If we are genuinely to take stock of what transpired during Covid with an eye toward transforming the systems—both ideological and institutional—responsible for the catastrophe of Covid World, a critical review of vaccine science and the institutions that generate, promote, and implement it would qualify as one essential point of departure. While I can hardly pretend to accomplish such a complex task in this postscript, I can nonetheless make a start by way of a preliminary examination of what I would like to call *the anatomy of pro-vax prejudice*.

In the aftermath of Covid, I think few would deny that those opposed to mass vaccination policies, whether we are speaking of Covid mRNA gene therapies or more traditional vaccines (the two classes of resistance may or may not overlap for any given individual[563]), have suffered the kind of social ostracism historically directed at other disfavored classes of persons.[564] What, after all, does it mean to label someone an anti-vaxxer? In today's parlance, the word itself typically functions as a kind of degrading epithet, one that can and often does operate in a manner roughly analogous to a racial slur. Both imply that the relevant person is in some wise inferior and so undeserving of the level of respect and attention awarded equals. Both can be associated with the perpetration of psychological, social, and physical violence.[565]

All forms of prejudice are comprised of a few distinct yet integrally related components which may be broadly described as *intellectual, affective, and moral* in nature. In the peculiar case of pro-vax prejudice, not only does the intellectual component possess a certain genetic priority, but the brand of intellectuality at play is specifically and exclusively scientific in nature.[566]

In this connection, it is crucial to note that the physical act of vaccination—inoculation by way of insertion of a needle—does not in and of itself qualify as any kind of moral good. Rather, the good associated with that material act depends upon the perceived medical and epidemiological *effects* of vaccination as such are observed, recorded, and interpreted for us by science. If one imagined a scenario in which the majority of the population believed that science had definitively established that vaccination did far more harm than good—that it sickened, injured, and killed people at a much higher rate than it prevented serious illness and death—the argument that citizens have a moral responsibility to vaccinate their children would be decisively rejected and the ethical equation radically reversed.

Because vaccination itself does not represent an intrinsic good, *the moral legitimacy of the pro-vax stance stands or falls with the validity of the science that grounds it.* The *seed* of pro-vax prejudice cannot therefore so much be found in the emotional hostility displayed toward anti-vaxxers, but rather inheres in forms of thinking—intellectual judgments—that fail the test of fact and reason in the very act of invoking the science that stakes its authority on rational, evidence-based processes and results.

More simply: *pro-vax prejudice begins with assuming*—on account of ideological dogmatism, ulterior motive, misplaced trust in expert authority, wishful thinking, willful ignorance, professional prestige, or other influences—*and asserting scientific justification when and where there is none.* Correlatively, it often imagines that is not I, but the Other—the anti-vaxxer—who is doing just that. Feelings of antipathy that fuel indignant moral condemnation frequently follow and fill out the character and force of the complex as a whole.

There could hardly be a more exemplary exhibition of the intellectual ground of pro-vax prejudice than the January 2022 YouTube medical lecture by Dr. Eric Strong. As indicated by its provocative title ("Is Anti-vaxxer an Offensive Slur?"[567]), Dr. Strong's lecture confronts the subject of this postscript head-on. Not only does he clearly articulate the *intellectual deficiency* he regards as inherent in the anti-vax stance, he does the great service of delineating, in detail, exactly what defines someone as an anti-vaxxer in the first place. He takes pains to do so because he wishes to differentiate genuine anti-vaxxers from persons who—while perhaps exhibiting hesitancy on the vaccine issue or opposing vaccine mandates on ethical grounds—nonetheless do not deserve the dreaded anti-vax label.[568]

Strong kicks off his analysis with a simple definition, one literally spelled out on the YouTube screen: "Anti-vaxxer: An individual whose opposition to vaccination is immutable to reason or evidence." (Doesn't he mean "impervious" rather than "immutable"?)

> In other words, an anti-vaxxer is incapable of being convinced to receive the vaccine, regardless of how much evidence is presented to them of its efficacy and safety and regardless of how reliable and trustworthy that data is.[569]

"Reason," "evidence," "data": Dr. Strong clearly speaks the language of science. He does not, however, make any effort to specify what might qualify data as "reliable and trustworthy." Nor does he seem to harbor any doubt as to what conclusion a reasonable person might draw from such data regarding the safety and efficacy of vaccines.

These are my qualms, not Strong's. As we shall soon see, however, they are crucial caveats.

After formulating his basic definition, Strong educates us as to how, exactly, to identify an anti-vaxxer. Confronted by someone advocating vaccination, the true anti-vaxxer will surely contend:

- That the Covid vaccines have not been sufficiently studied, *"despite the fact that they are the most studied medical intervention in history."*
- That the vaccines have not been studied for long enough, *"despite the fact that after eighteen months*[570] *and hundreds of millions of doses, there have been no safety signals to suggest the existence of delayed side effects."*
- That natural immunity is superior to vaccine-induced immunity, even though one must catch Covid to gain natural immunity, and despite

the fact that *"natural immunity plus vaccination definitely results in better immunity than either one alone."*

- That Big Pharma cannot be trusted, *"despite tremendous oversight of the Covid vaccines, and numerous independent analyses reaching the same conclusions on their safety and effectiveness as the pharmaceutical companies."*
- That if the vaccine manufactures had real faith in their products, they would not block lawsuits brought by the vaccine-injured, *"despite the fact that the vaccine-injured are still compensated. It's just that in the U.S. they're compensated by the federal government, not directly by the companies."*
- That the vaccines have killed thousands of people, *"despite this claim, which is based on a profound misunderstanding of the Vaccine Adverse Event Reporting System [VAERS], being repeatedly and thoroughly debunked."* [571]

In his initial definition, Strong puts his finger on the nature of the *intellectual* prejudice that colors contemporary attitudes about vaccination. A whole class of persons appear irrevocably convinced of the correctness of their position. They automatically regard any and all evidence that contradicts that position as unreliable, any source that supplies or cites such contradictory evidence as not creditable, and any argument that contests the prevailing view as inherently spurious.

Such rigid orthodoxy evidently precludes any impartial or objective—any real—scientific inquiry. No matter how well-established any given truth may appear,[572] such dogmatism qualifies as a singularly unenlightened stance. The strong irony inherent in Strong's argument, however, should be evident to any reader of this book. *It is not, after all, the anti-vaxxers that are guilty of such consequential bias, but self-assured vaccine proponents like Dr. Strong himself.*

To justify that counter-claim, one needs only to review the terms of Dr. Strong's own rebuttals of the typical anti-vaxxer's customary talking points. What Strong evidently views as established fact and irrefutable truths—as expressed in all those (in my transcription, *italicized*) prepositional phrases beginning with "despite"—are directly contrary to the full weight of fact and of reason marshaled in this book, if not simple common sense. To declare, for instance, that the experimental mRNA gene therapies rushed out after a few short months under the aegis of an EUA qualify as "the most studied medical interventions in history" is simply ludicrous.[573] Similary, for Strong to suggest—even in January 2020— that no warning signs of troublesome vaccine side effects had emerged, requires that he blithely disregard a whole trove of consequential data that tells a very different story.

And so it goes. Strong's point about the federal government stepping in to compensate the vaccine-injured entirely misses the point that such an arrangement does nothing to check Big Pharma's negligence or recklessness, but rather enables it while passing the bill on to taxpayers. Anyone at all familiar with the phenomena of regulatory capture will laugh—or cry—at Strong's assertion of the "tremendous oversight" exercised by federal agencies in their review of pharmaceutical products, or his reference to "independent analyses" (like that textbook example of scientific fraud, the famous *Nature* paper debunking the lab-leak theory?[574]) that confirm the credibility and authoritative expertise of scientists and public health officials. On what basis might Strong allege that the tens of thousands of deaths linked to vaccines by VAERS do *not* represent people killed by vaccines at all?

Because VAERS entries record correlation and do not prove causation, Strong *assumes* that the huge number of VAERS-recorded injuries and deaths are not due to vaccines, but to some ancillary cause. For many reasons discussed in *Two Roads*, however, it is highly probable that the prohibitive majority of deaths and injuries VAERS links to vaccines are indeed vaccine-related. Moreover, as Deb Conrad's story suggests, for anyone familiar with how VAERS operates and cognizant of the multiple means by which the public health system *discourages* VAERS filings, the notion that VAERS grossly *over-reports* actual vaccine injury and death is an absurdity. In presuming otherwise, Dr. Strong himself indulges in the very "magical thinking" he imputes to "irrational" anti-vaxxers.

There is one further reason to believe it is not the anti-vaxxers who hold "immutable" opinions impervious to fact and reason. It is those challenging the pro-vax establishment who call for robust debate and (like statistician Matthew Crawford, Dr. Madhava Setty, or RFK, Jr. himself) invite proponents to prove them wrong *not* by way of blanket statement or vapid generalization, but with specifics pertaining to particular points of contention. Leading vaccine proponents, on the other hand, avoid public debate with well-informed health freedom advocates like the plague.

The most recent and celebrated example of this phenomena involved podcaster Joe Rogan's offer to host a debate between Robert F. Kennedy Jr. and the well-known vaccine advocate Dr. Peter Hotez.[575] Predictably, Hotez—not

Kennedy—declined Rogan's offer. The terms in which MSNBC defended Hotez's refusal aptly characterize the tenor of much pro-vax prejudice.

In his June 20, 2023, opinion piece titled "Peter Hotez's Disinterest in Debating RFK Jr. on Vaccines Makes Perfect Sense: Why Would an Expert Want to Engage with a Remorseless Misinformation Peddler in a Poorly Designed Forum?" MSNBC editor Zeeshan Aleem writes:

> What Rogan is proposing is a debate between someone who has respect for the quest for truth and someone who doesn't. Hotez would be guided by an expert appraisal of empirical reality, while Kennedy would spread misinformation and disinformation about vaccines. How would that be edifying for the public?[576]

How, indeed? The public could not possibly be edified by any of the facts or reasons Kennedy might employ to substantiate his arguments since (secure in the unquestionable authority of experts like Hotez) these may safely be written off, *in advance,* as mis- and disinformation.

Who here is exhibiting a patent disrespect for "the quest for truth"?

So much for the widely recognized *intellectual* debility of anti-vaxxers whose views had best be suppressed entirely, even if doing so represents a course of action as thoroughly anti-scientific as it is anti-democratic. What of the anti-vaxxer's *moral* character and standing in society?

On this score, Eric Strong shows himself to be a tolerant soul not inclined to rush to judgment. Indeed, he goes so far as to imagine that even the benighted views of the anti-vaxxer may not in fact stem from inherent stupidity but rather devolve from forces beyond their control:

> Being an anti-vaxxer does not automatically make a person dumb or selfish. Aside from a tiny number who knowingly distort the truth for financial gain, the rest are simply promoting a sincerely held belief that was formed due to cognitive bias due to exposure to misinformation that was largely beyond their control. I do not blame the vast majority of anti-vaxxers for being anti-vax.[577]

I wonder if those in the anti-vax community could marshal sufficient empathy to maintain an equivalent position with respect to vaccine advocates such as Eric Strong himself.

Perhaps—although the idea that someone like Dr. Strong has little to no control over what he chooses to believe stretches credulity. At what point does "cognitive bias" bred of an entrenched system of belief become intellectual and social irresponsibility? If Dr. Strong is going to give public medical lectures touching on vaccine safety, should he not regard it as his civic as well as scientific duty to learn a thing or two about the realities of the VAERS system instead of merely parroting the talking points of the vaccine party line? Has Dr. Eric Strong never heard it said that people who live in glass houses had best not throw stones?

Be that as it may, whereas Dr. Strong generously declines to brand anti-vaxxers as inherently stupid and self-centered, a great many pro-vaccine persons display markedly less restraint. Disregarding the paramount fact that anti-vaxxers do *not* see a social benefit in vaccination but rather the opposite (negative medical outcomes and a degradation of public health), the enlightened anti-anti-vaxxer often feels entitled to brand those who disagree with them as inherently insensitive to the general welfare or, in plain terms, selfish and egotistical.

The anatomy of pro-vax prejudice in its dominant form today thus involves a destructive feedback loop between scientific truth claims, on the one hand, and ethical judgment, on the other. The intellectual superiority derived from belief in what is *uncritically* regarded as settled if not infallible "science" (even though no "science" that cannot brook disagreement and dissent can rightfully be so called) fuels a sense of moral superiority, and the complacent conviction confirming one's own more socially responsible and self-sacrificing humanity helps justify willful disregard of any scientific arguments advanced by anti-vaxxers.

Dr. Eric Strong's anti-vaxxer video dates from early 2022, when the deficiences of the Covid-19 program—though already recognized by some—were less glaringly evident than would be so further down the Covid road. One would hope that, in the almost two years intervening between then and now, the great majority of persons would have learned their Covid-19 vaccine lessons and thrown off the mantle of pro-vax prejudice like some old vermin-infested cloak. Many indeed have done so. Regrettably, however, a very sizable segment of American society (many if not most of whom are of a liberal persuasion) remain buttoned up in that vile old coat as if nothing untoward had transpired over the course of the last three or four years. Let me advance the argument of this second postscript by examining two more recent expressions of prejudice, the first from a book published in late 2022 and the second from a *New York Times* op-ed, printed just a week or so ago in mid-November 2023.

The title of best-selling author Andrea Wulf's recent *Magnificent Rebels: The First Romantics and the Invention of the Self*[578] promises courageous intellectual adventure, but one passage from Wulf's Prologue—the only one referencing the pandemic—can hardly be read without a sense of ironic letdown. In this passage, Wulf herself exhibits—no sort of rebellion, magnificent or not—but rather a textbook example of the moral as well as intellectual blindness inherent in pro-vax prejudice. Wulf:

> We've entered into a social contract with those who govern us. We've accepted laws that frame the society in which we live—though not in perpetuity. They are negotiable. Laws can be revised or changed in order to adapt to new circumstances....Take the global pandemic, for example, when millions of us voluntarily surrendered our basic rights and liberties for the greater good. For months, we didn't see our friends and families, and followed draconian rules because we believed it was the morally right thing to do. Other's didn't. They simply refused to obey these restrictions, insisting that their individual liberties were more important.[579]

The syntactical construction of Wulf's last three sentences is revealing. "We...followed draconian rules because we believed it was the morally right thing to do. Others didn't."

Didn't *what?* Follow the rules, or "believe it was the morally right thing to do"?

On first read, one may understand it either way. But Wulf's concluding sentence makes clear that she herself does not seem to be aware of the ambiguity and means simply to convey that those "others" did not follow the rules because they insisted that their "individual liberties" took precedence over the public good. Those others, to put it bluntly, were selfish and unwilling to make the personal sacrifice necessary to ensure the welfare of the community.

What Wulf's prejudice does not allow her even to see is that those others almost certainly believe—for reasons she does not seem to allow herself to consider or critically evaluate—that following those "draconian" rules does *not* in fact benefit public health. Those others also likely believe that infringing individual liberties—including the freedom of speech that permits fair public debate as to the objective merit of extraordinary measures such as lockdowns, masking, and mandates—is *morally* exactly the *wrong* thing to do. It is so because it violates principles that form the foundation of our democratic society and the "social contract" that underlies representative government rather than the exercise of arbitrary power.

Two Roads reveals that legitimation of the very policies Wulf supports and obeys depended upon a systematic and wide-ranging abrogation of the American people's civil rights.

In our constitutional democracy, jealous guardianship of the Bill of Rights is not extrinsic to moral and social responsibility but at its very core. The breaching of that law—including censorship of dissent under the indiscriminate aegis of "misinformation"—permits partisan and ill-informed opinions as to what does or does not serve the public good to rule unchallenged by reason, evidence, and the robust debate that defines a society as a free rather than tyrannically authoritarian. American citizens, Democratic or Republican, do not believe in the infallible or divine authority of a king or a pope or (is not this the lesson we need learn from Covid?) any cadre of public-health officials, no matter how "expert" they presume to be.[580]

Wulf's book concerns itself with a circle of philosophers and poets living in or near the small university town of Jena, Germany, in the wake of the French Revolution. As she notes in her prologue, this was a time when "most of the world was ruled by monarchs and leaders who controlled many aspects of their subjects' lives"[581]—a situation not unfamiliar to anyone who lived through the Covid era. In Jena, the idea of individual freedom accordingly served as the dynamic center of profound inquiry by the likes of Friedrich Schiller, Johann Gottlieb Fichte, the brothers Friedrich and August Wilhelm Schlegel, and Friedrich Schelling. To cite just one of the costly fruits that ripened on Jena's philosophic tree, Schelling's *Philosophical Investigations into the Essence of Human Freedom*[582] is considered by many the crowning achievement of that philosopher's prolific intellectual career.

If you are interested in what an *American* thinker[583] deeply influenced by German philosophical idealism in general and Schelling in particular might make of Covid World, I urge you to read volume 2 of *Reset or Renaissance.* If the French Revolution and the tremendous questions it posed for humanity, counts as the indispensable point of departure for the Jena Set's[584] meditations on truth, beauty, and (most urgently) freedom, so, in a similar and yet distinct guise, should the world-transformative phenomenon of Covid-19 pandemic mark a watershed in the intellectual as well as political history of our own time.

So much for literary preview. Let's return to the task at hand: examination of a second example of pro-vax prejudice in the contemporary world—this time, the world of American liberalism iconically represented by *The New York Times*.

David French's November 12, 2023, piece "The New Republican Party Isn't Ready for the Post-Roe World"[585] displays all too clearly how pro-vax prejudice has by now been baked into the system of establishment thought, especially on the Democratic side of the political spectrum. The gist of French's argument is simple: Republicans in the Trump era are losing post-Roe political battles because the pro-life position demands that others (chiefly, women interested in abortion) make dramatic sacrifices even while Republicans themselves typically refuse to take a similar burden upon themselves. Even in red Ohio (which Trump won by eight points, twice), a pro-choice referendum passed by more than thirteen points in the November 2023 election, lengthening the string of pro-choice victories recently chalked up in red states.

French does not rely solely upon blunt terms (like "selfish" or "egotistical") in making his argument, but translates the same ideas into a more sophisticated vocabulary that possess political as well as psychological resonance. He phrases the crux of the matter as follows:

> In the eight years since the so-called New Right emerged on the scene and Trump began to dominate the Republican landscape, the Republican Party has become less libertarian but more libertine, and libertinism is ultimately incompatible with a holistic pro-life worldview.[586]

French amplifies it thus:

> The difference between libertarianism and libertinism can be summed up as the difference between rights and desires. A libertarian is concerned with her own liberty but also knows that this liberty ends where yours begins. The entire philosophy of libertarianism depends upon a healthy recognition of human dignity. A healthy libertarianism can still be individualistic but it's also deeply concerned with both personal virtue and the rights of others. Not all libertarians are pro-life, but a pro-life libertarian will recognize the humanity and dignity of both mother and child.
>
> A libertine, by contrast, is dominated by his desires. The object of his life is to do what he wants, and the object of politics is to give him what he wants. A libertarian is concerned with all forms of state coercion. A libertine rejects any attempt to coerce him personally, but he's happy to coerce others if it gives him what he wants.[587]

French concludes his argument by returning to its predictable starting point, the person and (im)moral character of Donald Trump:

> Donald Trump is the consummate libertine. He rejects restraints on his appetites and accountability for his actions. The guiding principle of his

> worldview is summed up with a simple declaration: I do what I want. Any movement built in his image will be libertine as well.
>
> Trump's movement dismisses the value of personal character. It mocks personal restraint. And it's happy to inflict its will on others if it achieve what it wants. Libertarianism says that your rights are more important than my desires. Libertinism says my desires are more important than your rights, and this means that libertines are terrible ambassadors for any cause that requires self-sacrifice.[588]

After thus playing the Trump card, French proceeds to Exhibit A: the Republican response to Covid policy:

> I don't think the pro-life movement has fully reckoned with the political and cultural fallout from the libertine right-wing response to the Covid pandemic. Here was a movement that was loudly telling women that they had to carry unwanted pregnancies to term, with all the physical transformations, risks and financial uncertainties that come with pregnancy and childbirth, at the same time that millions of its members were also loudly refusing the minor inconveniences of masking and the low risks of vaccination—even if the best science available at the time told us that both masking and vaccination could help protect others from getting the disease.[589]

As if such personal intransigence weren't bad enough, French decries actions taken by certain red states to bend the law to accommodate the self-centered desires of its libertine Republicans:

> Even worse, many of the same people demanded that the state limit the liberty of others so that they could live how they wanted. Florida, for example, banned private corporate vaccine mandates.[590]

French's piece not only exposes the roots of pro-vax prejudice (unwarranted assumptions of intellectual and moral superiority), but displays a majestic oak of self-righteous judgment grown up from those roots. According to French, pro-lifers may or may not be libertine, but those who resisted masking and mass vaccinations *most certainly* are. In this case, no qualms or caveats need stand in the way of making direct translation between these persons' political stance and their moral and psychological fiber. Their opinions about masks and mandates grant French ready access to their inner life, sure insight into the quality of their soul, and certain knowledge as to whether that soul inclines to virtue or vice.

Nor is there much if any reason for doubt on that score—at least in French's mind. French confidently casts Covid dissidents (along with *libertine* pro-lifers) as nakedly selfish creatures dominated not by the combination of rational judgment and humane compassion characteristic of persons worthy of respect but by their own ungovernable desires. Freud in tow, French declares such types to be "dominated by...id."[591]

It is naturally very convenient that Donald Trump can be exhibited as the standard-bearer of the entire class of persons who (whether or not they happen to be pro-life) pushed back against the controlling Covid narrative and resisted masks, vaccine mandates, and the rest. Persons of sound mind and warm heart know, after all, that Donald Trump is just such a reprehensible libertine. If one can link the whole class of Covid dissidents to him (*despite* the fact that Trump consented to lockdowns, authorized Operation Warp Speed, and defended the mass vaccination program long after its evident failure), then one can surely be confident that they cannot possibly be right about anything or (given who they *are*) advance arguments that merit serious attention instead of blithe dismissal or outright suppression.

French's rush to moral as well as scientific judgment might be considered extreme, but I believe he merely gives frank expression to the mental and emotional currents characteristic of pro-vax prejudice generally. That prejudice packs the kind of strong emotional charge clearly evident in French's own impassioned rhetoric. Ironically, such dramatic affect *can* indeed suggest the sway of unconscious energies stemming from the id—the same primitive reservoir of primal desire French identifies as the source of Republican libertinism.

Why, after all, is David French so worked up about the moral character of Republicans today? He himself answers that question:

> An ethos that centers individuals' desires will bleed over into matters of life and death. It did during Covid, and it's doing so now, as even Republicans reject the pro-life cause.[592]

Although the first phrase above is less than perfectly lucid, French's overall meaning is clear enough. Covid concerns, as well as abortion, touch immediately upon matters of existential import—whether you, I, or another will live or die or suffer sore affliction. Nothing is more primal than that, so it is little wonder that matters public health policy, especially vaccination, generate (like abortion) passionate advocates on both sides. Not only liberty but life itself may be at stake. As most always in a social context, these two grave matters—life and liberty—are inextricably intertwined.

It is thus understandable that the vaccine question evokes strong passions and the moral judgments that usually accompany powerful feelings. Morality, after all, ultimately listens to the heart, the supreme court of human value. An "ethos" represents the translation between the sphere of value, centered in the heart, and the sphere of action responsive to the will. It is an internalized system of felt values that determines what we believe it is right and good to do, or not.

Can there be a sound or humane ethos *not* premised upon love and the affections that bond human beings to one another? I doubt it. Certainly no *liberal* ethos, like that informing French's op-ed, takes anything other than love as its principal foundation. The ethical core of liberalism has always been interpretable as a secularized form of the Christian ethos ("Love your neighbor as yourself") that sees self in other and vice versa.[593] An ethos contaminated by or (still worse) centered upon self-serving desires is thus anathema to liberal consciousness, and to the conscience we depend upon to discriminate right from wrongful action and so regulate the will.

Nothing I say in this postscript, or indeed anywhere in this book, should be understood to imply that I regard individuals such as Michael French or Andrea Wulf as more selfish than I or other Covid-resistant anti-vaxxers. I do not judge them as deficient with respect to their intellectual capacities or love for other human beings, or humanity in general. I do not know them personally and cannot presume to know the quality and character of their souls on the basis of one or another political stance they may take.

I do, however, request—if they do not wish to stand accused of an insidious type of prejudice corrosive of the social fabric they presume to honor—that they extend the same respect to me and to all those—including Robert F. Kennedy Jr.—they may consider anti-vaxxers.

That, however, is not the *only* favor I ask—for myself, for RFK Jr., for anti-vaxxers the world over, and, indeed, for humanity at large. For while I do not presume to judge the quality of their hearts or the conscientiousness of their wills, these are not, finally, the only soul faculties involved in these high stake questions of life, death, liberty, and love. World important matters are at hand—including the propriety of vaccination, especially of the compulsory sort—that call for *informed* judgment, and decisive verdict. The faculty that need be called upon to exercise efficient rather than deficient agency in this respect is an eminent one that that molds the feelings and steers the will, and surely guides both heart and hand.

I speak of the mind, the intellect, and the faculty of critical reason that empowers us—like those "magnificent rebels" Andrea Wulf celebrates—to think as *free* and independent agents, as is our *right* and our *privilege* and our *duty* as citizens of a democratic society. We do not live up to that charge if we eschew question, or uncritically accept edicts from on high, surrendering the prerogative to think and judge for ourselves to "expert" authorities whose means, methods, motives, and conclusions may—but also may not be—good or pure, but in any event should never be considered as beyond reasonable doubt, or immune to question. For it is in our capacity to seek and arrive at *truth,* and carefully and critically distinguish this from *illusion,* that our mind enables our feeling heart to hold steady in the midst of conflicting claims and diverse passionate emotions, and render a just verdict as to what, after all, serves love rather than fear, or hate, or power, and so may fairly and justly be accounted *good.*[594]

I earlier state that pro-vax prejudice consists of intellectual, moral, and affective components, but that the first serves as ground of the rest. In the course of the discussion that ensued, we have spontaneously touched upon each of these aspects and gained some sense of how each enters into the whole picture. Now, at this juncture, I wish to reassert (in the present context, at least) the priority of the mind and its signature quest for truth. I do so not because ideas are more important than feelings or actions, but because how and what we think inevitably frames the logic of the heart, and continually dictates the decisions of the will.

I have, throughout this book, sought to show the innumerable ways by means of which the matrix of pro-vax forces that produced Covid World spin webs of illusion. Let us move toward the conclusion of this postscript, and so this book, by looking for the signature of this diabolical work in the model pro-Covid-vax text under discussion, the *Times* op-ed by David French.

It is self-evident that French's moral judgment rest upon what he regards as rock-solid truth confirmed by "the best science." Yet is the science he relies upon any better than the *at best questionable* and *at worst fraudulent* variety so often encountered in this book? As French draws water from the same tainted well as most proponents of the controlling narrative, the answer to that question is regrettably all too predictable.

To his credit, French does attempt to supply some scientific substantiation for his pro-vax position. Continuing his discussion of the distinctly libertine character of the Republican resistance to the Covid-19 vaccination campaign, French writes:

> This do-what-you-want ethos cost a staggering number of American lives. A 2022 study found that there were an estimated 318,981 vaccine-preventable deaths from January 2021 to April 2022. Vaccine hesitancy was so concentrated in Republican America that political affiliation was more relevant than race and ethnicity as an indicator of willingness to take the vaccine. Now there's evidence from Ohio and Florida that excess mortality rates were significantly higher for Republicans than Democrats after vaccines were widely available.
>
> And this is the party that's now going to tell American women that respect for human life requires personal sacrifice?[595]

The number sounds impressive—318,981 vaccine-preventable deaths—and French presents it not as any kind of guess or speculative surmise that might reasonably be questioned but as proven fact. "This do-what-you-want ethos cost a staggering number of American lives." No conditional in that simple declarative sentence. 318,981 lives saved: a confidence-inspiring figure indeed—*until*, instead of swallowing the bait whole, you begin to *think* about it, and look a little more closely at how the researchers at the Brown School of Public Health arrived at it.

Despite the deceptive specificity, 318,981 is not a real number. Like the infamous Prof. Neil Ferguson (Imperial College) prediction that Covid would kill untold millions if the world did not lock down, the figure is the product—not of careful empirical observation and analysis—but of a *computer-generated model* (here, under the auspices of the Microsoft AI Health program) based on highly questionable if not demonstrably false assumptions.

To obtain a count of vaccine-preventable deaths *one must presume a set degree of vaccine effectiveness*. Is the Brown "study" transparent as to the presumed rate of vaccine effectiveness built into the model the researchers employ? Hardly. On the contrary, if an interested party like myself wants to find that out, he is in for a wild—and wildly revealing—ride.

I began, innocently, enough by clicking on the phrase "vaccine-preventable deaths" in French's op-ed, expecting to be directed to the relevant study. Revelation #1: I did *not* thereby access the relevant study, but rather found myself presented with the immediate source of the information relied upon by David

French—namely, the audio version, as well as written transcript of a May 13, 2022, *All Things Considered* spot from the Public Health series "Shots: Health News from NPR."[596] As the title ("This Is How Many Lives Could Have Been Saved with Covid Vaccination in Each State") of the four-minute listen indicates, *All Things Considered* is no more shy about the certitude implied by simple declaratives than is David French. The trend continues in the first sentence: "One tragic fact about the nearly one million people who died of COVID-19 in the U.S. is that a huge share of them didn't have to."[597]

The NPR piece, following the Brown model, provides extensive coverage of the many thousands of lives that could have been saved if states in the U.S.—especially those red states with vaccination rates hovering around fifty percent—had achieved an eighty-five, ninety-five, or even hundred percent vaccination rate. The 318,981 nation-wide figure correlates (as explicitly stated in the paper) with that hundred-percent mark. The article cites health expert Cynthia Cox's assessment of the value of the Brown study:

> I think this is a really clear way of demonstrating both the effectiveness of vaccines and also the need to continue to vaccinate more people and to make sure that they're up to date on those vaccines.[598]

Very well, but what was one piece of vital information that NPR did not provide? The Public Health Shot did *not* supply any information as to the rate of vaccine effectiveness *assumed and built into* the Brown/Microsoft model, or even any hint that one might want to consider the accuracy of such before advancing claims as to how the AI-Health–generated computer model supplies "a really clear way of demonstrating . . . the effectiveness of the vaccines."

The NPR piece, did, however, provide a link that I hoped would provide me immediate access to the study in question.

Clicking on the relevant link, I found myself face to face—not with a peer reviewed or preprinted study—but with a portion of the Brown University School of Public Health website dedicated to the role "VACCINES" play in confronting "GLOBAL EPIDEMICS." The Brown/Microsoft study did, however, feature prominently on the page, which confronts the reader with a glossy full-width photo of a life-sized needle being inserted into a woman's arm and a few choice sentences cut into that picture:

> Vaccines have proven to be spectacularly effective in preventing death from Covid-19, but throughout 2021 and 2022, the U.S. struggled to keep Americans up to date on vaccinations. Our Vaccine Preventable Deaths

> Dashboard shows that in that time when vaccines were widely available, every second Covid-19 death could have been prevented by vaccines.[599]

The "every second...death" figure is a variation or extrapolation of the 381,981 figure, which represents approximately half of the officially recorded Covid deaths that, as of April 2022, had transpired *after* the vaccines had become widely available in early 2021.

Below the cited sentence, your eye is greeted by a splay of data—including a large U.S. map, color coded by state—exhibiting the results of the model. As far as the original study is concerned, however, the site offers scant trace.

Below the information and map pertaining to the "Vaccine-Preventable Deaths" angle, the page features links to articles with titles such as "How to Talk about Vaccines for Our Youngest Children," "Covid-19 Vaccines: The Miracle That Fell Short," and "What is Vaccine Demand."[600] The content descriptions make perfectly clear that all the articles reflect intensive efforts to understand why vaccine uptake in the U.S. is not as robust as it could be, and what may be done to rectify that situation so as to maximize the number of shots delivered.

The website designers devote the last portion of the page to "Recommended Resources."

The first three of the five listed resources are a Brown document titled "Domestic Covid Vaccine Passports: Policy Options to Build Trust and Curtail Inequity;" a *Times* op-ed, "Four Ways to Fix the Vaccine Rollout"; and (my favorite) a "perspective" piece from the *Washington Post,* "Which Vaccine Should You Get? Whichever One You Can."[601]

One can search the entire web page without coming across the least sign that anybody involved with the Brown School of Public Health—or any of the media sources featured on the page—entertains any question as to either the efficacy or the safety of the Covid (or any other) vaccines, or even that such a question might merit attention. The one *Washington Post* article (the fourth in the "Recommended Resources" section) that may appear to do so, an op-ed titled "It's Time to Consider Delaying the Second Dose of Coronavirus Vaccine"[602] does not recommend delay on account of any questions pertaining to vaccine efficacy. On the contrary, the January 3, 2021, article cites the original Pfizer clinical trial data indicating (misleadingly[603]) that the efficacy of a single shot approaches eighty to ninety percent. Rather, the authors urge delay because they believe saving doses for a second shot prevents more people from getting their first one. A telling sentence from the article reveals its bottom line: "We need to vaccinate as many people as possible to save the most lives."[604]

By the way, the coauthors of this *Post* article will be familiar to the readers of this book. They are Dr. Robert Wachter of UCSF and Dr. Ashish Jha, majority (Democratic) witness at the November 2020 U.S. Senate hearing on early treatment chaired by Senator Ron Johnson. You may remember that Dr. Harvey Risch and Dr. Peter McCullough contested the veracity and integrity of Dr. Jha's testimony, Dr. McCullough going so far as to call it "reckless and dangerous to the nation."[605] It turns out that Dr. Jha, when not serving as the White House's Covid-19 response coordinator (a post he occupied in 2022 and 2023), or writing op-eds published in *The Washington Post,* serves as the dean of the Brown University School of Public Health.

Speaking, again, of Brown, the page we've been perusing does include a portion headed "THEPATHTOZERO / The Cost of Undervaccination," which contains a linked reference to the study in question described as "analysis by our team at the Brown School of Public Health." By this time, though, I had serious doubts as to whether clicking on that link would actually take me to the study itself.

Those doubts were justified. Rather than presenting me with the study, clicking that link brought up yet another newsy piece announcing "New Analysis Shows Vaccines Could Have Prevented 318,000 Deaths: National and State by State Data."[606] Near the top of the article, eye-catching links are provided that invite you to either "Explore the Dashboard" or "Read [the] NPR Story." Only if, after scrolling well down on the page, you click on a link for "methodology" (sandwiched between additional links to the Dashboard and NPR on one side, and one advertising "More on Vaccine Demand" on the other) can one access an *abstract* of the preprint of the relevant study itself on the MedRxiv Health Science Server, which page contains still another link that finally brings up the full text of the paper ("Estimating Vaccine Preventable COVID-19 Deaths under Counterfactual Vaccination Scenarios in the United States"[607]).

If you examine the main text of the paper to discover the assumptions as to vaccine effectiveness written into the Microsoft AI-Health-generated model, you will find scant mention of this all-important parameter, accurate estimate of which determines whether the model itself qualifies as a useful tool or falls into the category of what authorities themselves like to label misinformation. The fairly extensive introductory section contains a single sentence on the matter, declaring: "Clinical trials as well as large-scale observational data in the

U.S. demonstrate that vaccines are highly effective in preventing severe disease, hospitalization, and death from Covid-19 infection."[608] No figure for the assumed rate of vaccine effectiveness is given.

Nor is any such provided in any accessible and readily legible fashion in the "Statistical Methods" section. Here we learn that the model uses the weekly *average* of vaccine effectiveness (age stratifications in the original CDC data are conglomerated) as such can be derived from CDC data for the relevant period of time. Instead of citing any specific figure of such an average, the paper presents a CDC graph (labeled figure 3 in the paper) showing "Rates of Covid-19 Deaths by Vaccination Status / April 04, 2021–February 26, 2022." As far as I could tell, *at no point and in no place did the Brown study openly divulge the rate of vaccine effectiveness assumed in the paper.* Interested readers are rather left to their own devices to surmise the rate derived from the graph, information that (if Brown were at all interested in objectivity and transparency) should be readily available to all.

I am not a statistician, but can see that the CDC graph displayed shows virtually no deaths among the vaccinated population, but significant mortality for the unvaccinated—ten to twenty times that of the vaccinated for the latter part of 2021 and early months of 2022, the period covering the ascent and dominance of Delta and the initial Omicron surge. By my simple, homegrown math, if I work with the conservative estimate of ten times the number of deaths among the unvaccinated for every death in the vaccinated group, the estimated rate of vaccine effectiveness used in the Brown model would be ninety percent. That is, if one presumes a hundred persons who, if unvaccinated, would die of Covid, 90 of those would be saved by vaccination, yielding the (very conservative) ten-to-one ratio of unvaccinated to unvaccinated deaths indicated by the graph.

Such estimates track with virtually *none* of the comparable data presented in the course of this book and must be judged unreliable if not useless for multiple reasons documented in these pages, including radical distortion of counts of vaccinated versus unvaccinated Covid cases, hospitalizations and deaths leading to gross inflation of the latter and minimization of the former, as well as mass data disruption resulting from the conflation of deaths *with* Covid with deaths *by* Covid. Furthermore, the CDC information conflicts dramatically with data from generally more dependable international sources.

Nor, finally, does it track with experienced reality as such may be judged from the perspective of the present. I do not think that, at this juncture, anyone believes that, through the eight to ten months (say July 2021 through February 2022) following the vaccine roll out, the Covid-19 vaccines were so wonderfully effective that nine out of every ten persons who died from Covid was unvaccinated. *If* that were in fact the case, President Biden and all the public health would have been fully justified in declaring Covid "a pandemic of the unvaccinated" in the summer and fall of 2022, a story line that—not so very long after it was propagated—was completely and thoroughly discredited.

I need not cover this worn ground again, but will merely state the obvious. David French relies upon the Brown/Microsoft model to substantiate his claim that hundreds of thousands of lives could have been saved if more people—especially more Republicans!—had obeyed public health edicts and recommendations, and been vaccinated. Yet the model does absolutely nothing of the kind because it merely *assumes*—in a manner blatantly contrary to fact and reason—what it is presumed to demonstrate: namely, the fantastic efficacy of the Covid-19 vaccines. It does so even while going to great lengths to hide the grossly unwarranted assumption underlying its model's math.

To my mind, the Brown study does not qualify as real science at all, but rather should be regarded as disinformation. Correlatively, nothing in the study—or anything readily visible on the whole Brown Public Health School vaccine page—goes anywhere *near* the third rail of vaccine science: the problem of vaccine safety, the unresolved status of which renders studies such as this one moot from the outset.

What is most revealing about the little investigative excursion we have just taken is not any new information about the safety or efficacy (or lack thereof) of the Covid vaccines. Rather, following the trail of links leading from French's *New York Times* op-ed to the NPR *All Things Considered* spot, and thence to the website of the Brown School of Public Health, opens a window onto how government, academic institution, big tech, and mainstream media (with, of course, Big Pharma pulling strings in the background) collude to transform what could and should be genuine scientific inquiry into a form of state-sponsored propaganda—mis- and disinformation that passes as authoritative "expert" opinion not because of any real standard of excellence or devotion to impartial truth proper to real science but because of the pedigree of the institutions involved.

Why, though, am I speaking here of the government as well as Big Tech (Microsoft), academic institutions (Brown), and media (the *Times* and *Post*)? Not only because the Brown/Microsoft study relied upon (unreliable) government data, but because the entire Brown School of Public Health depends, heavily, upon government money. In 2021, the Brown School of Public Health received roughly fifty-five million dollars from the NIH—more than all but a handful of other Schools of Public Health in the country.[609] The NIH awarded Brown researchers nearly a hundred individual project grants in the same year.[610] Predictably, it is listed as a funding source for the Brown/Microsoft study itself—and, one might well imagine, innumerable kindred studies as disinterested in truth in science as this one.[611]

When one begins to catch a real glimpse of it, the power of the Matrix appears gigantic indeed, as no doubt the Philistine Goliath—garbed from head to toe in fearsome armor—did when he took the field to fight a shepherd boy armed with nought but a slingshot and invincible faith in God.

The same paragraph of David French's op-ed that cites the Brown/Microsoft vaccine-preventable deaths "research" mentions one other (supposedly) supportive scientific study. In this case, the link provided in French's piece brings one directly to the relevant material, a very recent (July 24, 2023) paper titled "Excess Death Rates for Republican and Democratic Registered Voters during the Covid-19 Pandemic."[612] After introducing its key question ("Was political party affiliation a risk factor associated with excess mortality during the COVID-19 pandemic in Florida and Ohio?"), the paper summarizes its chief findings:

> In this cohort study evaluating 538,159 deaths in individuals aged 25 years and older in Florida and Ohio between March 2020 and December 2021, excess mortality was significantly higher for Republican voters than Democratic voters after Covid-19 vaccines were available to all adults, but not before. These differences were concentrated in counties with lower vaccination rates, and primarily noted in voters residing in Ohio.[613]

As the authors of the paper themselves admit, the value of the study results remains limited because it could not control for a variety of confounding variables.[614] Even leaving these reservations aside, however, the results—despite the tone of the summary—seem to me singularly unimpressive. Of the two states studied (Ohio and Florida), the principal graph shows statistically significant differences in only one (Ohio). Moreover, of the four age-stratified groups studied (25–64, 65–74, 75–84, 85+), only two (75–84 and 85+) show *somewhat* higher excess death rates among Republicans, while one (the 65–74 age group) shows higher rates among Democrats, and one (25–64) show *no* statistical variance correlated with party affiliation. As one doctor who commented on the paper remarked "It may be premature for Republicans to rush to change their voter registration."[615]

Yet the most notable feature of the paper must be chalked up not to any differences it highlights, but to one *it not only ignores but* (whether deliberately or not) *hides and disguises.* The Brown study obscured disclosure of the assumed rate of vaccine effectiveness as if that crucial piece of information were nothing anybody need know or consider. In this paper—one that at least interprets empirical data sets rather than computer-model–generated extrapolations—the obfuscation or deception might well be considered even more egregious.

The paper deals with *excess mortality* and—although it does not explicitly say so or employ the term—excess mortality figures are (unless otherwise broken down and differentiated) *all-cause mortality* figures. Although the study implies that Covid-19 is largely responsible for the excess deaths it analyzes, it does not attempt any distinction between deaths purportedly caused by Covid and those due to other causes. The excess mortality figures it analyzes thus are all-cause mortality figures, and significant increases or decreases at any given time *may* be a consequence of, not Covid-19, but some other agency.

The principal figures and tables (graphs) provided with the paper present data pertaining to differences in excess mortality rates for Republicans and Democrats in Ohio and Florida. None of these, however, show simple all-cause mortality in the different age groups irrespective of political affiliation for the period under consideration. For that, one must to go to eFigure 1 in the "Supplemental Content" section (see page 395). Not only that, you must also scroll down through several pages of numeric analysis inscrutable to any non-statistician. If you do so, however, you will find "eFigure 1. Excess Death Rates by Age in Florida and Ohio: 2018–2021."[616]

At first glance, the four graphs—one for each of the four age groups—do not appear particularly remarkable, *especially* if one has been primed to understand the significant climb in excess mortality registered in the latter part of 2021 to reflect excess deaths due to Covid-19.

Yet wait a moment; wasn't Covid around and killing people (*lots* of people, we were told) already in 2020? If so, why do all the charts show excess mortality in Florida and Ohio as *either below the historically steady norm* for almost the whole of 2020 (the two lower age groups), *essentially flat or normal* (the sixty-five to seventy-four age group), or only trending quite gradually up toward the end of the year (the eighty-five-plus age group)?[617] Correlatively, if the Covid-19 vaccines were effective and thus *reducing* excess mortality (the premise of the study), why do the graphs show *steep rises in all age groups only in the third and fourth quarters of 2021*, precisely the time period when, after the initial rollout, millions and millions of people were first getting vaccinated?

Our Ohio–Florida study doesn't even ask, let alone try to answer that key question.

The readers of this book will find in its pages ready explanation for the facts just cited. But it is not one our pro-vax corps of public health experts—people who apparently take the *Post* and Wachter/Jha declarations ("Which Vaccine Should You Get? Whichever One You Can" and "We Need to Vaccinate as Many People as Possible to Save the Most Lives") as *articles of faith*—allow themselves to consider. No one likes waking up to nightmare.

The scandal signaled by the neglect of the steep rise in all-cause mortality in the latter half of 2021 has yet another dimension. This phenomenon, as represented in this set of CDC-based data, is not anomalous. It cannot be discounted as the effect of some strange malady afflicting only the people of Ohio and Florida because it is the same spectacular and extraordinarily disturbing phenomenon that Ed Dowd calls attention to in his book, *Cause Unknown.*

Dowd again:

> In 2021, the stats people expected went off the rails. The CEO of the OneAmerica insurance company publicly disclosed that during the third and fourth quarters of 2021, death in people of working age (18-64) was 40% higher than it was before the pandemic. Significantly, the majority of the deaths were not attributed to Covid.
>
> A 40% increase in deaths is literally earth-shaking, and not only for the devastated families and communities that directly experience the deaths. Even a 10% increase in excess deaths would have been a 1-in-200 year event. But this was 40%.
>
> And therein lies a story - a story that starts with obvious questions:
>
> What has caused his historic spike in deaths among young people?
>
> What has caused the shift from old people, who are expected to die, to younger people, who are expected to keep living?
>
> It isn't Covid, of course, because we know that Covid is not a significant cause of death in young people.[618]

What did the Florida–Ohio study say about the youngest (18–64) age group? Only that there was no significant difference between excess Republican and Democrat death in that age group for the relevant time period. A reasonable person, however, might think that fact entirely irrelevant in light of the more consequential one utterly neglected by the study: namely, the veritable tsunami of excess death afflicting eighteen- to sixty-four-year-olds—Republican and Democrat alike—during the latter half of 2021.

We thus have two related but distinct phenomena of special note: the significant rise in all-cause mortality for all age groups in the latter half of 2021, immediately after the vaccine rollout, *and* the disturbing fact that by far the greatest rise in excess death during that period involved younger working-age people. I've noted that the Democrat–Republican study graphs *do* reflect that first-named of the above phenomena. One would expect that the study graphs would reflect the second as well. Is this indeed the case?

The truthful, though puzzling answer, is both yes and no.

It *is* true that, upon *careful* scrutiny, the graphs—as one would expect—indeed reveal the rise in all-cause mortality in the younger age to be significantly steeper than that in any other group during the latter half of 2021. The study graphs thus are in fact generally consistent with the information conveyed in Dowd's book.[619] At first (or even second) glance, however, they do not *appear* to be so, because *the graphs are not portrayed in a standardized format and scale that makes comparison between different age groups visible.* Instead, they are presented in a variable format and scale that effectively hides these differences, making them virtually invisible to anyone casually perusing the data.

This is accomplished by scaling the graphs very differently. The first two demarcating lines on the vertical axis for the twenty-five-to-sixty-five age group are at twenty-five percent and fifty percent; those for the sixty-six-to-seventy-five group, though at similar heights on the page, are at fifteen percent and thirty percent; those for seventy-six to eighty-five are at 12.5 and twenty-five percent; those for the eighty-five-and-older group at ten and twenty percent. Because of these very significant differences in the visual presentation, the rise of the highly visible blue line that designates the *average* rise of excess mortality over time *looks roughly comparable in all groups,* with *the oldest group looking as if it shows the steepest rise when, in fact, the opposite is true.*

Whether or not this visual distortion represents a deliberate strategy to disguise the drastic rise in all-cause mortality in the youngest age group, or mere carelessness on the part of the researchers, I do not know. In any case, neither scenario is either scientifically or morally defensible. Indeed, I do not know which is worse, scientists deliberately hiding (covering up) a terrible truth so that the public remains unaware of facts that dramatically contradict the

eFigure 1. Excess Death Rates by Age in Florida and Ohio: 2018 – 2021

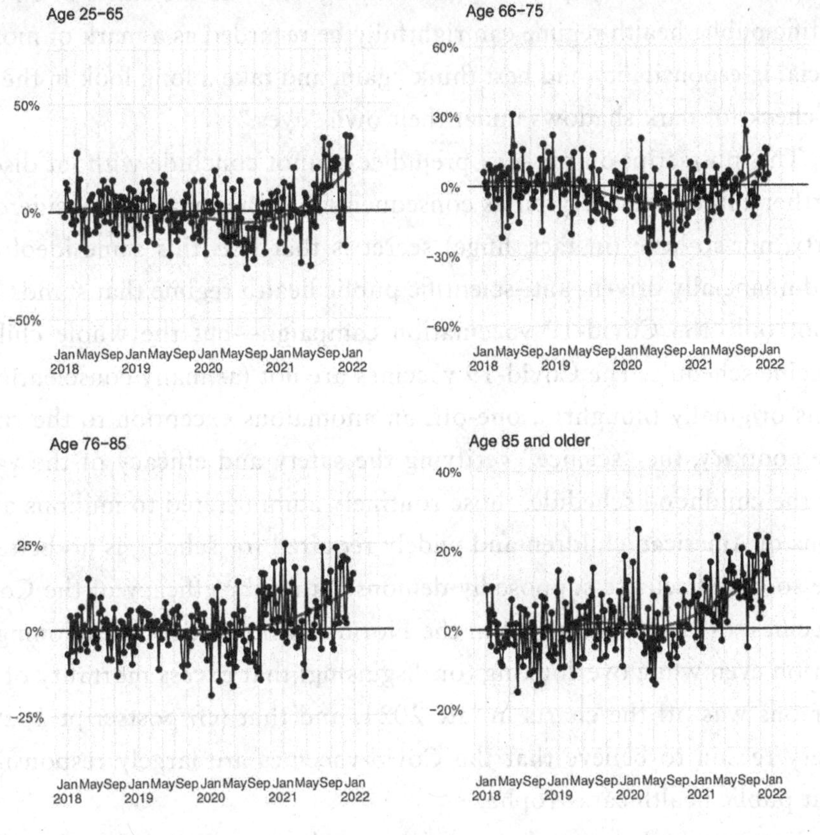

public health establishment's party line on the Covid-19 vaccines, *or* research scientists who are so wedded to a pro-vax orthodoxy that they themselves remain entirely blind to facts that contradict their suppositions, even when such facts are literally staring them in the face.

I think that, tragically, the history of public health with respect to vaccination consists of a toxic combination of both of the above. The Ohio–Florida study discloses the scientifically and ethically abysmal consequences of pro-vax prejudice. Here we have a study teasing out minor differences in excess mortality between Democratic and Republican voters while completely ignoring, and even hiding, the tsunami of death afflicting the population of persons under the age of sixty-five during precisely the period when Americans were undergoing mass vaccination and this younger population was widely subject to work-enforced mandates.

So it goes in the world of the so-called science that underlies the professional "expertise" of our present public health regime.[620] In view of the light shed upon the real facts of the case in this book, anyone—like David French or Andrea Wulf—who presumes that saying "nay" to the edicts of an anti-scientific public-health regime can rightfully be regarded as a mark of moral and social irresponsibility had best think again, and take a long look in the mirror to check for dark shadows under their own "ayes."

This postscript on pro-vax prejudice cannot conclude without disclosing further subterfuge every bit as consequential as that already considered. The dirty, not-so-little (in fact, huge) secret is that it is this same ideologically and financially driven, anti-scientific public health regime that stands behind —not only the Covid-19 vaccination campaign—but the whole childhood vaccine schedule. The Covid-19 vaccines are not (as many conscientious persons originally thought) a one-off, an anomalous exception to the rule. On the contrary, the "science" verifying the safety and efficacy of the vaccines on the childhood schedule, those routinely administered to millions and millions of American children and widely required for school, is no better than the so-called science supposedly demonstrating the efficacy of the Covid-19 vaccines, or that represented in the Florida–Ohio model championing vaccination even while overlooking (or disguising) that excess mortality of young persons was off the charts in late 2021, and that (cf. postscript 1) there is every reason to believe that the Covid-vaccines are largely responsible for that public health catastrophe.

Fortunately, I do not have to lay out the case supporting this position on childhood vaccines in detail here. The case has already been clearly and definitively made in a recent book fetchingly titled *Turtles All the Way Down: Vaccine Science and Myth.*[621] The anonymous authors cover all the important bases in eleven easy-to-read chapters full of facts and vital information. Home plate, though, surely must be the topic covered in the book's first chapter: the quality of the clinical trials that supposedly provide authoritative evidence that the "rigorously" tested vaccines are safe, and so *not* liable to kill or injure the very children whose health they are designed to safeguard.

The disturbing revelation here is that—in marked contrast to repeated statements by public health officials—*none* of the vaccines on the childhood schedule have been tested in RCTs (random control trials) employing a placebo control group, and most trials relied upon to secure government authorization are too short-lived (as brief as five days) to uncover most possible side effects. After a detailed discussion, the authors render a final verdict on the vaccine clinical trial system:

> It is virtually impossible to state the bottom line of the analysis presented above mildly, so here goes: **Vaccine trials in general, and childhood vaccine trials specifically, are purposely designed to obscure the true incidence of adverse events of the vaccine being tested.** [622]

The authors proceed to explain how that system works:

> How do they do this? By using a two-step scheme: First, a new vaccine (one which does not have a predecessor), is always tested in a Phase 3 RCT in which the control group receives another vaccine (or compound very similar to the experimental vaccine). A new pediatric vaccine is never tested during its formal approval process against a neutral solution (placebo). Comparing a trial group to a control group that was given a compound that is likely to cause a similar rate of adverse events facilitates the formation of a false safety profile. The rate of adverse events of the tested vaccine is said to be similar to the "background rate", hence it is considered safe. The researchers, and the vaccine manufacturers they work for, seem to "forget" that the compound they administered to the control group is a bioactive substance, carrying its own risks and side effects, and hardly represents the baseline or background rate that is essential to an RCT for a new vaccine.[623]

In a summary of their first chapter,[624] the authors supply a synopsis of the real-life consequence of this pseudo-science:

> As we have seen in this chapter, vaccine trials are designed and performed in such a way as to ensure that the true extent of adverse events is hidden from the public. There is not a single vaccine in the U.S. routine childhood vaccination program whose true rate of adverse events is known. The assertion that vaccines cause serious side effects in "one in a million" vaccinees contradicts the results of numerous clinical trials in which serious adverse events were reported in 1 in 40, 30, or even as few as 20 vaccinated infants. After becoming acquainted with the fine details of vaccine safety trials, hearing the familiar tune of "a similar rate of adverse events was reported in the control group" (which received another vaccine or similar compound) comes off as ludicrous, cynical, and patently immoral.[625]

After thus scientifically turning the pro-vaxxer's moral tables upside down, the authors comment on the broader significance of this finding:

> Current vaccine clinical trial methodology completely invalidates the claims that vaccines are safe and that they are thoroughly and rigorously tested. And pulling out that bogus card completely topples the childhood

vaccine program's house of cards, as officials' assurances of vaccine safety rely primarily on deliberately flawed, industry-sponsored clinical trials.[626]

Finally, they submit this succinct conclusion:

> Any reader looking for a quick and definitive understanding of the truth about vaccine safety—well, you can put this book down right now. You have your answer: The entire vaccine program is based on a deliberate cover-up of true vaccine adverse event rates.[627]

I expect the reader of *Two Roads*—a book featuring Deb Conrad's story as its formal and thematic center—would draw the same conclusion about *Covid-19* vaccine safety.

Nor are the authors of *Turtles All the Way Down* by any means the only ones onto this story, dispelling the myth and promoting the truth about vaccine science. Indeed, as if the program were made to order for this postscript, on Thanksgiving Day *The Highwire* hosted a segment called "Vaccine Experts under Oath" that covers some of the same territory explored in *Turtles.* Host Del Bigtree's introduction to the segment echoes one of the central themes of this postscript:

> We've talked a lot about the Covid vaccines, and the issues that are becoming apparent to everybody, but one of the big questions really is: "What about the other vaccines...we've been giving our children? We recognize that the Covid vaccine wasn't tested very long, was kind of raced out, and didn't end up being effective, but that's an anomaly right?"
>
> The truth is...all Covid was, was a rehash of how all these vaccines have been approved. You just finally watched how the sausage was made with your own eyes.
>
> For those of you who are asking questions...or are hearing about the huge debate around whether Robert F. Kennedy Jr. is telling the truth or not, we thought we would give you some of the evidence we've collected in our work.[628]

I recommend watching the hour-long show whether you are a confirmed anti-vaxxer, a vaccine skeptic, someone who has simply gone along with the mainstream position trusting "the experts" without thinking too much about it, or if you are a vaccine advocate disdainful of anti-vaxxers. Those in the latter category should, at the very least, take intellectual, moral, and civic responsibility for getting the facts on vaccine "science" straight now that the thick ice is breaking, and—despite the longstanding efforts to suppress highly inconvenient truths—"reliable" information is finally surfacing.

I can in no wise report upon all the issues addressed in "Vaccine Experts under Oath," an episode which includes video clips of ICAN attorney Aaron Siri soliciting testimony (the legal term is *deposing*) from eminent vaccinologists in the context of one or another vaccine-injury lawsuit brought by ICAN. Perhaps I can, however, whet your appetite by sharing a select slice of the program's treatment of what—until Covid—undoubtedly qualifies as the most high-profile vaccine-injury issue of all.

When we speak of injuries or diseases that have allegedly been caused by vaccination, one has received inestimably more public attention than any other. Countless parents (especially mothers) have claimed that their previously healthy child suddenly fell into an autistic condition within days or a few short weeks after receiving one or another of a select group of the childhood vaccines, including the DTaP (diphtheria, tetanus, and acellular pertussis) vaccine. The medical establishment, however, unequivocally rejects the notion that there may be any truth to the parental allegations, continually insisting that extensive and rigorous scientific study has thoroughly disproven the hypothesis (first suggested by Dr. Andrew Wakefield[629]) of a causal connection between vaccination and autism. Yet those debunking counter-claims turn out to be, not a matter of fact, but rather yet another sterling example what might well be called "science fiction."

Below, you will find ICAN attorney Aaron Siri reporting on ICAN's attempt to procure the studies representing the science that has presumably settled the autism question. We catch up with Siri well into the episode's exploration of the topic, and shortly after he has demonstrated that *neither an official institute of medicine (IOM) review nor the world's foremost vaccinologist*, Dr. Stanley Plotkin (the man who literally wrote the textbook on vaccines and whom we have just seen Siri deposing) *could identify a single scientific study disproving the alleged causal link between vaccines and autism.* Aaron Siri:

> Maybe the Institute of Medicine couldn't find [such studies], maybe the leading vaccinologist in the world [Plotkin] doesn't have the studies, but the CDC surely should have these studies. The CDC on its website says vaccines don't cause autism. So we submitted a Freedom of Information Request to the CDC asking them, "Please, provide all studies relied upon by the CDC to claim that DTaP vaccines don't cause autism." We did the same for the HepB vaccine, Prevnar, Hib, and the inactivated polio vaccine, as well as all the vaccines combined. We said, "Please give us the studies."

Guess what? They didn't give it to us. So we had to sue them in federal court. And here is the conclusion to that federal lawsuit.

The CDC finally listed twenty studies that they rely upon, they say, to claim that vaccines don't cause autism for the vaccines given in the first six months of life... So we read the twenty studies. Here's the thing about them: eighteen of them involved thimerosal, an ingredient not in any of the vaccines we asked about, or the MMR vaccine not given until at least one year of life. One of them involved antigen... that study even says it can't tell you whether vaccines cause autism because it didn't study them, just studied a compound of them. And, finally, the last thing it provided, incredibly, was a review from 2012, the one we looked at before... The only review or study they provided us that actually involved a single one of the vaccines given in the first six months of life was a study by the Institute Of Medicine that found "we don't have a single study of whether DTaP does or doesn't cause autism!"

I had an opportunity to depose maybe the second or third leading vaccinologist in the world, Dr. Kathryn Edwards, in a case specifically about vaccines and autism. You can hear when I confronted her about this issue, what she had to say about the state of the science with regard to whether vaccines cause autism—again, the issue they say they have studied more thoroughly and robustly than any other claimed vaccine injury.[630]

Let's pick up the dialogue between Aaron Siri and Dr. Kathryn Edwards after a few preliminary questions serve to confirm Dr. Edwards' comprehensive knowledge of the relevant science:

AS: In your opinion, did the clinical trials relied upon to license the vaccines... many of which are still on the market today; were they designed to rule out that the vaccine causes autism?

KE: No. You've badgered me into answering the question the way you want me to, but I think that's probably the answer.

AS: Is that your accurate and truthful answer?

KE: Yes.

If one cannot trust the oft-repeated, supposedly authoritative claims that science has disproved the possibility that vaccines may cause autism, can one trust *anything* the medical establishment has to say about vaccines?

Let me add a footnote to the vaccine/autism story. It is not that vaccinologists and other knowledgeable personnel simply and repeatedly lie about what has or has not been proven. If one listens carefully to the claims made about the alleged connection between vaccines and autism, one will often hear some authority declaring, not that science has positively demonstrated that vaccines do not cause autism, but rather (and usually with emphatic flourish) that *there is no study, and so no scientific evidence, providing evidence of that causal link.* At one point in *The Highwire* episode, Aaron Siri remarks:

> In my experience deposing vaccinologists and immunologists, pediatricians and infectious disease specialists—particularly vaccinologists—when there isn't any evidence one way or another, their conclusion is, it doesn't cause it. I've not experienced that in any other area of science.

One needs to add here that, as Aaron Siri well knows, there *is* evidence that vaccines cause autism: namely, the allegations of innumerable parents who, in their view, have experienced the phenomena themselves, and whose lives have been irrevocably altered by it. Such testimony, however, can be considered merely anecdotal, and—insofar as it cannot prove any causal link (formal physiological or comparative studies are required for that[631])—does not qualify as "scientific." One may ask why, given the witness borne by parents (parents who, as Bigtree clarifies, are *not* naturally inclined to attribute their child's illness to vaccination, because doing so identifies the parents themselves as agents complicit in the drastic harm done to their own child), relevant studies have *not* been done, so that science might in fact arrive at a definitive conclusion? The answer, unfortunately, is all too obvious: *if* such studies were done, they might very well confirm the causal link, so that no scientist or physician or public health official or man or woman on the street could any longer say: "There are no scientific studies that provide any evidence that vaccines cause autism."

Where would the vaccine program that absolutely depends on parents' trust in the safety of the shots administered to their children be then?

Meanwhile, the incidence of autism in society continues to skyrocket. The rise has been most dramatic in recent decades, especially since the dramatic expansion of the childhood vaccine schedule in the 1980s. A little over a half-century ago, autism was an exceptionally rare event. Rates of autism in the U.S. in the 1960s and 1970s were approximately one per two thousand. Those rates rose to roughly one per thousand in the 1980s.[632] Today, according to CDC MMWR data published in March 2023, "One in thirty-six (2.8%) eight-year-old children have been identified with autism spectrum disorder."[633] That amounts to *a more-than-fifty-fold increase* over the last sixty years or so.[634]

Nor is autism by any means the only chronic illness on the rise—and dramatically so—in the U.S. On the contrary, it is emblematic of a deeply disturbing and widely recognized trend. The title of a *Forbes* article from *last* Thanksgiving couples frank announcement with pugnacious query: "Our Nation's Chronic Disease Epidemic Is Getting Worse. So Who's Responsible?"[635]
All parties agree with the declarative part of the Forbe's title. The piece itself states: "Today almost half of the U.S. population or 133 million Americans, are living with one chronic condition and forty percent of adults suffer two or more."[636] That figure is up from the already high twenty-seven–percent 2018 figure for multiple chronic conditions quoted in a CDC research brief.[637] The distressing trend, moreover, has been ongoing for some time. A 2008 Kaiser Family Foundation study found that chronic disease among working age adults in the U.S. increased twenty percent over the course of the prior decade.[638]

If there's broad consensus as to the nature of the phenomena, there's none as to its cause. Perhaps the only point agreed upon by most public health experts is that the increase has nothing whatsoever to do with the nation's burgeoning vaccine program. *Never mind* the fact that most of that rise has occurred in the aftermath of the huge expansion of the childhood vaccine schedule initiated in the late 1980s, a development that spectacularly increased (by as much as sevenfold or more) the number of vaccinations typically received by American children.[639]

The medical establishment does not seem to know what to make of the frightening rise of chronic disease in the U.S., a rise so steep, that—if the trend continues—it may well eventually constitute an existential threat to the physical and socioeconomic integrity of the nation.[640] Its position on autism typifies mainstream thinking with respect to the more general issue. An NBC news piece floats the common—yet factually, rationally, and experientially insupportable—notion that more discriminating diagnostic techniques are merely *identifying* many cases of autism spectrum disorder that previously flew under the radar, and alludes (vaguely) to undefined genetic and environmental factors, before making the report's one unequivocal statement:

> Precisely what those [genetic and environmental] factors are is still unknown, but researchers are at least clear on one fact: Autism has nothing to do with vaccines.[641]

NBC turns to Penn State Professor Girirajan for official confirmation:

> We know for sure, for so many years now, that vaccines don't cause autism, said Santhosh Girirajan, an associate professor at Pennsylvania State University.[642]

Robert F. Kennedy Jr., coauthor of the just published *Vax-Unvax: Let the Science Speak*[643] is not so sure.

The hypothesis (more or less explicitly proposed in *Vax-Unvax*) that excessive vaccination acts as one principal cause of the increase in chronic disease in the U.S., is not so difficult to test. One could, for instance, conduct broad-ranging epidemiological studies comparing the incidence of chronic disease among the vaccinated, on the one hand, and the unvaccinated on the other. Our public health and medical research establishment do not, however, deliberately perform such studies, because doing so may demonstrate that unvaccinated children are significantly less subject to chronic disease than vaccinated children, and indeed that the number of vaccinations received tends to be *directly* related to a child's susceptibility to chronic disease. In other words, contrary to current dogma the *more* vaccinations a child receives the *less* healthy he or she is likely to be.[644]

Even if studies deliberately designed to settle this question are, for political reasons, as scarce as fountains in a desert, it does not mean that information along these lines cannot be culled from high-quality studies that may have been performed with other ends in mind. *Vax-Unvax* offers an exhaustive compilation of data from such studies, even while winnowing out all data the reliability of which may be subject to question. I will not steal the book's thunder but expect you can guess the results arrived at when, in fact rather than name, science—not money, ideology, politics, and entrenched prejudice—is finally allowed to speak.

To cite just one telling example: studies compiled in *Vax-Unvax* reveal that *autism diagnoses in vaccinated children are four to five times higher than those for unvaccinated children.*[645] That correlation may not qualify as definitive proof of causality, but to deny that it constitutes a result that justifies concern and highlights a need for further investigation defies reason and common sense.

As a consequence of Covid, more and more persons—including eminent medical professions once staunchly supportive of the mainstream position—are waking up to the truth that industrial society's religious worship of vaccination is grounded in myth rather than science. Dr. Pierre Kory, a veteran of the Covid wars and never one to mince words, has this to say about Kennedy and Hooker's *Vax-Unvax:*

> In *Vax-Unvax,* Kennedy and Hooker shine a blinding light on the appalling lack of research and blatant propaganda behind the entire inflated and ever-expanding childhood vaccine schedule. The author's painstaking investigation and rigorous analyses are rivaled only by their bravery in exposing the depth and breadth of the lies we've been told.[646]

The "depth and breadth of the lies we've been told"—the lies or half-truths ("there are no scientific studies showing that vaccines cause autism") that are the coin of Lucifer's kingdom.

By now, I hope it will be clear that pro-vax prejudice only *pretends* to be pro-science. In fact, as books like *Turtles* and *Vax-Unvax* show, the opposite is consistently and emphatically the case. The pro-vax position must be judged an anti-science position not only because "the best science" suggests that mass vaccination (whether we are speaking of the Covid vaccines or the bloated childhood schedule) does more harm than good. It is so as well, and still more conclusively, because the pro-vax platform today depends upon *blocking* the science that would allow more definitive answers to a host of urgent questions, and the *suppression* of public debate (as in the case of the proposed Kennedy-Hotez dust-up, which can stand for *all* the debates that should but do not take place) on the basis of the false premise that "science" has already settled the burning questions.

Insofar as reason or intellect is allowed into the precinct of opinion, the stubborn refusal to reflect critically upon the assumptions underlying one's own judgments qualifies as the very root of prejudice. Pro-vax prejudice, perhaps more than almost any other kind, is intimately linked to the secular enlightenment mentality of the modern temperament. The powerful moral and affective components of the prejudice are grounded in and derivative of the *intellectual* premise that science has definitively proven mass vaccination to be a principal means by which humanity allays the threat of illness and death always knocking at the door of life. Coincidently, and in a manner likewise integral to the modern worldview, vaccination is valued as a ritual display of one's love of and responsibility toward one's fellow human beings. Many persons awed by the godlike power of science and devoted to a communitarian ethos exhibit a positively religious investment in both the rightness and righteousness of the pro-vax position.

Yet, as with all systems of beliefs (including, of course, organized religion), the living truth that may have inspired conviction in the first place tends, in time, to be deadened and occluded by dogma that no longer reflects the creative genius that originally birthed a cherished initiative. It is the peculiar strength of science that, in principle, "science" cannot be identified with any given substantive position—not a heliocentric universe, not Newtonian physics, not the idea of evolution by natural selection, and certainly not the safety and efficacy of manufactured vaccines. Rather, the essence of science inheres in the *method* of impartial and open-ended inquiry that provokes question, depends upon dissent, and acknowledges the possibility of error as the precondition of genuine truth.

What pro-vax proponents need realize is that revisiting the issue and (if fact and reason so dictate) changing their minds about vaccines does not entail abandoning the enlightened reverence for science that kindled the Age of Reason and its overthrow of the "hag of superstition" that—still today—fuels religious intolerance; nor does it constitute a betrayal of the social contract that serves the Party of Humanity. *On the contrary,* it is the means of redeeming and revivifying commitment to ideals and principles that have hardened into dogmatic ideology, and suffered corruption and betrayal by the very institutions (scientific, governmental, informational, and more) supposed to uphold and represent them.

The kind of radical critical praxis implicit in these perspective may well be the stuff—not merely of reform within the limited domain of public health—but systemic change profound enough to be judged nigh revolutionary. Purgative, cathartic transformation of real magnitude is very much needed in America today, a nation in which corporate industry, science, technology, media, and government have—as the story of Covid told in *Two Roads* vividly reveals—formed an unholy alliance corrosive of truth and destructive of democracy. This matrix is naturally comprised of powerful parties invested in their own special interests (their wealth, their authority, their prestige, their power, their ideology, their righteousness) more than Truth, the elusive character of which has a peculiar way of consorting with respect for the sovereign individual and the essence of human freedom.

If the kind of change I augur here is not permitted to proceed by way of democratic processes consonant with enlightened principles and ends, reaction against systems of power and authority that no longer hear the people's voice, no longer represent the people's interest, and no longer serve the people's needs will almost certainly take more violently destructive, regressive rather than progressive forms, the force of which may go so far as to shatter the foundations of the nation.

The story of Covid, as I tell it in *Two Roads,* is a scandal. If you've read this book through, I hope there is a very good chance you will agree that

Robert F. Kennedy Jr.—far from spreading intellectually and morally irresponsible misinformation—was one of many courageous souls who stood up to speak truth to power, and who did—and continues to do—whatever he can to shred the web of illusion in which the whole world was—and many respects remains—hopelessly caught.

Branding RFK Jr. an anti-vaxxer and demeaning him on that score stands as the first line of defense against the truths he tells. The crumbling of the "vaccine wall" prompts the question: What else may he get right that the "trusted news" that runs interference for the Matrix will tell you, again and again, is so very, very wrong?

Be then not abused by those who deal in the shades of truth, rather than the thing itself, nor allow yourself to be deceived by false prophets whose very being is imposture.

> The wind bloweth where it listeth, and thou hearest the sound thereof, but canst not tell whence it cometh, and whither it goeth: so is every one that is born of the Spirit.
>
> He that hath ears to hear, let him hear.[647]

So turn the page. For, in truth, apocalypse is coming.

That is no country for old men.

PART VIII

CODA

"PRAGUE" (A POEM)

It may strike my reader as a strange choice to end this *Covid Chronicle* with a poem, especially one set in Prague that appears to have nothing to do with either Covid or America. Several allusions—to Rilke, to Jan Hus, to Yeats' "Sailing to Byzantium" (the first line of which concludes Postscript II)—do form a tentative connection between the texts of *Two Roads* and "Prague," but the real reasons for ending with the poem are naturally deeper.

Artificial boundaries are anathema to the American spirit. Emerson famously wrote, "A foolish consistency is the hobgoblin of little minds,"[648] and the catholic spirit of the Sage of Concord would surely warn us against any overly myopic construction of Covid. The cataclysmic affair that transfigured the world can, after all, not be reduced to little more than an extended quibble over masks, mandates, and spike proteins. Such matters are, to be sure, critical—Covid World did and still does revolve around them—but the concrete particulars point as well to more profound and far-reaching concerns. Masks and vaccine vials, the icons of Covid public health policy, are the symbols and characters of no mere kitchen quarrel but an epic saga.

Two Roads aspires to sketch not only the map of Covid country but also (even as it marks a fateful fork) a path to freedom. It endeavors to detail the ways in which the dark forces behind Covid World constricted the liberty of the American people to the point of strangulation, as well as the intellectual and moral means by which we may strive to throw off the chokehold that—despite the lessening of pressure—has by no means been released. The fight for the personal liberty that grounds human dignity, whether fought with swords or words, is always a spiritual as well as material battle. American revolutionaries like Adams and Jefferson (whom we will encounter in volume 2) knew that truth in the marrow of their bones, and it was the faith and courage bred of that knowledge that led to victory in a war these magnificent rebels had little military business winning, and thus midwifed the birth of this nation.

I will write a good deal about the idea of freedom or liberty in volume 2 (*Covid and the Apocalypse of the Modern Mind*) and do so in a more philosophical and intellectual–historical guise than in *Two Roads*. Even so, the essence of human freedom (Schelling, again) qualifies as the underlying theme of both books, and the spiritual battle to which I've referred inevitably involves engagement with inner as well as outer adversaries. That battle—as the postscript you have just read reveals—necessitates throwing off the yoke of obedience to unworthy masters and breaking the ideological chains that bind the mind to dogma and the spectral images that imprison it in illusion.

As Emerson tells us in so many words, the living insight born of truth is the gift of spirit and the badge of freedom, because it is the Spirit that is and makes us free.

Even so: the terrain of spirit itself, formally assigned to the realm of religion, is no less fraught with traps that would catch and hold the seeker than any other. Indeed, precisely because religion professes to speak the language of spirit, its tropological jaws can close with still more deadly force upon the pilgrim life of the mind.

I do not mean thus to imply that the wisdom inscribed in ancient books cannot be trusted or is inherently deceptive. The consciousness of anyone who imagines that the sacred texts and stories that come down to us through the ages are nought but figments of diseased imagination and devoid of any real revelation will find their own faculties impoverished by such indolence. Nonetheless, if it is foolish to regard the wisdom of tradition as easily outraced by the shiny car of progress, it is no less unsound to believe that the modern soul can complacently rest upon the merit of esteemed ancestors and all they have said and done. Emerson would certainly not have us leave Plato or our Bible behind as we walk toward the future, but would admonish us that we, as citizens of a new world, must learn to read them with fresh eyes, trusting that the immortal spirit that rejuvenates the dead letter is the same that animates the genius of our own individual soul.

This need for renewal, for drawing new water from the well of the past so as to look forward to a future of our own more original design—a future not stamped in the mold of illusion, fear, and servile ignorance but in that of truth, freedom, love, reverence, and courage—constitutes the main theme of *Reset or Renaissance*.

Against that background, perhaps you will understand why "Prague" may, after all, be a fit ending to *Two Roads*, and, perhaps, a still better prelude to all that is to come.

Prague [649]

I cannot conceive that the cross *should* remain, *which was, after all, only a cross-roads. It certainly should not be stamped on us on all occasions like a brand mark. For is the situation not* this: *he intended simply to provide the loftier tree, on which we could ripen better....*

We should not always talk of what was formerly, *but the* afterward *should have begun.*

—Rilke, *The Young Workman's Letter*

Hus, the Clock, the turrets of Our Lady
before Tyn (where Brahe's entombed); the bridge
over the Charles peopled by stone figures.
The philosophical and theological libraries
at Strahov. Prague Castle and St. Vitus's
towering cathedral; the tiny rooms
of smiths on Golden Lane. Rudolf II's
alchemical chambers hidden underground;
gravestones crowded in the Jewish Cemetery.
Café Slavia near the National Theatre
where Rilke palavered, and Jindrisska Ulice
where he lived as a child near Wenceslas Square.
The Velvet Revolution of 1989.
History goes on and on, labyrinthine
as the streets of Staré Mêsto, where I walk
in the midst of a human tide surging,
every hour, toward Old Town Square
to see Time marked on the face of the Clock.

~

The show begins with Death. A skeleton tolls
the hour, turning a timeglass upside-down.
Greed, Vanity, and Sensual Pleasure shake
foppish heads, signaling refusal that changes
nothing. The gawkish crowd watches twelve apostles
appear and disappear in two small windows
opening briefly above the clock face.
When all are gone and the hour struck, we hear
the crow of a golden cock. Yet if it sings
of what is past, or passing, or to come

we do not listen. Christ is not yet risen
in our hearts. This court is no Byzantium.

~

In the Basilica of St. George (circa 920),
there is a sculpture titled: *Kristus
kmene Stromu* or *Christus aus dem Baumstamm.*
The Czech-born German artist Otto Herbert Hajek
created the work in 1947/48, gifting it,
as a sign of reconciliation, to Vaclav Havel
and the Czech people in the aftermath
of the Velvet Revolution. The work portrays
the death of Christ in sorrow, and yet there is
no cross. Instead, Jesus himself becomes
the Tree. Which? Both. Knowledge *and* Life.
Because once the forbidden fruit is bitten
and history begins, there is no way back
but forward. Being is nothing if not forgiveness.

~

Crucifixions—painted, sculpted—are everywhere
in Prague. Everywhere, the image of Jesus
nailed to the cross is a chief object
of veneration, an icon the faithful worship
in thought and prayer. Even so, here,
contemplating Hajek's kindred yet different
(deeply different) symbol, I, who am
Jewish by birth and just recently come
from bearing witness to drawings and poems
by children at Theresienstadt, most of whom
were soon dead (one poem likens a yellow
flicker of wings to tears of the sun and ends:
"Butterflies don't live here / In the ghetto")
—I, sunk in reverie before Hajek's
Christus aus dem Baumstamm, ask myself: *Why?*

~

Rilke, compelled as a child to kiss the feet
of a wooden Jesus in the church
on Jindrisska, asked the same question.
To worship a man—any man—as God
when the soul itself did not know divinity

seemed to him vain delusion. And yet, spiritual
nomad that he was, he reckoned *an old*
picture of Christ I have had standing before me
since boyhood among his few treasured possessions.
Until the War, when, cut off from his home
in Paris, the poet lost all he'd left there.

~

I myself am a kind of wandering Jew.
Not that I have ever deliberately
scoffed at the sight of the human soul
bearing the awful weight of mortal strife.
Even so, have I ever *known* what I have *seen*
making my pilgrim way through history?
Recognized the shrine, the mecca of the quest?
If there is such a holy place or person;
alpha and omega, origin and end.

~

I am standing, still, in front of *Christus*
aus dem Baumstamm. No nails, no cross, no crowd,
no spear, no mother, no son; no thief, no
Roman soldier. No human being undergoing
the agony of death at the impolitic hands
of others; no half-clad body tragically torn
but the trunk turned, like fleeing Daphne,
into a tree; one no longer nailed
to its place in history, but dark wood
one with the mythic substance of the soul,
with love and death and metamorphosis.
Crowned—not by thorns—but invisible laurel.

~

This is an act of pure imagination.
The features of the face (deep frown,
downcast eyes) remain all-too-human, as does
the terror remembered in the giving of the gift.
But *how* do we remember history?
Why give an image, any image, of Christ
in remembrance of the horror of the holocaust?

~

No nails, no cross, no crowd
In time, the symbol of the cross becomes
no thief, no spear
not icon but false idol. In time, the symbol
no mother, no son, no soldier
of the cross becomes a crusade against infidels.
No nails, no cross, no crowd
In time, the symbol of the cross is twisted
no thief, no spear
into a tool of white supremacy. In time,
no mother, no son, no soldier
the symbol of the cross comes to mean
no nails, no cross, no crowd
the reverse of what it means. In time, the image
no thief, no spear
of dolorous Jesus dying for our sins
no mother, no son, no soldier
eclipses human history. In time,
no nails, no cross, no crowd
belief in a redeemer that dwells outside
no thief no spear
the soul's own time bars the soul's redemption.
no mother, no son, no soldier
In time, the tender plant of human being
no nails, no cross, no crowd
drinks the tears of sun that rain on us
no thief, no spear
in a shower of light, the spirit of
no mother, no son, no soldier
not a dying Jesus, but a living Christ.

NOTES

1 EUA stands for Emergency Use Authorization, the legal aegis under which expedited Covid-19 vaccine development went forward.
2 Charles Dickens, *A Tale of Two Cities*. The Dickens Project, https://dickens.ucsc.edu/programs/dickens-to-go/best-of-times.html.
3 Ralph Waldo Emerson, "Lecture on the Times" in *Emerson: Essays and Lectures* (New York: Library of America, 1983).
4 Max Horkheimer & Theodor W. Adorno, *Dialectic of Enlightenment: Philosophical Fragments* (Stanford, CA: Stanford University, 2002).
5 Patrick J. Deneen, *Why Liberalism Failed* (New Haven, CT: Yale University, 2018).
6 Robert N. Bellah, *Religion in Human Evolution: From the Paleolithic to the Axial Age* (Cambridge, MA: Harvard University, 2011).
7 Klaus Schwab and Thierry Malleret, *COVID-19: The Great Reset* (Geneva: WEF, 2020).
8 Both postscripts toward the end of *Two Roads* ("Covid World," Aug. 2023, and "The Kennedy Candidacy and the Anatomy of Pro-Vax Prejudice") were written well *after* almost all of vol. 2 (*Covid and the Apocalpyse of the Modern Mind*) was written.
9 PBS NewsHour: WATCH: "Senators Hear Update on Early Outpatient Treatment for Covid-19," Nov. 19, 2020: https://www.youtube.com/live/EJpxcbTAuk8?si=1HrwfTyRGiihf5cq.
10 Ibid.
11 Ibid.
12 Ibid.
13 Ibid.
14 Nor did Dr. McCullough hesitate to point out that Dr. Jah's professional credentials, as judged by his lack of publication in the areas of concern, were far inferior to his own.
15 Mateja Cernic, *Ideological Constructs of Vaccination* (Newcastle Upon Tyne, UK: Vega Press, 2018), p. 395.
16 Ibid., p. 402.
17 Sarah Maslin, "Johnson and Johnson to Pay New York $230 Million to Settle Opioid Case," *New York Times*, June 26, 2021, https://www.nytimes.com/2021/06/26/nyregion/johnson-johnson-opioid-lawsuit-new-york.htm.l
18 Sara Randazzo, "States Announce $26 Billion Settlement to Resolve Opioid Lawsuits," *Wall Street Journal*, July 21, 2021, https://www.wsj.com/articles/states-announce-26-billion-settlement-to-resolve-opioid-lawsuits-11626890613.
19 "Johnson & Johnson to Pay $5bn in Landmark 26 bn US Opioid Settlement," *The Guardian*, July 21, 2021, https://www.theguardian.com/us-news/2021/jul/21/us-opioid-settlement-state-attorneys-general-johnson-and-johnson.
20 Cernic, *Ideological Constructs*, p. 393.
21 Ibid., p. 399.
22 Alexander Polikoff and Elizabeth Lassar, *A Brief History of the Subordination of African Americans in the U.S.: Of Handcuffs and Bootstraps* (New York: Routledge, 2020).
23 Daniel Joseph Polikoff, *Rue Rilke* (Asheville, NC : Chiron, 2016).
24 I believe these two were Dr. Dan Erikson and Artin Massihi. See Jeffrey A. Tucker, "How Lockdowns Make us Sicker," *Brownstone Institute*, Dec 13, 2022, https://brownstone.org/articles/how-lockdowns-made-us-sicker.
25 In fact, the article cited in the prior note contends that the Erickson–Massihi position was fully in accord with established

scientific understanding and that the contrary position amounted to a rash and unjustified overthrow of basic, previously widely accepted immunological and epidemiological principles.

26 See previous note. The Jeffrey A. Tucker article, like my text, also calls attention to the extreme nature of the reaction to the doctors' statement.

27 Children's Health Defense Team, "Graduate Student Tells RFK Jr. How She Took on Her School's COVID Vaccine Policy—and Won," *The Defender*, June 28, 2021, https://childrenshealthdefense.org/defender/rfk-jr-the-defender-podcast-cait-corrigan-earlham-college-covid-vaccine.

28 "Canadian MP Derek Sloan Raises Concerns about Censorship of Doctors and Scientists," June 17, 2021, https://youtu.be/4cVSMyTYBjo?si=ARet21oqxR-Zh6Ju.

29 Ibid.

30 Ibid.

31 Ibid.

32 Ibid.

33 Ibid.

34 Ibid.

35 Ibid.

36 Ibid.

37 Ibid.

38 Ibid.

39 Ibid.

40 Ibid.

41 Ibid.

42 Ibid.

43 Ibid.

44 Ibid.

45 Ibid.

46 Ibid.

47 Ibid.

48 Ibid.

49 Megan Redshaw, "Nearly 11,000 Deaths After Covid Vaccines Reported to CDC, as FDA Adds New Warning to J + J Vaccine," *The Defender*, July 16, 2021, https://childrenshealthdefense.org/defender/vaers-deaths-injuries-reported-cdc-covid-vaccines-moderna-pregnant-women.

50 Ibid.

51 Ibid.

52 Joseph Mercola, "To Prevent Three Deaths, COVID Jab Kills Two," July 5, 2021, https://articles.mercola.com/sites/articles/archive/2021/07/05/covid-shots.aspx?

53 "Safety of COVID-19 Vaccines," Nov. 3, 2023, https://www.cdc.gov/coronavirus/2019-ncov/vaccines/safety/safety-of-vaccines.html.

54 It later came to light that these figures, while not outright fraudulent, are profoundly misleading. The figures as cited imply that for every 100 people vaccinated, 85 to 90 persons who may have contracted the disease if they were not vaccinated did not do so, so that the vaccines confer very high protection. The actuality is nothing of the sort.

The figures represent relative rather than absolute risk reduction and do not reflect a meaningful reduction in any given individual's chance of serious disease. The absolute risk reduction for the Pfizer test is .084%. One way of understanding this is to know that it means over 100 persons would have to be vaccinated to prevent one person from testing positive (not even contracting symptomatic Covid!) for Covid. It is also the case that, when all facts were accounted for, there were more deaths in the vaccine group than the placebo group on account of a much greater risk of cardiac failure in the vaccine group. The trial results were presented as representing great success.

The sober truth is rather the opposite. The whole case is an instructive instance of how easy it is to manipulate numbers and technical terms to disguise the truth. For one representative later analysis of the data, see Aseem Malhotra, "Curing the Pandemic of Misinformation on Covid-19 mRNA Vaccines through Real Evidence-based Science," *Journal of Insulin Resistance*, 5 (1): 71, Sept. 26, 2022, https://www.ncbi.nlm.nih.gov/pmc/articles/PMC9557944.

55 Joseph A. Lapado and Harvey A. Risch, "Are Covid Vaccines Riskier Than Advertised?" *Wall Street Journal,* June 22, 2021, https://www.wsj.com/articles/are-covid-vaccines-riskier-than-advertised-11624381749.

56 Public Health Ontario, "Explained: COVID-19 PCR Testing and Cycle Thresholds," https://www.publichealthontario.ca/en/About/News/2021/Explained-COVID19-PCR-Testing-and-Cycle-Threshold.s

57 Dr. Madhava Setty, "Want to Get to 70% Vaccine Coverage, Mr. President? Here's How You Do It," *The Pulse,* July 27, 2021, https://thepulse.one/2021/07/27/want-to-get-to-70-vaccine-coverage-mr-president-heres-how-you-do-it/

58 CDC COVID-19 Vaccine Breakthrough Case Investigation Guidelines, cited in Joseph Mercola, "To Prevent Three Deaths, COVID Jab Kills Two," *Technocracy News and Tech*: https://www.technocracy.news/mercola-to-prevent-three-deaths-covid-jab-kills-two.

59 Cited in Joel S. Hirschhorn, "Reducing Data on Breakthrough Covid Infections Not in Public Interest," *TrialSite News,* June 24, 2021, https://trialsitenews.com/reducing-data-on-breakthrough-covid-infections-not-in-public-interest.

60 Ibid.

61 Ibid.

62 Ibid.

63 Ibid.

64 Cited in James Fetzer, "Four New Discoveries About Safety and Efficacy of Covid Vaccines," *Principia Scientific International,* July 17, 2021, https://principia-scientific.com/four-new-discoveries-about-safety-and-efficacy-of-covid-vaccines.

65 "mRNA Inventor Shares Viral Thread Showing COVID Surge in Most-Vaxxed Countries," *Algora Blog,* July 17, 2021, https://www.algora.com/Algora_blog/2021/07/17/mrna-vaccine-inventor-shares-viral-thread-showing-covid-surge-in-most-vaxxed-countries-2.

66 @RWMaloneMD, "This Is Worrying Me Quite a Bit," Twitter, July 16, 2021, https://twitter.com/RWMaloneMD/status/1416188314701475844?

67 @holmenkollin, "Something Really Odd Is Going On," Twitter, July 16, 2021, https://threadreaderapp.com/thread/1415989536933490688.html.

68 Lapado and Risch, "Are Covid Vaccines Riskier than Advertised?", *Wall Street Journal,* June 22, 2021.

69 Megan Redshaw, "Cleveland Clinic: Already Had Covid? Vaccine Provided No Added Benefit," *The Defender,* June 9, 2021, https://childrenshealthdefense.org/defender/cleveland-clinic-previous-covid-infection-vaccine-no-benefit.

70 Ibid.

71 Megan Redshaw, "Dad: My Son's School Made Him Get a COVID Vaccine, Now He Has a Heart Condition," *The Defender,* July 6, 2021, https://childrenshealthdefense.org/defender/teen-heart-condition-pfizer-covid-vaccine-fabio-berlingieri-fox-friends.

72 Dr. Ros Jones' testimony, "166th Meeting of the FDA Vaccines and Related Biologic Products Advisory Committee," June 10, 2021, https://youtu.be/YepMK2jkwrk?si=tsyAYknWLUHGGUzn.

73 E.g., Dr. Janci Chann Lindsay's public comment before the CDC's Advisory Committee on Immunization Practices (ACIP), April 23, 2021 (YouTube video no longer available).

74 National Institute of Health, U.S. Library of Medicine, "Moderna Covid-19 Vaccine mRNA-1273 Observational Pregnancy Outcome Study," June 12, 2021, https://clinicaltrials.gov/ct2/show/NCT04958304.

75 Mercola.com. More detail cannot be provided as Mercola.com now regularly deletes content after initial posting.

76 Megan Redshaw, "Federal Lawsuit Seeks Immediate Halt of COVID Vaccine, Cites WhistleBlower

Testimony Claiming CDC is Under-Counting Vaccine Deaths," *The Defender*, July 20, 2021, https://childrenshealthdefense.org/defender/americas-frontline-doctors-federal-lawsuit-halt-covid-vaccines-cdc-vaccine-deaths.
77 Ibid.
78 Ibid.
79 Madelyn Resse, "Santa Clara County revises total Covid deaths by over 20%," *San Jose Spotlight,* July 8, 2021, https://sanjosespotlight.com/santa-clara-county-revises-total-covid-deaths-by-over-20.
80 America's Frontline Doctors, etc. et al v. Becerra et al., case# 2:2021cv-00702-CLM, July 19, 2021, U.S. District Court for the Northern District of Alabama, https://dockets.justia.com/docket/alabama/alndce/2:2021cv00702/177186.
81 Ibid.
82 Ibid.
83 Robert Langreth, "Are mRNA Covid Vaccines Risky? Here's What the Experts Say," *Bloomberg*, March 21, 2021, https://www.bloomberg.com/news/articles/2021-03-22/are-mrna-covid-vaccines-risky-what-the-experts-say-quicktake.
84 Ibid.
85 Megan Redshaw, "U.S. Surgeon General, Rockefeller Foundation, Announce Big Initiative to Address 'Urgent Threat' of Vaccine Misinformation," *The Defender,* July 16, 2021, https://childrenshealthdefense.org/defender/surgeon-general-ockefeller-foundation-initiatives-vaccine-misinformation.
86 Matt Taibbi, "If Private Platforms Use Government Guidelines to Police Content, Is that State Censorship?" *Racket News*, July 2, 2021, https://taibbi.substack.com/p/a-case-of-intellectual-capture-on.
87 Ibid.
88 Ibid.
89 Ibid.
90 Ibid.
91 Ibid.
92 Ibid.
93 Ibid.
94 The Informed Consent Action *Network, and Del Bigtree, Plaintiffs, v. YOUTUBE LLC and FACEBOOK, INC, Defendants*, suit filed Dec. 30, 2020, in the United District Court for the Northern District of California, San Jose Divison. *ICAN* member mailing, Jan., 2021.
95 Ibid.
96 Ibid.
97 Ibid.
98 Charlotte Tobit, "Journalists Claim Alternative Covid-19 News 'Has Been Censored' to Create 'One Official Narrative,'" *PressGazette,* July 26, 2021, https://www.pressgazette.co.uk/journalists-claim-alternative-covid-19-news-censorship-create-one-official-narrative.
99 Ibid.
100 Ibid.
101 Ibid.
102 https://quoteinvestigator.com/2015/06/01/defend-say.
103 Paul Feyerabend, *Against Method* (London: Verso, 2010).
104 Paul Feyerabend, *Science in a Free Society* (London: Verso, 1987).
105 Dr. Joseph Mercola and Ronnie Cummins, *The Truth About COVID-19,* (White River Junction, VT: Chelsea Green, 2021), p. 115.
106 @eh_den, "Pfizer Leak: New Contract/New Country," Twitter, July 27, 2021, https//threader.app/thread/1419992103116025858 (account suspended).
107 Ibid.
108 Mercola and Cummins, *The Truth about COVID-19*, p. 112.
109 Merritt, "SARS-CoV2 and the Rise of Medical Technocracy," D. G. Rancourt, "All Cause Mortality During COVID-19," and Yanni Gu, "A Closer Look at US Death Due to COVID-19," cited in Mercola and Cummins, *The Truth About COVID-19*, p. 112.
110 Mercola and Cummins, *The Truth About COVID-19,* p. 113.
111 Ibid.
112 Ibid. p. 114.
113 Ibid. pp. 113–114.

114 Ibid. p. 114.
115 Dr. Madhava Setty, "Want to Get to 70% Vaccine Coverage, Mr. President? Here's How You Do It," *The Pulse,* July 27, 2021, https://thepulse.one/2021/07/27/want-to-get-to-70-vaccine-coverage-mr-president-heres-how-you-do-it.
116 Ibid.
117 Ibid.
118 Ibid.
119 Ibid.
120 Ibid.
121 Megan Redshaw, "Conflict of Interest: Reuters 'Fact Checks' COVID-Related Media Posts, But Fails to Disclose Ties to Pfizer, World Economic Forum," *The Defender,* Aug. 11, 2021, https://childrenshealthdefense.org/defender/reuters-fact-check-covid-social-media-pfizer-world-economic-forum.
122 Ibid.
123 Ibid.
124 Ibid.
125 Ibid.
126 Ibid.
127 Ibid.
128 Ibid.
129 Ibid.
130 Ibid.
131 "Rand Paul Presses Senate Witness on Covid-19 Vaccine Policy," U.S. Senate hearing, June 23, 2021, https://www.youtube.com/watch?v=ogA-U3Fy6ww.
132 Suri Kinzbrunner, "No, the Unvaccinatted Aren't Selfish or Ignorant. Here's Why I'm Not Vaxxed," *Newsweek,* Aug. 10, 2021, https://www.newsweek.com/no-unvaccinated-arent-selfish-ignorant-heres-why-im-not-vaxxed-opinion-1617993
133 Megan Redshaw, "Exclusive Interview: Mom Whose 14-Year-Old Son Developed Myocarditis after Pfizer Vaccine No Longer Trusts the CDC, Public Health Officials," *The Defender,* Aug. 11, 2021, https://childrenshealthdefense.org/defender/emily-jo-14-year-old-son-aiden-myocarditis-pfizer-vaccine/
134 Ibid.
135 Ibid.
136 Ibid.
137 Ibid.
138 Ibid.
139 Jeffrey A. Tucker, "WHO Deletes Naturally Acquired Immunity from Its Website," American Institute for Economic Research, Dec. 23, 2020, https://www.aier.org/article/who-deletes-naturally-acquired-immunity-from-its-website.
140 Robert Frost, "The Road Not Taken" (1915), https://www.poetryfoundation.org/poems/44272/the-road-not-taken.
141 Press Briefing by the White House COVID-19 Response Team, Aug. 5, 2021, https://www.whitehouse.gov/briefing-room/press-briefings/2021/08/05/press-briefing-by-white-house-covid-19-response-team-and-public-health-officials-48.
142 Suri Kinzbrunner, "No, the Unvaccinated Aren't Selfish or Ignorant," *Newsweek,* Aug. 10, 2021, https://www.newsweek.com/no-unvaccinated-arent-selfish-ignorant-heres-why-im-not-vaxxed-opinion-1617993.
143 Lindsay Kalter and Ralph Ellis, "CDC: COVID-19 Is a Pandemic of the Unvaccinated," July 16, 2021, https://www.webmd.com/lung/news/20210716/delta-variant-rising-covid-case-counts-every-state.
144 Press Briefing, "White House COVID-19 Response Team," Aug. 5, 2021. https://www.whitehouse.gov/briefing-room/press-briefings/2021/08/05/press-briefing-by-white-house-covid-19-response-team-and-public-health-officials-48.
145 Ibid.
146 Dr. Joseph Mercola, "How the CDC Manipulated Data to Create 'Pandemic of the Unvaxxed' Narrative," Aug. 16, 2021, *The Defender,* https://childrenshealthdefense.org/defender/cdc-manipulated-data-create-pandemic-unvaxxed-narrative.
147 "Doctor Who Did Early Research on Covid Vaccine: This Is Not a Pandemic of the Unvaccinated," *The Ingraham Angle,* Fox News, Aug. 6, 2021, https://video.foxnews.com/v/6266738894001#sp=show-clips

148 Ibid.
149 Ibid.
150 Ibid.
151 Ibid.
152 https://www.voiceforscienceand solidarity.org
153 Geert Vanden Bosch, "To All Authorities, Scientists, and Experts around the World, Whom This Concerns," open letter, Mar. 6, 2021, https://www.geertvandenbossche.org; https://37b32f5a-6ed9-4d6d -b3e15ec648ad9ed9; this website is defunct as of Oct. 12, 2023; another version is posted at https://twitter.com /GVDBossche/status /1368232172872732675. Meanwhile, more material from Vanden Bossche is available on his Voice for Science and Solidarity website (see prior note). However, I am unable to locate the quoted material on the new sites.
154 Ibid. (see above notes).
155 Ibid. (see above notes).
156 Geert Vanden Bossche, "Not Covid-19 Vaccine-induced Immunity but Naturally Acquired Immunity Enables Herd Immunity," July 14, 2021, https://www.voiceforscienceand solidarity.org/search?query=blog +not+covid-19-mediated-but -naturally-acquired-immunity-enables.
157 Ibid.
158 Ibid.
159 Geert Vanden Bossche, "Urgent Call to WHO: Time to Switch Gears," YouTube, March 11, 2021, https:// www.youtube.com/watch?v =mUlDeCRDLnU&t=19s
160 Bret Weinstein and Dr. Pierre Kory, "The Joe Rogan Experience #1671," June 22, 2021, https://open.spotify .com/sode /7uVXKgE6eLJKMXkETwcwoD.
161 Front Line, "COVID-19 Crtical Care Alliance Website, Treatment Protocols/Ivermectin," https: //covid19criticalcare.com/ivermectin.
162 Kevin Dunleavy, "With 1.2B Deal for Molupiravir, U.S. Bets on Merck's COVID-19 Oral Antiviral," *Fierce Pharma,* June 9, 2021, https://www .fiercepharma.com/pharma/1-2b -deal-for-molnupiravir-u-s-bets-merck -to-finally-provide-effective-covid-19 -treatment.
163 Ibid.
164 U.S. Senate Committee on Homeland Security and Governmental Affairs, "Early Outpatient Treatment: An Essential Part of a COVID-19 Solution. Part II," Dec. 8, 2020, https://www.hsgac.senate.gov /hearings/early-outpatient-treatment -an-essential-part-of-a-covid-19 -solution-part-ii.
165 Ibid.
166 Ibid.
167 Ibid.
168 Ibid.
169 Ibid.
170 Ibid.
171 Ibid.
172 Ibid.
173 Ibid.
174 Ibid.
175 Ibid.
176 Ibid.
177 Ibid.
178 Ibid.
179 Bret Weinstein and Dr. Pierre Kory, *The Joe Rogan Experience* #1671, June 22, 2021, https://open .spotify.com.
180 Nanette Asimov, "You Are Not a Horse: Bogus COVID Craze for Ivermectin Vexes Bay Area Feed Stores," *San Francisco Chronicle,* Sept. 3, 2021, https://www.sfchronicle. com/bayarea/article/You-are-not-a -horse-Bogus-COVID-craze-for -16430581.php.
181 Ibid. p. C1.
182 Ibid.
183 Ibid. p. C7.
184 @grahamwalker, "The Snti-vax and Misinformation People," Twitter, Sept. 3, 2021; this reference no longer exists.
185 Asimov, "You Are Not a Horse," *San Francisco Chronicle,* C7.
186 Bryant A, Lawrie TA, et al. "Ivermectin for Prevention and Treatment of COVID-19 Infection: A Systematic Review, Meta-analysis, and Trial Sequential Analysis to Inform Clinical Guidelines," *American Journal of Therapeutics,*

28 (4): e434–e460, June 21, 2021. https://doi.org/10.1097/MJT.0000000000001402.

187 Front Line Covid-19 Critical Care Alliance, https://covid19criticalcare.com

188 Ibid., "Summary of the Evidence"; article no longer posted by FLCCC Alliance: covid19criticalcare.com.

189 Ibid.

190 Asimov, "You Are Not a Horse," *San Francisco Chronicle,* C7.

191 Vladimir Zelenko interview with Del Bigtree, in "A Feast of Consequences," *The HighWire,* #231, Sept. 2, 2021, https://thehighwire.com/videos/episode-231-feast-of-consequences.

192 The author feels obliged to note that later in the course of the pandemic, the efficacy of monoclonal antibody treatment declined dramatically so that, as of 2023, this treatment method is no longer generally employed. The decline in efficacy is an effect of viral evolution and the emergence of mutant strains with different properties. Cf. Lisa O'Mary, "Covid-19 Monoclonal Antibody Treatment No Longer Effective," WebMD, Dec. 4, 2022, https://www.webmd.com/covid/news/20221204/covid-19-monoclonal-antibody-treatments-no-longer-effective.

193 Dr. Richard Bartlett interview with Del Bigtree, "A Feast of Consequences," *The HighWire,* #231, Sept. 2, 2021, https://thehighwire.com/videos/episode-231-feast-of-consequences/

194 Ibid.

195 Ibid. Fauci clip inserted in interview," A Feast of Consequences," *The HighWire,* episode 231, Sept. 2, 2021, https://thehighwire.com/videos/episode-231-feast-of-consequences.

196 Ibid.

197 U.S. senate hearing, "Dr. Anthony Fauci to Sen. Rand Paul at Hearing: You Do Not Know What You're Talking About," YouTube, July 20, 2021, *YouTube,* https://www.youtube.com/watch?v=Pnb2Yxri6eY

198 Ibid.

199 See note 195.

200 See the postscript, "Covid World," Aug. 2023, for an update on this issue.

201 *The Joe Rogan Experience* #671.

202 Dr. David Brownstein, "The Right Way to Fight Viruses," *Natural Way to Health* newsletter, vol. 14, no. 8, Aug. 2021, p. 1.

203 Ibid., p. 7.

204 Ibid., p. 2.

205 Ibid., p. 3.

206 Ibid., p. 5.

207 Ibid., p. 3.

208 David Brownstein, MD, et al., "A Novel Approach to Treating COVID-19 Using Nutritional and Oxidative Therapies," *Science, Public Health Policy and the Law, 2: 4–22,* July 7, 2021, https://www.publichealthpolicyjournal.com/clinical-and-translational-research.

209 David Brownstein, *A Holistic Approach to Viruses* (West Bloomfield, MI: Medical Alternatives, 2021).

210 Brownstein, "The Right Way to Treat Viruses," p. 5.

211 Ibid., pp. 5, 7.

212 David Brownstein, *Iodine: Why You Need It, Why You Can't Live without It* (West Bloomfield, MI: Medical Alternatives, 2009).

213 David Brownstein, "The Right Way to Fight Viruses," *Natural Way to Health Newsletter*, Aug. 2021, p. 5.

214 Ibid.

215 Kate Dalley, "Our First Hand ICU Story – What Is Actually Killing People in the Hospital," Rumble, Aug. 6, 2021, https://rumble.com/vktdpt-our-first-hand-icu-story-what-is-actually-killing-people-in-the-hospital.

216 Ibid.

217 Ibid.

218 "Covid-19 Treatment Guidelines: Supplements: Summary Recommendations," Dec. 20, 2023, *NIH Website*, https://www.covid19treatmentguidelines.nih.gov/therapies/supplements/summary-recommendations.

219 See note 215.

220 See note 215.
221 Tom Porter, "How a New York Billionaire-funded Anti-vax Group Is Contributing to the Vaccine Hesitancy that's Crippling the U.S. Recovery," *Business Insider*, Aug. 24, 2021, https://www.businessinsider.com/ican-billionaire-funded-antivax-group-trump-fans-ties-2021-8.
222 Ibid.
223 Ibid.
224 Ibid.
225 "Del Bigtree's Full Interview with *Insider* Reporter, Tom Porter," *The HighWire*, Aug. *17, 2021*, https://thehighwire.com/videos/del-bigtrees-full-interview-with-insider-reporter-tom-porter.
226 Porter, "How a New York Billionaire-funded Anti-vax Group..." *Business Insider.*
227 See note 225.
228 David Cole and Daniel Mach, "We Work at the ACLU. Here's What We Think about Vaccine Mandates," *The New York Times*, Sept. 2, 2021, https://www.nytimes.com/2021/09/02/opinion/covid-vaccine-mandates-civil-liberties.html
229 Ibid.
230 Cathrine Axfors and John P.A. Ioannidis, "Infection Fatality Rate of COVID-19 in Community-dwelling Populations with Emphasis on the Elderly: An Overview," https://pubmed.ncbi.nlm.nih.gov/35306604.
231 Robert F. Kennedy Jr., interview with Dr. Peter McCullough, "What Fauci Should Have Done," *The Defender Podcast*, Aug. 24, 2021, https://open.spotify.com/episode/27CRxt52ntiS79YsLI4b4V.
232 Nguyen Van Vinh Chau, "Transmission of SARS-CoV-2 Delta Variant among Vaccinated Healthcare Workers, Vietnam," *Lancet*, Aug. 10, 2021, https://papers.ssrn.com/sol3/papers.cfm?abstract_id=3897733#.
233 Ibid.
234 RFK Jr., "What Fauci Should Have Done," interview with Dr. Peter McCullough.
235 Ibid.
236 Ibid. Unfortunately, the name of the author of the cited paper is inaudible.
237 Ibid.
238 Ibid.
239 Sivan Gazit, et al., "Comparing SARS-CoV-2 Natural Immunity to Vaccine-induced Immunity: Reinfection Versus Breakthrough Infections," *medRxiv/BMJ Yale*, Aug. 25, 2021, https://www.medrxiv.org/content/10.1101/2021.08.24.21262415v1; https://doi.org/10.1101/2021.08.24.21262415.
240 Cited in Tyler Durden, "'This Ends the Debate'—Israeli Study Shows Natural Immunity 13x More Effective Than Vaccines at Stopping Delta," *Zero Hedge*, Aug. 28, 2021, https://www.zerohedge.com/covid-19/ends-debate-israeli-study-shows-natural-immunity-13x-more-effective-vaccines-stopping
241 Gazit et al., "Comparing SARS-CoV-2 Natural Immunity To Vaccine-induced"
242 Cited in Durden, "This Ends the Debate."
243 Ibid.
244 Ibid.
245 Levi's work cited on Bigtree, "A Feast of Consequences," *HighWire* #231.
246 Ibid.
247 "We've Never Seen Vaccine Injuries on This Scale — Why Are Regulatory Agencies Hiding COVID Vaccine Safety Signals?" *The Defender*, Aug. 12, 2021, https://childrenshealthdefense.org/defender/vaccine-injuries-regulatory-agencies-hiding-covid-safety-data.
248 RFK Jr. interview with Dr. Peter McCullough, "What Fauci Should Have Done."
249 Ibid.
250 Ibid.
251 Ibid.
252 See note 247.
253 Mathew Crawford, "Defining Away Vaccine Safety Signals," *Rounding the Earth Newsletter*, July 27, 2021, https://roundingtheearth.substack.com/p/defining-away-vaccine-safety-signals
254 Ibid.

255 Ibid. If you are wondering about what that last phrase ("another false COVID statistic") refers to, you can read another piece by Crawford disclosing that VAERS-registered *vaccine-related deaths* are routinely (that means, so far as Crawford can tell, without exception) counted as deaths *caused by Covid,* even if under 5% of such persons had a test-confirmed current Covid infection. cf. Mathew Crawford, "Probable Misclassification of Vaccine Deaths as Covid-19 Deaths," *Rounding the Earth Newsletter,* July 27, 2021, https://roundingtheearth.substack.com/p/probable-misclassification-of-vaccine

256 Ibid.

257 RFK Jr. interview with Dr. Peter McCullough, "What Fauci Should Have Done."

258 Ibid.

259 Ibid.

260 Ibid.

261 Ibid.

262 Ibid.

263 President Joseph Biden, presidential address on Covid-19, Sept. 9, 2021, https://www.youtube.com/watch?v=IA2SCoYl8_U&t=10s.

264 Ibid.

265 Ibid.

266 Ibid.

267 Ibid.

268 Nina Pierpoint, "Covid-19 Vaccine Mandates Are Now Pointless," *The Defender,* Sept. 9, 2021, https://childrenshealthdefense.org/wp-content/uploads/Pierpont-Why-mandated-vaccines-are-pointless-final-1.pdf.

269 Ibid.

270 Catherine M. Brown et al., "Outbreak of SARS-CoV-2 Infections, Including COVID-19 Vaccine Breakthrough Infections, Associated with Large Public Gatherings, Barnstable County, Massachusetts, July 2021," *CDC Morbidity and Mortality Weekly Report,* Aug. 6, 2021.

271 Koen B. Pouwels et al. on the COVID-19 Infection Survey Team, 2021, "Impact of Delta on Viral Burden and Vaccine Effectiveness against New SARS-CoV-2 Infections in the UK," medRxiv, posted Aug. 24, 2021, https//doi.org/10.1101/2021.08.18.21262237.

272 Pierpont, "Covid-19 Vaccine Mandates," p. 5.

273 Ibid.

274 Ibid.

275 Ibid. pp. 6–7.

276 Ibid. p. 9. This turns out to have been a prescient warning. Two years later, many relevant lawsuits have been brought (see the postscript for some update on this score). Many more are likely to follow in due course.

277 Erin Banco, "Biden Covid Team Sees Vaccine Efficacy Waning in Unpublished Data from Israel," *Politico,* Sept. 9, 2014, https://www.politico.com/news/2021/09/14/covid-israel-data-vaccine-efficacy-511777.

278 Nathan Jeffay, "Portugal, Sweden Slap COVID Entry Ban on Israelis, Including Vaccinated," *Times of Israel,* Sept. 3, 2021, https//www.timesofisrael.com/portugal-sweden-slap-covid-entry-ban-on-israelis-including-those-vaccinated.

279 Kim Iversen, "Israel Cases SPIKE as country REQUIRES 3rd Jab," *Kim Iversen Show,* Sept. 16, 2021, https://www.youtube.com/watch?v=4ZyYQrw6rao.

280 Erica Carbajal, "Nearly 60% of Hospitalized COVID-19 Patients in Israel Fully Vaccinated," *Becker's Hospital Review,* Aug. 19, 2021. https://www.beckershospitalreview.com/public-health/nearly-60-of-hospitalized-covid-19-patients-in-israel-fully-vaccinated-study-finds.html.

281 Ibid.

282 Kim Iversen, "Israel Cases SPIKE."

283 Ibid.

284 Ibid.

285 Banco, "Biden Covid Team Sees Vaccine Efficacy Waning," Politico.

286 Ibid.

287 Iversen, "Israel Cases SPIKE."

288 Retsef Levi, public comment, "FDA Vaccine-Related Biological Products Advisory Committee," Sept. 17, 2021,

https://www.youtube.com/watch?v=WFph7-6t34M&t=15495s.
289 Dr. Jessica Rose, public comment in YouTube video, ibid.
290 Ibid.
291 Steve Kirsch, public comment in YouTube video, ibid.
292 Dr. Joseph B. Fraiman, public comment in YouTube video, ibid.
293 President Joseph Biden, public address, Sept. 9, 2021. https://www.youtube.com/watch?v=IA2SCoYl8_U&t=10s.
294 Tracy Beth Hoeg, et al., "SARS-CoV-2 mRNA Vaccination-Associated Myocarditis," medRxiv, https://www.youtube.com/watch?v=IA2SCoYl8_U&t=10s; https://doi.org/10.1101/2021.08.30.21262866.
295 Del Bigtree, "The VAERS Scandal," *The Highwire* #233, Sept. 16, 2021, https://thehighwire.com/videos/episode-233-the-vaers-scandal.
296 TikTok video clip from *The Highwire,* ibid. (posted Sept. 6, 2021, on TikTok by John Stokes).
297 President Joseph Biden, public address, Sept. 9, 2021, https://www.youtube.com/watch?v=IA2SCoYl8_U&t=10s.
298 World Tribune Staff, "Unexpected and Heartbreaking: Thousands Flood ABC Affiliate's Facebook Page with Vaccination Horror Stories," *World Tribune,* Sept. 13, 2021, https://www.worldtribune.com/unexpected-and-heartbreaking-thousands-flood-abc-affiliates-facebook-page-with-vaccination-horror-stories.
299 *World Tribune* staff: "Unexpected and Heartbreaking: Thousands flood ABC Affiliate's Facebook Page with Vaccination Horror Stories," *World Tribune,* Sept. 13, 2021. https://www.worldtribune.com/unexpected-and-heartbreaking-thousands-flood-abc-affiliates-facebook-page-with-vaccination-horror-stories.
300 Ross Lazarus, "Electronic Support for Public Health Vaccine Adverse Event Reporting System," Harvard Pilgrim Healthcare submission to the U.S. Dept. of Health and Human Services (grant ID: R18 HS 017045), inclusive dates December 1, 2017–Sept. 30, 2010, https://digital.ahrq.gov/sites/default/files/docs/publication/r18hs017045-lazarus-final-report-2011.pdf.
301 Video clip on "The VAERS Scandal," *The Highwire* #233.
302 Ibid.
303 Ibid.
304 WECT News staff, "Novant Health Issues Statement on Leaked Internal Discussion of Covid-19 Patient Numbers," WECT News 6, Sept. 10, 2021, https://www.wect.com/2021/09/10/novant-health-issues-statement-leaked-internal-discussion-covid-19-patient-numbers.
305 David Zweig, "Our Most Reliable Pandemic Number Is Losing Meaning," *The Atlantic,* Sept. 13, 2021, https://www.theatlantic.com/health/archive/2021/09/covid-hospitalization-numbers-can-be-misleading/620062.
306 Ibid.
307 Peter Doshi, public comment, FDA Sept. 17, 2021 meeting. https://www.youtube.com/watch?v=WFph7-6t34M.
308 Deborah Conrad on "The VAERS Scandal," *The Highwire* #233, Sept. 16, 2021, https://thehighwire.com/videos/episode-233-the-vaers-scandal.
309 Ibid.
310 Ibid.
311 Ibid.
312 Ibid.
313 Ibid.
314 Ibid.
315 Ibid.
316 Ibid.
317 Ibid.
318 Ibid.
319 Ibid.
320 Ibid.
321 Ibid.
322 Ibid.
323 Ibid.
324 Ibid.
325 Ibid.
326 Ibid.
327 Ibid.
328 Ibid.
329 Ibid.
330 Ibid.

331 Ibid.
332 Ibid.
333 Ibid.
334 Ibid.
335 Video clip, Deborah Conrad, "The VAERS Scandal," *The Highwire,* #233, https://thehighwire.com/ark-videos/the-vaers-scandal.
336 Ibid.
337 Julie Washington, "UH, Cleveland Clinic CEOs worry COVID-19 Vaccine Mandate Could Lead to Staff Reduction, Endangering Patient Care," *University Health,* Aug. 26, 2021, https://www.cleveland.com/coronavirus/2021/08/uh-cleveland-clinic-ceos-worry-covid-19-vaccine-mandates-could-lead-to-staff-reduction-endangering-patient-care.html.
338 Robert King, "AHA Concerned Federal Vaccine Mandate Could Exacerbate Severe Worker Shortage," *Fierce Healthcare,* Sept. 10, 2021, https://www.fiercehealthcare.com/hospitals/aha-concerned-federal-vaccine-mandate-could-make-workforce-shortages-worse.
339 Ibid.
340 Kristen Hwang, "Nurse Shortages in California Reaching," *CalMatters,* Aug. 5, 2021, https://calmatters.org/health/coronavirus/2021/08/california-nurses-shortage/
341 Bob D'Angelo, "NY Hospital to Pause Baby Deliveries after Staffers Quit over Vaccine Mandate," *Kiro 7 News,* Aug. 16, 2021, https://www.kiro7.com/news/trending/ny-hospital-pause-baby-deliveries-after-staffers-quit-over-vaccine-mandate/nnmbmq6vtfft5ddamxv46dq5tq/
342 Alyssa Lukpat and Lauren McCarthy, "Nebraska Is Recruiting Unvaccinated Nurses to Plug a Staffer Shortage," *New York Times,* Aug. 26, 2021, https://www.nytimes.com/2021/08/26/us/nebraska-delta-nurses-unvaccinated.html
343 Grant Schulte, "Nebraska State Job Ad Touts Lack of Vaccine Requirement, *US News*, Aug. 24, 2021, https://www.usnews.com/news/best-states/nebraska/articles/2021-08-24/nebraska-state-job-ad-touts-lack-of-vaccine-requirement.
344 *The Highwire,* #233.
345 Walt Whitman, "Song of Myself, 15," https://poets.org/poem/song-myself-15.
346 Walt Whitman, "Song of Myself, 1," https://poets.org/poem/song-myself-1-i-celebrate-myself.
347 Eleanor Roosevelt, from "10 Inspiring Eleanor Roosevelt Quotes," United Nations Foundation, https://unfoundation.org/blog/post/10-inspiring-eleanor-roosevelt-quotes.
348 Thousands of medical professionals declare Covid policies "Crimes against Humanity," *The Desert Review,* Sept. 28, 2021, https://www.thedesertreview.com/news/thousands-of-medical-professionals-declare-covid-policies-crimes-against-humanity/article_e2863f70-2074-11ec-8212-abe09d13e222.html.
349 Ibid. The original declaration, as well as an updated version, may also be viewed at https://doctorsandscientistsdeclaration.org.
350 George Fareed, "Dr. Fareed Addresses Italian Senate at COVID Summit, *The Desert Review*, Sept. 16, 2021, https://www.thedesertreview.com/news/local/dr-fareed-addresses-italian-senate-at-covid-summit/article_75ef29c2-16ff-11ec-9560-1b32c7c0d4a0.html.
351 Joselito N. Villero, "Dr. Fareed Awarded Branding Iron," *The Desert Review,* Sept. 26, 2021, https://www.thedesertreview.com/news/dr-fareed-awarded-branding-iron/article_e9a02b9e-1e45-11ec-9c7e-931e2e5b9f4f.html.
352 "Meeting of the COVID-19 Giants," Dr. Philip McMillan interviewing Robert Malone and Geert Vanden Bossche, *Vejon Health,* Sept. 25, 2021, https://www.youtube.com/watch?v=qP31cfD3YOY.
353 Ibid. In that interview, Vanden Bossche speaks about discrimination on the basis of vaccination status "the ultimate example of scientific nonsense" because, in any given case, there is no way of knowing who may

be more likely to transmit the disease.

354 "Fauci Blasts Critics in Fiery TV Appearance," *MTP-Daily*, June 9, 2021, https://www.independent.co.uk/news/world/americas/us-politics/fauci-interview-today-science-covid-b1862899.html.

355 PBS NewsHour, "Senators Hear Update on Early Outpatient Treatment for Covid-19," Nov. 19, 2020, https://www.youtube.com/watch?v=EJpxcbTAuk8&t=5513s

356 The course of events may appear to discredit my arguments: the U.S. did not fundamentally alter its Covid policy, and—while Covid remains a health threat in 2023—by now, in November, most everyone is comfortable regarding the pandemic as over. I would contend, however, that the U.S. (along with most of the rest of the world) finally emerged from the pandemic *in spite of rather than because of* official policy. The development that seemed to prove decisive was the emergence of a variant (Omicron) both more infectious and less virulent than Alpha or Delta, and which fortunately accelerated the natural transition of Covid-19 from a pandemic to an endemic state of disease. This means that a combination of *a lessening of disease virulence* and *widespread infection that engenders significant natural immunity in the population at large* has resulted in many fewer cases of serious disease or death, despite the ongoing persistence of Covid-19.

Correlatively, I would argue (a) that the terrible toll taken by Alpha and Delta (and even the lesser toll attributable to Omicron) could have been largely averted by more responsible policy; (b) that the mass vaccination campaign probably impeded rather than enhanced the transition to endemicity; and (c) that the true and ongoing crises faced now, in the wake of Covid, are not attributable to the disease itself but to the pandemic of injury and death caused by massive use of the unsafe mRNA vaccines. See, especially, postscript 1 (Covid World, Aug. 2023) for further information on that score. Last, I would suggest that the ideas or principles elucidated in the current and next chapter remain keenly relevant to any future "pandemic planning."

357 "Meeting of the COVID-19 Giants," Dr. Philip McMillan interviewing Robert Malone and Geert Vanden Bossche, *Vejon Health*, Sept. 25, 2021, https://www.youtube.com/watch?v=qP31cfD3YOY. I take my focus on strategy and tactics from Vanden Bossche's comments in this interview. Here is one choice passage: "I mean, nobody talks anymore about herd immunity. What is the objective still of the mass vaccination campaign? Can anybody tell me what is the objective? I mean, if there is no objective, well then there is also no strategy, of course. And there is no strategy. There is only tactics, right?...Everybody is doing something. But there is no common objective and every country is doing their own thing. So this is really a disaster, because the only way to solve this still, I mean, we don't change virology. We don't change immunology. It's still the interplay between the virus and the immune system. It's still herd immunity. So how, where are we going to get herd immunity from? *Certainly not, certainly not* from the vaccination. And even less when we do mass vaccination."

358 cf. "Rand Paul Roasts Heads of HHS," *The Highwire* #236 ("WHO is the Blame"), Oct. 7, 2021, https://thehighwire.com/videos/rand-paul-roasts-head-of-hhs.

359 Ibid.

360 Senator Paul, himself, *is* an MD.

361 Ibid.

362 "Meeting of the COVID-19 Giants," Dr. Philip McMillan interviewing Robert Malone and Geert Vanden Bossche, *Vejon Health*, Sept. 25, 2021, https://www.youtube.com/watch?v=qP31cfD3YOY

363 Hospital treatment of the seriously ill—the third pillar—may act as a safety net but itself serves as an indication of system *failure.*

364 Alfred Bourla, Interview on *ABC News This Week*, Sept. 26, 2021, https://abcnews.go.com/ThisWeek/video/fizer-ceo-albert-bourla-80242255.

365 Pfizer's real agenda, one suspects, has little to do with human health and welfare but aims to turn the whole of humanity into users, compelled by force if not inclination to shoot up with a never-ending stream of Pfizer products, year after sad, sad year.

366 Declaration of Independence. July 4, 1776. From the National Archives of the United States, https://www.archives.gov/founding-docs/declaration-transcript.

367 *PBS NewsHour,* "Senators Hear Update on Early Outpatient Treatment for Covid-19." Nov. 19, 2020, https://www.youtube.com/watch?v=EJpxcbTAuk8&t=5513s.

368 CDC website, accessed first week of Nov. 2021, https://www.cdc.gov/coronavirus/2019-ncov/vaccines/recommendations/children-teens.html.

369 "Meeting of the COVID-19 Giants," Dr. Philip McMillan interviewing Robert Malone and Geert Vanden Bossche, *Vejon Health,* Sept. 25, 2021, https://www.youtube.com/watch?v=qP31cfD3YOY. Why is protecting younger persons (first and foremost, children and teenagers, and young adults) so critical? Because, as Vanden Bossche explains, it is precisely the robust and flexible form of natural immunity (both innate and acquired after infection) possessed by this population that constitutes society's strongest and most important line of defense against the evolution of more infectious and virulent viral strains. The younger population's natural resilience supplies the broad-based immunological resources society can draw upon to reduce the infectious pressure that drives viral evolution. Here is Vanden Bossche's own words on the topic from this same interview: "This is the buffer. The younger age groups, you bring them in unvaccinated, you're going to see a *diminishment* in infectious pressure. They are the vaccuum cleaners. If we start vaccinating these people, they lose this potential.... When people get vaccinated, they are going to breed, in fact, those infectious, more infectious strains, and through immune selection pressure, there is no longer this elimination. We lose completely this buffer."

370 See the prior note.

371 CDC website, accessed first week of Nov. 2021, https://www.cdc.gov/coronavirus/2019-ncov/vaccines/recommendations/children-teens.html.

372 Senator Ron Johnson, remarks before Expert Panel on Vaccine Mandates, Nov. 2, 2021, https://www.youtube.com/watch?v=lkVN3KwDfvI.

373 Ibid.

374 Ibid.

375 "Who Will Help Us?" *The Highwire* #240 ("A Strike at the Heart"), Nov. 4, 2021, https://thehighwire.com/videos/who-will-help-us.

376 Aidin Vaziri, "State's Covid-19 Rate at 'Worrisome' Levels," *San Francisco Chronicle,* Nov. 10, 2021.

377 "Province Raises Covid-19 Alarm," *San Francisco Chronicle,* Nov. 10, 2021, p. A4.

378 "WHO Says Cases Ebb Everywhere Except Europe," *San Francisco Chroncle,* Nov. 11, 2021, p. A5.

379 Vaziri, "States Covid-19 Rate at 'Worrisome' Levels," *San Francisco Chronicle,* Nov. 10, 2021, p. A9.

380 Servellita et al., "Predominance of Antibody-resistant SARS-CoV-2 Variants in Vaccine Breakthrough Cases in the San Francisco Bay Area, California, *MedRxiv,* Aug. 25, 2021, https://www.medrxiv.org/content/10.1101/2021.08.19.21262139v1; https://doi.org/10.1101/2021.08.19.21262139.

381 Ibid.

382 Ibid.

383 Ibid.
384 Ibid.
385 Ibid.
386 David Leonhardt, "Good Morning. Is It Time to Start Moving back to Normalcy?" *The New York Times,* Nov. 12, 2021; weblink for the same piece under the title "How Does This End? Thinking about Covid and Normalcy," https://www.nytimes.com/2021/11/12/briefing/when-will-covid-end.html.
387 Monica Gandhi, "Don't Worry, Covid Outbreaks Are New Normal," *San Francisco Chronicle,* Nov. 13, 2021, p. A10.
388 Leonhardt, "Good Morning. Is It Time to Start Moving Back to Normalcy?" (or "How Does This End?").
389 Vaziri, "State's Covid-19 Rate at 'Worrisome' Levels," *San Francisco Chronicle,* Nov. 10, 2021.
390 Gandhi, "Don't Worry."
391 Ibid.
392 Ibid.
393 Scott Ostler, "Packer's Rodgers Cancels Himself," *San Francisco Chronicle,* Nov. 6, 2021, p. B1.
394 Chase Goodbread, "Vikings OL Dakota Dozier Hospitalized Due to Covid-19 Complications, *NFL News,* Nov. 10, 2021, https://www.nfl.com/news/mike-zimmer-vaccinated-vikings-player-in-er-after-contracting-covid-19.
395 Gandhi, "Don't Worry, COVID Outbreaks Are New Normal."
396 Charles Eisenstein, "Elements of Refusal," Nov. 11, 2021, https://charleseisenstein.substack.com/p/elements-of-refusal.
397 @KlausK, "Threadreader," Sept. 19, 2021, https://threadreaderapp.com/thread/1439691439227670534.html.
398 Del Bigtree, "Sins of Science," *The Highwire* #241, Nov. 11, 2021.
399 Dzevad Mesic, "Jerremy Chardy: I Regret Getting Vaccinated. I Have a Series of Problems Now," *Tennis World,* Sept. 25, 2021, https://www.tennisworldusa.org/tennis/news/Tennis_Interviews/102836/jeremy-chardy-i-regret-getting-vaccinated-i-have-series-of-problems-now.
400 "Pedro Obiang, 29-Year-Old Professional Footballer, Suffers Myocarditis after COVID-19 Vaccine, Possible End of Career," *The COVID World,* Aug. 22, 2021, https://thecovidworld.com/pedro-obiang-29-year-old-professional-footballer-suffers-myocarditis-after-covid-19-vaccine.
401 Adan Salazar, "Watch: Two Cricket Players Collapse, Convulse On Field Just Days After Team Fully Vaxxed," *CloudHedges,* July 5, 2021, https://cloudhedges.com/2021/07/05/watch-two-cricket-players-collapse-convulse-on-field-just-days-after-team-fully-vaxxed.
402 Ibid. The story was carried by multiple sources.
403 "Roy Butler: Healthy 23-Year-Old Soccer Player Dies 4 Days after Receiving Johnson & Johnson COVID-19 Vaccine, *The COVID World,* Aug. 19, 2021, https://thecovidworld.com/roy-butler-healthy-23-year-old-footballer-dies-4-days-after-receiving-covid-19-vaccine.
404 Ibid.
405 Ibid.
406 Brian Wallstin, "Vermont Leads Nation in New COVID Cases and Vaccination Rate," *ABC News* 10, Nov. 16, 2021, https://www.news10.com/news/coronavirus/vermont-leads-nation-in-new-covid-cases-and-vaccination-rate.
407 John Ingold, "What Is Driving Colorado's Covid Surge? Not Even the Experts Are Sure," *The Colorado Sun,* Nov. 5, 2021, https://coloradosun.com/2021/11/05/coronavirus-case-surge-hospitalizations-why.
408 Ibid.
409 Stephen Murphy, "COVID-19: Ireland's Co Waterford Has One of the Highest Vaccinaation Rate in the World—So Why Are Cases Surging?" *Sky News,* Nov. 6, 2021, https://news.sky.com/story/covid-19-irelands-co-waterford-has-one-of-the-highest-vaccination-rates-in-the-world-so-why-are-cases-surging-12461642.

410 Mollie Cooke, "Gibraltar Cancels Christmas Celebrations Amid Covid Spike," *UK Express,* Nov. 17, 2021, https://www.express.co.uk/news/uk/1521786/Gibraltar-news-covid-cases-rise-Christmas-lockdown.

411 Joshua Cohen, "Austria Locks Down Most of the Unvaccinated, Unleashing Heated Discussions across Europe about How to Tackle the Latest Covid-19 Surge," *Forbes,* Nov. 15, 2021, https://www.forbes.com/ sites/joshuacohen/2021/11/15/austria-locks-down-most-of-the-unvaccinated-unleashing-heated-discussions-across-europe-about-how-to-tackle-the-latest-covid-19-surge/?sh=1e6316124315.

412 Like most all such claims, this one is open to distortion on account of any number of factors. As I have noted previously, classification of unvaccinated and vaccinated persons may be conducted in a manner that artificially inflates counts of the former while deflating counts of the latter.

413 Murphy, "COVID-19: Ireland's Co Waterford."

414 As reported by Jeffrey Jaxen on *TheHighwire,* #242, "The Vanden Bossche Interview," Nov. 18, 2021, https://thehighwire.com/watch.

415 Alexander Zhang, "Brits Will Need 3 Jabs to Be Considered 'Fully Vaccinated,'" *The Epoch Times,* Nov. 15, 2021, https://www.theepochtimes.com/brits-will-need-3-jabs-to-be-considered-fully-vaccinated-uk-prime-minister-johnson_4105147.html.

416 "An Interview with Dr. Anthony Fauci," *The Daily,* a *New York Times* podcast, Nov. 12, 2021, https://www.nytimes.com/2021/11/12/podcasts/the-daily/anthony-fauci-vaccine-mandates-booster-shots.html.

417 Jacqueline Howard, "Some 'Frustrated' States Don't Wait for FDA, Expand Covid-19 Vaccine Booster Eligibility to All Adults," *CNN Health,* Nov. 17, 2021, https://www.cnn.com/2021/11/16/health/states-allow-booster-shots-for-all-adults-wellness/index.html.

418 Apoorva Mandavilli, "New Study of Covid Booster Shots Fans Debate over Benefits," *The New York Times,* Sept. 15, 2021, https://www.nytimes.com/2021/09/15/health/covid-booster-shot-data.html.

419 Robert F. Kennedy Jr., *The Real Anthony Fauci: Bill Gates, Big Pharma, and the Global War on Democracy and Public Health* (New York: Skyhorse, 2021), xiii, xxiii.

420 Ibid., p. 4.

421 Ibid., pp. 6–7.

422 Ibid., pp. 7, 8.

423 Ibid., p. 9.

424 Ibid.

425 Ibid., p. 11.

426 Ibid., p. 13.

427 Ibid., pp. 70–71.

428 Ibid., p. 72.

429 Ibid.

430 Ibid., p. 75.

431 Ibid., pp. 75–76

432 Ibid., p. 76.

433 Ibid., p. 82.

434 Ibid., p. 87.

435 Ibid., p. 75.

436 Ibid., p. xv.

437 Mercola and Cummins, *The Truth about COVID-19* (White River Junction, VT: Chelsea Green, 2021), xiii.

438 Ibid., xvii, xviii.

439 Josh Holder, "Tracking Coronavirus Vaccination Around the World," *The New York Times,* updated Dec. 4, 2021, https://www.nytimes.com/interactive/2021/world/covid-vaccinations-tracker.html.

440 Kennedy, *The Real Doctor Fauci,* p. 1.

441 Ibid.

442 Ibid., p. 18.

443 Ibid., p. 3.

444 Alex Gutentag, "The War on Reality," https://www.tabletmag.com/sections/news/articles/the-war-on-reality-gutentag.

445 Kennedy, *Fauci*, pp. 2–3.

446 Ibid., p. 7.

447 Charles Eisenstein, "The Human Family," Dec. 4, 2021, https://charleseisenstein.substack.com.

448 Today, a little over a month later (Aug. 29), this statement requires qualification. A purported uptick in the count of Covid cases (Covid-related deaths, however, have not risen) and associated media hoopla has once more stirred the Covid pot, and controversy revolving around mask mandates and other potential restrictions has been heating up once again.

449 This means that not only can I not cover all developments related to the six above-listed categories, but also there are important topics treated in my Covid Chronicle that do not fit readily in any of those and thus will not be addressed in this postscript: for instance, the present plight of workers in many fields who lost jobs on account of Covid mandates and ongoing work shortages created or exacerbated by those mandates.

450 The one possible caveat on this score of which I myself am aware involves Geert Vanden Bossche's speculation that Covid vaccination might drive the evolution of variants that were not only more transmissible but more virulent. While it appears that this frightening scenario has not so far materialized, on the August 17 airing of *The Highwire,* Vanden Bossche argued that deep concern remains on this score, not because a variant threatening to all may emerge but because vaccinees with diminished immune resistance may be rendered peculiarly vulnerable to one or more new variants, which then may indeed constitute a serious and even lethal threat to that class of persons. "Inescapable," *The HIghwire*, Episode #333, Aug. 17, 2023, https://thehighwire.com/ark-videos/inescapable/

451 Max Maza and Nicholas Yong, "FBI Chief Christopher Wray Says China Lab Leak Most Likely," *Fox News*, March 1, 2023, https://www.bbc.com/news/world-us-canada-64806903.

452 "COVID Origins Hearing Wrap Up: Facts, Science, Evidence Point to Wuhan Lab Leak," House Committee on Oversight and Accountability Press Release, March 8, 2023, https://oversight.house.gov/release/covid-origins-hearing-wrap-up-facts-science-evidence-point-to-a-wuhan-lab-leak

453 Ibid.

454 Ibid.

455 U.S. Senate Committee on Health, Education, Labor, and Pensions hearing, July 20, 2021. Relevant clip from *The Highwire,* episode 329, "Cause and Effect," July 20, 2023, https://thehighwire.com/watch.

456 Ibid., screen-shot of relevant email at time marker 33:09

457 The full text of the letter is included in Brianna Herlihy, "Fauci Referred to Justice Department for Criminal Investigation for Allegedly Lying under Oath to Congress," *Fox News,* Aug. 9, 2023, https://www.foxnews.com/politics/fauci-referred-justice-department-criminal-investigation-allegedly-lying-under-oath-congress.

458 Ibid.

459 Ibid., Earhardt–Markson interview, video clip.

460 Robert F. Kennedy Jr., *The Wuhan Cover-Up and the Terrifying Bioweapons Arms Race* (New York: Skyhorse, 2023).

461 Riley Griffin, "US Stops Funding to Chinese Lab at Center of Covid Controversy," *Bloomberg News,* July 18, 2023, https://www.bloomberg.com/news/articles/2023-07-18/us-suspends-wuhan-institute-funds-over-covid-stonewalling#xj4y7vzkg.

462 Ibid.

463 Monica Dutcher, "Families of COVID Victims Sue Eco-Health Alliance Alleging Gain-of-Function Research Caused 'Undue Risk' and 'Harm,'" *The Defender,* Aug. 14, 2023, https://childrenshealthdefense.org/defender/covid-gain-of-function-ecohealth-lawsuit.

464 Front Line Covid Critical Care Alliance website, Aug. 4, 2023 update, https://covid19criticalcare.com/two-leading-covid-19-doctors-are-facing-accusations-of-spreading-misinformation-by-american-board-of-internal-medicine-abim-committee.

465 Robert Apter, et al., Plaintiffs v. U.S. Department of Health and Human Services, et al., Defendants, United States District Court for the Southern District of Texas, Galveston Division, No. 3:22-ev-184, Dec. 6, 2022, Memorandum Opinion and Order, https://assets.childrenshealthdefense.org/fpx75ohbqjq3/4r84UdVWT77QyGfyGmqxjA/20f9a011f9fb818b508d595f41e82f83/2022.12.06_Order_Dismiss_Apter_Bowden_Marik_v._HHS_Becerra_Califf.pdf.

466 Ibid.

467 Proceedings, United States Appellate Court for the Fifth Circuit, Priscilla Richman presiding judge, Aug. 8, 2023, https://twitter.com/TheChiefNerd/status/1688965831294652437.

468 U.S. FDA tweet, Aug. 21, 2021, https://twitter.com/US_FDA/status/1429050070243192839.

469 Appellate Court for the Fifth Circuit, Aug. 8, 2023, proceedings.

470 The statements additionally virtually concedes that the FDA did not have a sound scientific basis for its uncompromising and singularly aggressive stance on ivermectin.

471 FLCCC data aside, commentator Roman Balmakov details how the weight of the evidence drawn from the studies cited *on the FDA's own informational website*—the very one featuring the famous "You are not a horse" caption—supports the efficacy of ivermectin for the prevention and/or treatment of Covid-19. Of 32 completed studies listed on the website, 16 showed significant benefit; 6 showed mixed results; and 10 showed no benefit. This, remember, for a drug that, when used in approved dosage, has a stellar safety record, with its risk of harm less than that posed by aspirin or tylenol. Roman Balmokov, "Exposing the FDA's Orwellian Lie About Ivermectin," *Facts Matter, Epoch Times TV*, June 8, 2023, https://www.ganjingworld.com/video/1ftl6vgsasltcQmJCQWRjIyn71u61c.

472 Ibid.

473 Jonas Herby, Lars Jonung, and Steve H. Hanke, "A Literature Review and Meta-analysis of the Effects of Lockdowns on COVID-19 Mortality," (Johns Hopkins) Studies in Applied Economics (SAE) no. 200, Jan. 2022, https://sites.krieger.jhu.edu/iae/files/2022/01/a-literature-review-and-meta-analysis-of-the-effects-of-lockdowns-on-covid-19-mortality.pdf. A recent study (Aug. 2023), one that focuses special attention on the multiple ways in which the imposition of lockdowns violated basic premises of established medical and public health ethics, confirms the Hopkins study conclusion. "In the face of another pandemic, there must be a much higher bar to implement an extended lockdown, with high-quality evidence that the benefit would substantially exceed the harm. Such evidence does not presently exist." Daniel Miller and Alvin Moss, "Rethinking the Ethics of Covid-19 Pandemic Lockdowns," *Hastings Center Report,* 53, no. 4 (2023): 3–9. DOI: 10.1002/hast.1495.

474 Tom Jefferson, et al., "Physical interventions to interrupt or reduce the spread of respiratory viruses," Cochrane Library Reviews, Jan. 30, 2023, https://www.cochranelibrary.com/cdsr/doi/10.1002/14651858.CD006207.pub6/full.

475 Vinay Prasad interview with Tom Jefferson and Carl Heneghan, "Will EBM survive?" Youtube, https://www.youtube.com/watch?v=P_JTBftjQuA.

476 Perhaps the most consequential counter-statement was presented by *New York Times* columnist Zeynep Tufekci, "Here's Why the Science Is Clear that Masks Work," *New York Times,* March 10, 2023, https://www.nytimes.com/2023/03/10/opinion/masks-work-cochrane-study.html.

477 https://www.cochrane.org/news/statement-physical-interventions-interrupt-or-reduce-spread-respiratory-viruses-review

478 See the Prasad interview with Jefferson as cited above.

479 Cited in Joseph Mercola, "Mask Study Imploding Cochrane Collaboration in Latest Debacle," *Epoch Times,* April 5, 2023, https://www.theepochtimes.com/audio/health/mask-study-imploding-cochrane-collaboration-in-latest-debacle_5172668.html.

480 Tracy Beth Hoeg, Alyson Haslam, and Vinay Prasad, "An Analysis of Studies Pertaining to Masks in Morbidity and Mortality Weekly Report: Characteristics and Quality of All Studies from 1978 to 2023," *MedRxiv*, July 11, 2023, https://www.medrxiv.org/content/10.1101/2023.07.07.23292338v1.full.

481 Ibid.

482 Ibid.

483 Ibid.

484 It is not only the authors of the July 23 paper (Hoeg, Haslam, and Prasad) who express deep concern about the CDC's misinterpretation and misrepresentation of mask science. Very recently, a FOI (Freedom of Information) request turned up a letter to federal health officials written and signed by scientists from several top research institutions. As reported in the August 21 edition of the Epoch Times (Megan Redshaw, "Secret Letter to CDC: Top Epidemiologist Suggests Agency Misrepresented Scientific Data to Support Mask Narrative," *Epoch Times*, Aug. 21, 2023), "In a recently obtained letter sent in November 2021 to the... CDC, top epidemiologist Michael Osterholm, director of the Center for Infectious Disease Research and Policy at the University of Minnesota, and seven colleagues informed the agency it was promoting flawed data and excluding data that did not reinforce their narrative." The emphatic letter itself declares: "We strongly urge IDSA [Infectious Disease Society of America] to remove the suggestion that masking prevents serious disease from its webpage on Masks and Face Coverings for the Public. In addition, the podcast by Dr. Monica Ghandi where such irresponsible claims are made should be removed from the website. We also recommend that IDSA reconsider its statements about the efficacy of masks and face coverings for preventing transmission of SARS-CoV-2. We do not agree that the evidence for their efficacy has strengthened throughout the pandemic, as the website suggests," https://img.theepochtimes.com/assets/uploads/2023/08/21/id5477758-Letter-on-deadly-risks-on-CDC-IDSA-website.

485 Stephen Petty, "Effectiveness of Masks," Testimony before the New Hampshire Senate Health and Human Services, March 30, 2022, https://www.youtube.com/watch?v=J3dnkbKoj4A.

486 For instance, Bundgaard (lead author), "Effectiveness of Adding a Mask Recommendation to Other Public Health Measures to Prevent SARS-CoV-2 Infection in Danish Mask Wearers," *Annals of Internal Medicine,* 174 (3): 335–343, March 2021, https://pubmed.ncbi.nlm.nih.gov/33205991.

487 Petty, "Effectiveness of Masks."

488 Ibid.

489 It only stands to reason that restricting breathing, often for extended periods, would have negative consequences. One particularly disturbing study on the topic appeared in March, 2023 (Kai Kisielinski, et al., "Possible Toxicity of Chronic Carbon Dioxide Exposure Associated with Face Mask Use, Particularly in Pregnant Women, Children, and Adolescents—A Scoping Review," *Heliyon*, March 2, 2023 (https://pubmed.ncbi.nlm.nih.gov/37057051/). The paper notes that mask wearing, even for short periods, can dramatically increase carbon dioxide intake; indeed, a mask wearer may inhale as much as 80 times the concentration of carbon dioxide as someone breathing fresh air. Animal research reveals even much lower levels as positively toxic. The paper's discussion section states:

"Circumstantial evidence exists that extended mask use may be related to current observations of stillbirths and to reduced verbal motor and overall cognitive performance in children born during the pandemic. A need exists to reconsider mask mandates."

490 Petty, "Effectiveness of Masks"

491 Petty shared that, in addition to the many podcasts he has made available, he has sent a 27-page letter to the CDC detailing his views.

492 Dr. Yaakov Ophir, "The COVID Vaccine Efficacy Narrative Is Falling Apart," *The Defender,* April 11, 2023, https://childrenshealthdefense.org/defender/covid-vaccine-efficacy-narrative.

493 Yaakov Ophir, et al., "The efficacy of COVID-19 Vaccine Boosters against Serious Illness and Deaths: Scientific Fact or Wishful Myth?, *Journal of the American Physicians and Surgeons,* vol. 28, no. 1, spring 2023, https://jpands.org/vol28no1/ophir.pdf.

494 Recently, leprosy (now often called Hansen's disease to soften the stigma of the older term) has been added to the list of serious illnesses potentially associated with or triggered by Covid-19 vaccination. See, for instance, Barbara de Barros, et al., "Covid-19 Vaccination and Leprosy—a UK Hospital-based Retrospective Cohort Study," *PLOS Neglected Tropical Diseases*, 17 (8): e0011493, Aug. 4, 2023, https://doi.org/10.1371/journal.pntd.0011493.

495 Gretchen Vogel and Jennifer Conzin-Frankel, "Rare Link between Coronavirus Vaccines and Long Covid-like Illness Starts to Gain Acceptance," *Science*, 381 (6653), July 7, 2023, https://www.science.org/toc/science/381/6653.

496 ICAN attorney Aaron Siri discusses the V-safe data in numerous interviews. One that took place immediately after release of the data is "Why Did this Take Numerous Legal Demands before the CDC Handed over the Data?" *Fox News @ Night,* Oct. 4, 2022, https://www.foxnews.com/video/6313218294112. For more extended treatment, see "Justice For All," Del Bigtree, *The Highwire,* Episode #288, Oct. 6, 2022. https://thehighwire.com/ark-videos/justice-for-all/. The most convenient place to access relevant V-safe data is the interactive dashboard provided by ICAN at ICANdecide.org/V-safe.

497 The V-safe program provided three boxes one could check in the case of an adverse event, one for medical help, one for missing school or work, and the third for the inability to perform daily functions.

498 Siri, "Why Did this Take Numerous Legal Demands before the CDC Handed over the Data?"

499 ICANdecide.org/V-safe.

500 "Justice For All," Del Bigtree, *The Highwire,* Episode #288, Oct. 6, 2022, https://thehighwire.com/ark-videos/justice-for-all/. For the Aaron Siri clip, see also https://thehighwire.com/ark-videos/exclusive-aaron-siri-breaks-down-cdcs-v-safe-data.

501 Prof. Dr. Konstantin Beck, "Women and Children First!—Baby Gap and Young People's Excess Mortality in Switzerland," University of Lucerne, Doctors For Covid Ethics Town Hall Meeting, June 22/July 11, 2023, https://rumble.com/v32h4l6-women-and-children-first-baby-gap-and-young-peoples-excess-mortality-in-swi.html.

502 Ibid.

503 The alpha and delta strains, which preceded the more transmissible but less dangerous omicron strain, which gained prominence around Nov. 2022.

504 Beck, "Women and Children First!"

505 Edward Dowd, *"Cause Unknown": The Epidemic of Sudden Deaths in 2021 and 2022* (New York: Skyhorse, 2022).

506 "Excess mortality" is mortality in excess of expected all-cause mortality. All-cause mortality, as Dowd explains, is a readily available and non-controversial statistic, one that actuarial insurers habitually

work with and break down in various ways. In the context of Covid, it is revealing because it is generally quite constant, though naturally rising proportionately with population increase. For instance, in 1955 as well as 1956, roughly 1.5 million Americans died; in 2017 through 2019, roughly 2.8 million each year. 2020 saw a small but unspectacular spike. It was in 2021 that, according to Dowd, "the stats people expected went off the rails." As reported by the CEO of OneAmerica, deaths in people of working age (18–64) went up by an unheard-of 40%. A 10% increase would constitute a 1-in-200 year event, and the majority of deaths were not attributable to Covid. Dowd, "*Cause Unknown,*" p. 2.

507 Ibid., p. 1

508 Owing, in part, to the low susceptibility of this age group to death from Covid-19, data does not support the idea that it was Covid itself that caused the dramatic rise in excess mortality in young adults in the U.S., or (in Beck's analysis) Germany or Switzerland.

509 Alexandra Bruce, "Video: Shocking Findings in the CDC Data on Excess Mortality: Edward Dowd, *Global Research/Forbidden Knowledge TV,* March 10, 2022, https://www.globalresearch.ca/edward-dowd-future-recession-shocking-findings-cdc-covid-data-democide/5773944.

510 Phinancetechnologies.com/humanities project.

511 Megan Redshaw, "mRNA Covid Vaccines May be Triggering 'Turbo Cancers' in Young People: Experts," *Epoch Times,* July 28, 2023, https://www.theepochtimes.com/health/mrna-covid-vaccines-may-be-triggering-aggressive-turbo-cancers-in-young-people-experts.

512 Ibid.

513 Ibid.

514 Michael Palmer, et al., *mRNA Vaccine Toxicity,* D4CE.org, https://doctors4covidethics.org/mrna-vaccine-toxicity.

515 https://doctors4covidethics.org/mrna-vaccine-toxicity.

516 This, of course, is likely the result of myocarditis. The high exertion associated with athletic activity puts significantly additional demands on heart function, and if any (even subclinical) vaccine-induced heart-tissue damage has occurred, cardiac arrest may result.

517 Nicolas Hulscher, et al., "A Systematic Review of Autopsy Findings in Deaths after COVID-19 Vaccination," *Lancet,* July 5, 2023, removed July 6, 2023, reposted in Will Jones, "Lancet Study on Covid Vaccine Autopsies Finds 74% Were Caused by Vaccine—Study Is Removed within 24 Hours," *The Daily Sceptic,* July 6, 2023, https://dailysceptic.org/2023/07/06/lancet-study-on-covid-vaccine-autopsies-finds-74-were-caused-by-vaccine-journal-removes-study-within-24-hours.

518 Ibid.

519 Obviously, if the vaccine were at all efficacious in preventing death, one should expect a negative, not positive, correlation between vaccination and all-cause mortality. To put the matter bluntly, the actual result means that the more people vaccinate, the more people die.

520 Ibid. The multiple citations provided in the original paper can be traced by finding the paper on the Daily Sceptic; see citation above.

521 Ibid.

522 Thomas Paine, *Common Sense and Selected Works of Thomas Paine* (San Diego: Word Cloud Classics, 2014), 335. The citation is from *The Age of Reason,* which dates from 1793, shortly before Paine's imprisonment in France.

523 Lucia Sinatra, "Rutgers Set to Kick Out Students Today Unless They Comply With Covid Vaccine Mandate," *The Defender,* August 15, 2023, https://childrenshealthdefense.org/defender/rutgers-disenroll-students-covid-vaccine-mandate.

524 Ibid.

525 Ibid.

526 Brenda Baletti, "Judge to Rule on NY Vaccine Mandate Case—1 Day Before Schools Starts," *The Defender,* August 14, 2023, https://childrenshealthdefense.org/defender/judge-rule-new-york-teacher-covid-vaccine-mandate-case.

527 Ashton Pittman, "Mississippi Must Grant Religious Exemptions For Childhood Vaccines, Federal Judge Rules," April 20, 2023, https://www.mississippifreepress.org/32683/mississippi-must-grant-religious-exemptions-for-childhood-vaccines-federal-judge-rules

528 Mississippi State Department of Health News Release, July 14, 2023, https://msdh.ms.gov/page/23,25673,341.html.

529 Ibid.

530 Much of the legal jockeying in the case revolves around the point that the state retains secular or medical exemptions, so that the complete exclusion of any category of religious exemptions therefore constitutes unlawful discrimination against religious interests. If no exemptions of any sort were granted—a radical step I am not sure any state is willing formally to take, and one subject to its own legal scrutiny—a different argument would be required.

531 Judge Joseph F. Bianco, 2nd Circuit Concurrence and Dissent, Case 22–249, document 109, Aug. 04, 2023, 3551654, https://drive.google.com/file/d/1wwvXmNyYyuDOvh6PSEXZlz9X8uc4ian_/view.

532 Ibid.

533 "Second Circuit Upholds Dismissal of Challenge to Connecticut's Religious Exemption Repeal; We the Patriots USA Vows to Appeal to the U.S. Supreme Court," *We the Patriots USA Legal Newswire*, Aug. 4, 2023, https://www.law.com/legalnewswire/news/?id=3058068.

534 In this connection, the most relevant portion of the March 3, 2023, memo from chair of the Department of Medical Education and Clinical Sciences and the interim dean of Elson S. Floyd College of Medicine reads: "There were components with the roundtable that were inconsistent with the expectations of the evidence based medical education expected in developing a future generation of physicians. *The expressed views will require us to review your teaching assignments in the frame of the education of our students* (emphasis mine, DJP). As cited in Informed Choice Washington, "WSU Ends Six Year Employment of Dr. Reni Moon, a Board-certified Pediatrician, for Providing Testimony at a U.S. Senate Fact-finding Roundtable," July 25, 2023, https://informedchoicewa.org/news/pediatricians-contract-terminated-by-wsu-after-reporting-to-senate-roundtable-on-covid-shot-harms.

535 According to ICWA article cited above, "The termination letter says nothing about Dr. Moon's past involvement with WSU's medical school. She has worked or volunteered for the WSU Floyd College of Medicine since 2015, starting with contributions to the accreditation effort before the school even launched. For three years, she volunteered on both the Admissions Committee and the Diversity Equity Committee. She was the founding faculty sponsor for the school's Pediatric Interest Group while she taught at the school as an Associate Clinical Professor. Dr. Moon appeared to be a significant contributor to the founding of the school itself, making her termination far from routine (emphasis ICWA).

536 ICWA article, cited above.

537 Michael Shellenberger, "The Censorship Industrial Complex," testimony before the House Select Committee Hearing on the Weaponization of the Federal Government, March 9, 2023, https://judiciary.house.gov/sites/evo-subsites/republicans-judiciary.house.gov/files/evo-media-document/shellenberger-testimony.pdf.

538 Matt Taibbi, Written Statement, House Select Committee Hearing on the Weaponization of the Federal Government on the Twitter Files, March 9, 2023, https://judiciary.house.gov/sites/evo-subsites/republicans-judiciary.house.gov/files/evo-media-document/taibbi-testimony.pdf.

539 AG Schmitt, "Missouri and Louisiana File Suit Against President Biden, Top Administration Officials for Allegedly Colluding With Social Media Giants to Censor and Suppress Free Speech," *AG Schmitt Webpage*, May 5, 2022, https://archive.ph/fXN4V.

540 Judge Terry A. Doughty, "Memorandum Ruling on Request For Preliminary Injunction," State of Missouri et al vs. Joseph R. Biden et al, Case No 3:22 – CV - 01213, July 4, 2023, https://ago.mo.gov/docs/default-source/press-releases/missouri-v-biden-ruling.pdf.

541 Ibid.

542 Ibid.

543 Alex Gutentag, Leighton Woodhouse, and Michael Shellenberger, "Free Speech to the Supreme Court and Beyond," *Public,* Aug. 11, 2023, https://public.substack.com/p/free-speech-to-the-supreme-court.

544 Ironically enough, the Democratic Party evidently does not in the least see matters in this light. On July 20, 2023, and so in the wake of Judge Doughty's decision, the House Select Subcommittee convened another session of its hearings on the weaponization of the federal government. The hearing proved a shameful display of partisan vitriol on the part of the Democratic members of the committee, who appeared intent, not upon looking the specter of state-sponsored censorship in the face or addressing the constitutional concerns registered in Judge Doughty's decision but in crucifying Robert F. Kennedy Jr., who had been called as one of the three majority witnesses. Many noted the irony that, in a hearing on censorship, the Democrats' chief aim appeared to be to silence/censor one of the witnesses. It is also the case that the attorneys general of 21 states have filed amicus briefs in support of the government's position. (see https://oag.ca.gov/news/press-releases/attorney-general-bonta-joins-multistate-amicus-brief-supporting-federal). All but a handful of these are blue; the rest are purple. While it may be true that the scope of Judge Doughty's injunction raises legitimate questions, Democrats as a class appear singularly and frighteningly oblivious to the grave civil liberty issues raised by the case, as if the mere fact that a Democratic administration was charged automatically means that government authority is legitimate authority, and all criticism thereof mere partisan fury on the other side. In other instances, of course, Republicans are guilty of the same kind of uncritical hyper-partisanship, which clearly cripples responsible governance.

545 Aaron Kheriaty, *The New Abnormal: The Rise of the Biomedical Security State* (Washington, DC: Regnery, 2022).

546 Suzanne Burdick, "'So Many Pitfalls: Feds Push School-based Health Centers as Critics Sound Alarm Over Lack of Parental Consent," *The Defender,* Aug. 9, 2023, https://childrenshealthdefense.org/defender/school-based-health-centers-vaccines-mental-health-counseling.

547 https://www.gcvcadvocates.org.

548 Cited in Burdick, "So Many Pitfalls."

549 https://childrenshealthdefense.org/wp-content/uploads/georgia-highlands-school-center-consent-form.pdf.

550 Cited in Burdick, "So Many Pitfalls."

551 Ibid.

552 Ibid.

553 Ibid.

554 World Health Organization.

555 James Roguski, "100 Reasons," Substack, Jan. 5, 2023, https://jamesroguski.substack.com/p/100-reasons. In addtion to supplying relevant information, Roguski's

substack includes links to the whole relevant set of WHO documents, the historic International Health Regulations as well as the proposed amendments, and multiple drafts of the so-called Pandemic Treaty.

556 Ibid.

557 Ibid.

558 Aaron Kheriaty, *The New Abnormal: The Rise of the Biomedical Security State* (Washington, DC: Regnery, 2022).

559 Medical Countermeasures.

560 Roguski, "100 Reasons" and associated links to original WHO documents.

561 One of the reasons for the delay was that I had written well into volume 2 before I realized that I was working on a multivolume project. Also, an agreement that fell through postponed publication.

562 "2024 Presidential Race Stays Static in the Face of Major Events, Quinnipac University Poll Finds; RFK Jr. Receives 22% as Independent Candidate in Three-way Race," *Quinnipac University Poll*, Nov. 1, 2023, https://poll.qu.edu/poll-release?releaseid=3881.

563 In the latter part of this postscript, I offer evidence that the reasons for resistance to the Covid vaccine apply, as well, to the more traditional vaccines to a far greater extent than is commonly supposed.

564 A few points of difference require recognition here. I acknowledge that the kind and degree of violence historically inflicted upon African Americans may well be considered to comprise a class of its own. I do not know of unvaccinated persons enslaved or lynched on account of their convictions (though abusive quarantines did transpire during Covid). As well, the calculus of kind and degree of violence changes when one is speaking about an unalterable aspect of one's identity—such as skin color—and a belief or position that can potentially be changed. Prejudice based on the latter, however, is not necessarily any less egregious or deadly, as the extraordinary violence historically associated with religious intolerance shows. And the psychological, social, and material violence inflicted by vaccine mandates (in many Covid-era cases resulting in loss of livelihood, and, in the case of school mandates, constituting a life-altering form of social exclusion) and even milder forms of medical and social coercion can be immensely consequential.

565 See prior note.

566 One could think of other types of prejudice in which context the intellectual component may likewise be accorded priority but possess a very different character. We are not, for instance, dealing here with theological disputation and the religious intolerance too often a deadly consequence thereof.

567 Eric Strong, "Is Anti-vaxxer an Offensive *Slur?*" *Strong Medicine YouTube video*, Jan. 16, 2022, https://www.youtube.com/watch?v=swG-3zm5wlE.

568 Contrary to the drift of my discussion, Strong himself argues that the "anti-vax" label should not be regarded as a slur because he, at least, employs it as a descriptive rather than pejorative label. Yet while Strong himself may not exhibit the emotional vitriol often directed at anti-vaxxers, his own presentation illustrates multiple ways in which he regards anti-vaxxers as displaying certain intrinsically negative characteristics, including irrational mental inflexibility.

569 Strong, "Anti-vaxxer."

570 Although most persons were vaccinated no earlier than spring of 2021, Strong evidently takes the first clinical trials run in July 2020 as the starting point of the "eighteen month" span he cites.

571 All (italicized) quotations are from Strong, "Anti-vaxxer."

572 One might well here think of the geocentricity of the universe before Copernicus, but the history of science is naturally chock-full of

cases in which an established truth is questioned and ultimately partially or wholly repudiated. Indeed, one could well argue that such instances point to the very essence of science itself as—not a set of dogmas—but a creative enterprise. Several of the scientists featured in the pages of this book (beginning with Dr. Welsh) have insisted that without acknowledgment of error and openness to change, there is no true science at all.

573 It is so especially if one means to imply that such was the case before the roll-out of the vaccines. It's conceivable that by January 2022, the Covid vaccines had indeed received a fair bit of scientific attention. Even then, however, it seems to me wildly implausible that they would fit Strong's description, especially since the history of science includes studies that last for many, many years. Even if the quantity of science devoted to the Covid vaccines by 2022 had been considerable (although still, I suspect, hardly comparable to many other interventions), the lack of longevity would disqualify such science from representing satisfactory review of the phenomenon in question.

574 Kristian G. Andersen, et al., "The Proximal Origin of SARS-CoV-2," *Nature Medicine,* 26: 450–452, 2020. https://doi.org/10.1038/s41591-020-0820-9. As discussed in the text, as well as postscript 1, definitive evidence has emerged that this paper was deliberately manipulated so as to misrepresent known scientific facts so as to serve a specific political end: namely, discrediting the lab leak hypthosesis that would incriminate Fauci and others as agents of the illegal gain-of-function research that precipitated the pandemic.

575 After Kennedy appeared on the *Joe Rogan Experience* in mid-June 2023, Hotez posted a (June 17) tweet criticizing spotify for hosting Rogan and providing him with a platform for anti-vaccine advocates such as Kennedy to disseminate "nonsense." Rogan immediately replied, "Peter, if you claim what RFK Jr. is saying is 'misinformation,' I am offering you $100,000 to the charity of your choice if you're willing to debate him on my show with no time limit." https://twitter.com/joerogan/status/1670196590928068609. Others subsequently added a great deal more money to sweeten the pot. Kennedy accepted the offer to debate; Hotez did not.

576 Zeeshan Aleem, "Peter Hotez's Disinterest in Debating RFK Jr. on Vaccines Makes Perfect Sense," MSNBC, June 20, 202, https://www.msnbc.com/opinion/msnbc-opinion/joe-rogan-rfk-jr-vaccine-debate-podcast-hotez-rcna90201.

577 Strong, "Anti-vaxxer."

578 Andrea Wulf, *Magnificent Rebels* (New York: Random House, 2022). In books such as this one as well as her bestseller *The Invention of Nature,* Wulf brings popular attention to previously little known figures of great importance to our intellectual and cultural history. If she happens to read this book, I hope she receives my criticism in the spirit of truth-seeking that she so admirably celebrates in hers.

579 Ibid., 3. One could argue that Wulf here does not really exhibit pro-vax prejudice per se, but rather criticizes those who resisted all or most public health edicts, especially lockdowns. It is indubitably true, however, that those who did not wish to vaccinate were roundly and aggressively condemned on the basis of just this logic, which rests upon two foundational assumptions: 1) the edicts of public health officials are lawful and not violative of essential rights or liberties—or, even if they may be construed as so violative, are nonetheless justified by exceptional emergency circumstances; 2) the policies enacted by public health officials enhance rather than endanger the health and welfare of the community as a whole. A third assumption follows

logically from these two, namely that (3) a largely unquestioning obedience to the "expert" authority of health officials qualifies as the only socially responsible and morally defensible stance. These are the key assumptions underlying the narrower phenomenon of pro-vax prejudice per se. As an alternative to Dr. Strong's definition, one might propose that an anti-vaxxer is one who contests one if not both of the two primary assumptions and so—naturally—the third as well.

580 I know nothing of Andrea Wulf's own political leanings, and (if her biography is a trustworthy index) she is a European rather than American citizen. Even so, the attitude she expresses in her prologue is typical of left-of-center Americans who identify as liberal or progressive. There are, of course, numerous exceptions, including particularly notable ones like RFK Jr. himself. In fact, many citizens chastened and educated by the debacle of Covid World find themselves (and here I believe I borrow a term from Del Bigtree) politically "marooned"—i.e., deeply alienated from both major parties, each of which appears to be undergoing transformations that render them all but unrecognizable to prior adherents. The Democratic Party's unblinking allegiance to the authoritarian overreach on the part of the government stands out as one manifestation of this trend on the leftward side of the political spectrum. RFK Jr.'s decision to run, not as a Democrat, but as an Independent, may well be considered emblematic of the present lamentable situation. Unprecedented partisanship and polarization render the government largely incapable of the constructive civil debate essential to good governance, casting a bright spotlight upon the worst deficiencies of the reigning two-party system—a system in which allegiance to a particular party too often trumps allegiance to truth.

581 Wulf, *Rebels,* p. 10.

582 F. W. J. Schelling, *Philosophical Investigations Into the Essence of Human Freedom*, translated by Jeff Love and Johannes Schmidt (Albany: SUNY, 2007). Schelling published the German original in 1809, after the heyday of the Jena years, which nonetheless were seminal for his whole philosophical career.

583 Ralph Waldo Emerson.

584 After introducing all the characters ("dramatis personae") whose stories she tells in her book, Wulf writes: "Each of these great intellects lived a life worth telling. More extraordinary than their individual stories, however, is the fact that they all came together at the same time in the same place. That's why I've called them the 'Jena Set.'" *Magnificent Rebels* (New York: Vintage, 2022), p. 10.

585 David French, "The New Republican Party Isn't Ready for the Post-Roe World," *New York Times*, Nov. 12, 2023, https://www.nytimes.com/2023/11/12/opinion/ohio-abortion-republicans.html.

586 Ibid.

587 Ibid.

588 Ibid.

589 Ibid.

590 Ibid.

591 Ibid.

592 Ibid.

593 Of course, it is not quite so simple at that. As explored in detail in volume 2, the liberal ethos includes the interplay of a number of distinct elements, including a strong emphasis on individuality. It is also part of my argument that individuality and community are, if rightly construed, complementary rather than contradictory characteristics. That perspectives allows the statement made in this text to stand.

594 Volume 2 centers on the constructive as well as destructive legacy of Enlightenment thought. As highlighted in that book, Kant's phrase (borrowed from Horace) "*sapere aude*" is often regarded as the motto of the Enlightenment.

Roughly translated as "have the courage to trust your own intellect," the phrase captures the gist of one of the most constructive and indeed truly liberating initiatives of Enlightenment thought, one that paved the way for those magnificent Romantic rebels that form the subject of Wulf's book. All of the philosophy she writes about assumes Kant as a foundation, even when critical of Kantian premises.

595 Ibid.

596 Selena Simmons-Duffin and Koko Nakajimo, "This Is How Many Lives Could Have Been Saved with Covid Vaccinations in Each State," *All Things Considered,* National Public Radio Health News, May 13, 2022, 5:01 pm, https://www.npr.org/sections/health-shots/2022/05/13/1098071284/this-is-how-many-lives-could-have-been-saved-with-covid-vaccinations-in-each-state.

597 Ibid. As argued in *Two Roads,* the declaration of needless death is true, but it is so because of the government's repressive lockdowns, sabotage of early treatment options, and mass administration of an unsafe vaccine.

598 Ibid. As reported in the NPR piece, Cynthia Cox is director of the Peterson-Kaiser Health System Tracker and coauthor of an earlier study estimating the number of vaccine-preventable deaths in the U.S.

599 Brown School of Public Health, https://globalepidemics.org/vaccinations.

600 Ibid.

601 Ibid.

602 Robert M. Wachter and Ashish K. Jha, "It's Time to Considering Delaying the Second Dose of Corona Virus Vaccine," *Washington Post,* Jan. 3, 2022, https://www.washingtonpost.com/opinions/2021/01/03/its-time-consider-delaying-second-dose-coronavirus-vaccine/

603 The impression given by the announcement of the Pfizer data is that the vaccine was indeed tremendously protective. The figure cited leads one to believe that, of 100 persons who contracted Covid all of them had been vaccinated, only roughly ten would have gotten sick. It soon emerged, however, that the Pfizer figure represented relative not absolute risk, which is a very different matter, as it is only the latter that really represents the level of protection afforded by any given individual. The absolute risk figure from the trial was .084. This means, roughly, that 119 persons would have to be vaccinated in order to prevent one case of—not even serious illness—but a positive PCR Covid test. It's also the case that in the trial itself more vaccinated persons died than did unvaccinated persons in the control group, largely because the risk of cardiac arrest among the vaccinated was much higher. Aseem Malhotra is just one of many physicians/researchers who dissects the Pfizer data. His two Covid-related articles in the *Journal of Insulin Resistance* are very well worth reading, as they cover not only this topic but also some of the most basic scientific and sociopolitical questions pertaining to Covid World. It's the first that covers this particular issue. Aseem Malhotra, "Curing the Pandemic of Misinformation on Covid-19 mRNA Vaccines Through Real Evidence-based Medicine," part 1, *Journal of Insulin Resistance,* Sept. 26, 2022. https://www.ncbi.nlm.nih.gov/pmc/articles/PMC9557944.

604 Ibid.

605 PBS NewsHour, "Senators Hear Update on Early Outpatient Treatment for Covid-19," Nov. 19, 2020, https://www.youtube.com/watch?v=EJpxcbTAuk8&t=5513s.

606 Brown University School of Public Health website, https://globalepidemics.org/2022/05/13/new-analysis-shows-vaccines-could-have-prevented-318000-deaths.

607 Ming Zhong, Meghana Kshirsagar, Richard Johnston, Rahul Dodhia, Tammy Glazer, Allen Kim, Divya Michael, Sameer Nair-Desai, Thomas C. Tsai, Stefanie Friedhoff, Juan M.

Lavista Ferres, "Estimating Vaccine Preventable Covid-19 Deaths under Counterfactual Vaccination Scenarios in the U.S., medRxiv, May 21, 2022, https://org/10.1101/2022.05.19.20227531o.

608 Ibid.

609 "NIH Awards by Location and Organization," *NIH Research Portfolio Online Reporting Tool,* Dec. 22, 2022 data release, https://report.nih.gov/award/index.cfm?ot=10&fy=2022&state=US. Brown is proud of its NIH funding. The page detailing its research centers declares, "With nearly $55 million in annual external funding, the Brown School of Public Health ranks among the top ten schools of public health for NIH funding." Though I did not research the matter, this website and the one from the Yale School of Public Health (connected with the Ohio-Florida paper I discuss next) produce the distinct impression that most large schools of public health in the U.S. are largely dependent upon NIH funding. It would naturally follow that the research funded in these institutions is, to a significant degree, controlled by NIH directives. To take it a step further, the Brown site conveys the sense that the entire culture of public health education at such institutions is determined by government positions and prerogatives. Given the influence of industry on government, the notion that objective science can, as a rule, emerge from these institutions seems wildly implausible. Perusal of the site also makes clear the force of the truth that public health policy is largely directed not by doctors with extensive medical practice and know-how or independent expertise but by those indoctrinated in this culture chained to predetermined industry/government agendas.

610 Ibid.

611 To me, it looks as if the hard truth of the matter is that the institutions and organs implicated in this story—the Brown School of Public Health, NPR, the NIH itself—are not at all serving their appointed purpose in a fashion consonant with a democratic society. On the contrary, they are functioning much more like what Louis Althusser, in his classic essay "On Ideology" (in Louis Althusser, *On the Reproduction of Capitalism / Ideology and Ideological State Apparatuses,* New York: Verso, 2014) calls "ideological state apparatuses" (ISAs), the function of which is not to conduct impartial science or engage in independent journalism but to produce, support, and transmit a certain ideologically saturated story line prescribed by the powers that be. Althusser speaks of the state, but in the contemporary context the state and its agencies may well be serving the interests of that global network of power I've called the matrix. In any event, the chief point is that at present, the academic, media, and government institutions that are supposed to serve the people certainly cannot be blindly trusted and that persons who—like David French and Andrea Wulf—believe they are acting as free moral and intellectual agents while uncritically depending on these sources for information and direction with respect to, for instance, the vaccination issue, are operating under an illusion. Rather than independent citizen-agents, their very subjectivity—the basis of their moral and intellectual judgment—has been largely controlled and determined for them by the system in which they are embedded. The Althusserian term for this kind of ideologically controlled constitution of subjectivity is "interpellation," or the process by which the political or social subject is produced and controlled by—in Althusser's versions—ISAs and RSAs ("repressive state apparatuses," such as the police and other enforcement agencies). The only way out of this kind of entrapment and control is constant exercise of critical reason as a means of resistance to undue social, ideological, and material control. It

should also be mentioned—without the suspicion that this mention itself reveals one as a Marxist—that the class(ist) dimensions of the ideological warfare staged by the matrix should not be overlooked. It is, on the other hand, somewhat playfully interesting what the word *matrix* spells when the "t" and "i" are omitted.

612 Jacob Wallace, et al., "Excess Deaths for Republian and Democratic Registered Voters During the Covid-19 Pandemic," *JAMA Internal Medicine,* 183 (9): 916–923, July 24, 2023, https://doi.org/10.1001/jamainternmed.2023.1154.

613 Ibid.

614 The authors state: "One alternative explanation is that political party affiliation is a proxy for other risk factors (beyond age, for which we adjusted) for excess mortality during the Covid-19 pandemic, such as rates of underlying medical conditions, race and ethnicity, socioeconomic status, or health insurance coverage, and these risk factors may be associated with differences in excess mortality by political party, even though we only observed differences in excess mortality after vaccines were available to all adults." Ibid.

615 Binh Ngo, MD, July 25, 2023, comment attached to the Wallace et al "Excess Deaths" paper by the "Comments" link.

616 Wallace et al., "Excess Deaths," Supplemental Content link, eFigure 1.

617 One ready explanation for this fact is that the number of people actually killed by Covid-19 was exaggerated, and perhaps grossly so, because of the conflation of deaths *with* Covid with deaths *by* Covid. There is, as well, the notable contributing factor that, as a general rule, Covid-19 killed people who were sick or unhealthy already, typically suffering from several comorbidities, the class of persons who, over the course of a year, were already most vulnerable to demise. The lack of excess mortality in the youngest age group certainly makes sense, as this class of person was not highly susceptible to death by Covid.

618 Dowd, *"Cause Unknown," p.* 2.

619 It is true that Dowd reports a 40% increase in all-cause mortality among young people for the said period, whereas the Florida-Ohio study show peaks of 35%, and so—while both increases are dramatic and of roughly comparable scale—there is a not entirely insignificant discrepancy. Two plausible reasons for that discrepancy immediately come to mind. First, Florida and Ohio results may differ slightly from those reflecting a nationwide account. Secondly, and perhaps more persuasively, the Florida-Ohio study excludes all 18- to 25-year-olds. A significant increase in excess deaths among this (one would presume usually very healthy) age group could hike the figure for the whole group.

620 cf. footnote 42 above. Research for the Ohio-Florida study stems in part from the (heavily NIH-funded) Yale School of Public Health.

621 Zoey O'Toole and Mary Holland (eds.), *Turtles All the Way Down: Vaccine Science and Myth,* Washington, DC: Children's Health Defense, 2022. The book was published anonymously, for obvious reasons.

622 Ibid., p 52.

623 Ibid.

624 Each chapter in *Turtles* includes a succinct but thorough summary, making assimilation of the substance of the book that much easier.

625 Ibid., pp. 81–82.

626 Ibid., p. 82.

627 Ibid.

628 "Vaccine Experts under Oath," *The Highwire*, episode #347, Nov. 23, 2023, https://thehighwire.com/ark-videos/vaccine-experts-under-oath.

629 Wakefield published an infamous 1998 paper in *The Lancet* suggesting the possibility of a link (via mechanisms of inflammation of the digestive tract) between autism and the MMR vaccine. He did not assert that

his research proved such a link, but did suggest that his results indicated that the question should be further investigated. His integrity and credibility were challenged in the wake of that paper, and his mainstream medical career was efficiently destroyed. Wakefield to this day stands behind his work (which was retracted by the journal). Perhaps history will one day tell whether the attacks on Wakefield were justified and whether his hypothesis of a link between certain vaccines (whether the list includes the latest form of the MMR vaccine or not) and autism may be borne out after all. In any event, his treatment to date qualifies him to stand as a posterboy victim of pro-vax prejudice. The same medical establishment that discredited him has declined to perform the kind of studies that could reliably offer more definitive proof (or disproof) of his hypothesis.

630 "Vaccine Experts Under Oath," *The Highwire,* Episode #347.

631 Wakefield also pointed to a possible physiological basis for linkage. I do not know whether any further work has either substantiated or disproved the physiological link (via digestive tract inflammation) he suggested or explored other physiological mechanisms. Given what happened to Wakefield, one need not wonder why this may be terra incognita.

632 See Wikipedia entry: "Epidemiology of Autism."

633 "Autism Prevalence Higher, According to Data from 11 ADDM Communities," *CDC Newsroom*, March 23, 2023, https://www.cdc.gov/media/releases/2023/p0323-autism.html.

634 The autism epidemic (and I believe it should be viewed as such) affects boys at four times the rate it does girls. According, again, to the CDC itself, one in every 25 boys suffers from autism, and one in every 100 girls does so. "Autism Prevalence," *Autism Speaks,* https://www.autismspeaks.org/autism-statistics-asd.

635 Rita Numerof, "Our Nations Chronic Disease Epidemic Is Getting Worse. So Who's Responsible?" *Forbes,* Nov. 22, 2022, https://www.forbes.com/sites/ritanumerof/2022/11/22/our-nations-chronic-disease-epidemic-is-getting-worse-so-whos-responsible/?sh=38c784365263.

636 Ibid.

637 Peter Boersma et al., "Prevalence of Multiple Chronic Conditions among U.S. Adults, 2018," CDC Research Briefhttps://www.cdc.gov/pcd/issues/2020/20_0130.htm.

638 Whitney Blair Wyckoff, "Study: Chronic Disease Increased by 25% Over Last Decade," *Commonwealth Fund Newsletter,* July 28, 2008, https://www.commonwealthfund.org/publications/newsletter-article/study-chronic-disease-increased-25-percent-over-last-decade.

639 That expansion was triggered by the passage of the National Childhood Vaccine Injury Act of 1986. Among other things, the act provided immunity from prosecution for vaccine manufacturers, who had previously suffered tremendous losses on account of lawsuits holding them responsible for unsafe medical products. The most relevant clause of the act reads: [The act] "provides that no vaccine manufacturer shall be liable in a civil action for damages arising from a vaccine-related injury or death: (1) resulting from unavoidable side effects; or (2) solely due to the manufacturer's failure to provide direct warnings." It is this act that provides for the government compensation for injury to which Dr. Eric Strong alludes. The system, however, is deficient and (as previously noted) does nothing to inhibit pharmaceutical development and marketing of unsafe products. Rather, it is a green light for pharmaceutical company's recklessness and greed.

640 If, for instance, incidence of severe autism continues its rapid climb, there are multiple reasons why the social and economic burden

represented by this often long-lived population could eventually become, if not insupportable, close to that extreme. This does not gainsay the value or human dignity of any given autistic individual or the special gifts such persons may represent for their family and community.

641 Aria Bendix, "Autism Rates Have Tripled. Is It More Common, or Are We Just Better at Diagnosis?" *NBC Health News,* Jan. 25, 2023, https://www.nbcnews.com/health/health-news/autism-rates-rising-more-prevalent-versus-more-screening-rcna67408.

642 Ibid.

643 Robert F. Kennedy Jr. and Brian Hooker, *Vax-Unvax: Let the Science Speak* (New York: Skyhorse, 2023).

644 This represents the gists of the study results compiled in *Vax-Unvax*. One need add, too, that there are many reasons to consider the threat of deadly or debillitating epidemics of infectious disease today to be overblown, and—correlatively—the role of vaccines in curtailing such disease likewise to be greatly exaggerated with respect to both the past and the present. The subject is too complex to enter into in detail here, but one may find relevant discussion in a number of sources, including chapter 8, "The Disappearance of Disease" in *Turtles All the Way Down.* A relevant section from that book discusses how sanitation, better nutrition enabled by advances in transportation, and other engineering and lifestyle improvements played the primary role in curbing the infectious disease epidemics that followed extensive urbanization in the 19th century. The passage reads: "Improvements in living conditions led to dramatic decrease in infectious disease mortality between the mid-19th and mid-20th centuries, as well as a sharp decline in morbidity to the point that some were virtually eliminated. Effective medical drugs and vaccines, however, only became available in the 1930s and 1940s, after most of the reduction in infectious disease mortality had already been realized. Historically, vaccination contributed marginally to reductions in a small number of diseases, which were trending downward anyway.... Although they are well aware that the bulk of the reduction in the burden of infectious disease cannot be attributed to vaccines and that extensive research literature and rock-solid scientific evidence have proven that fact, health authorities around the world continue to promote the largely false 'vaccines eradicated the great diseases of yore' myth. At the same time, they feed the public another misleading myth—'our health has never been better'—while ignoring the surge of chronic morbidity that has plagued the Western world since at least the mid-20th century. This huge wave or morbidity continues to gain momentum even now." *Turtles All the Way Down*, pp. 305–306. As far as our contemporary situation is concerned, treatment of infectious disease is more sophisticated and effective today than in the past. Moreover, many contemporary vaccines, including the measles and polio vaccines, do not guarantee immunity or preclude transmission. The combination of these factors means that the popular notion that it is only mass vaccination that prevents infectious diseases from again breaking out and causing deadly epidemics today is open to serious question. In general, I think it is safe to say that promotion of the vaccine agenda has relied far more on ignorance and fear than upon science, truth, and real moral and social responsibility.

645 Kennedy and Hooker, Vax-Unvax, fig. 2.2, p. 15; fig. 2.6, p. 23.

646 Ibid., blurb.

647 The Holy Bible, King James version, John 3:8 and Matt. 11:15.

648 Ralph Waldo Emerson, "Self-Reliance," in *Essays and Lectures* (New York: Library of America, 1983), p. 265.

649 The poem is based upon the author's first trip to Prague in the summer of 2017, the city of Rilke's birth representing the last of many locales important to the poet visited by the author (see the author's account of his initiatory Rilke pilgrimage in *Rue Rilke* (Chiron, 2016), which explores the theme of the encounter of New and Old World sensibilities implicit in "Prague." To give the reader unfamiliar with Prague and its history some background information without peppering the poem with footnotes, I provide some of that information here.

•

* Hus (Jan): c. 1370–1415. Czech theologian considered by many the first reformer of the church and forerunner of Protestantism. On account of his speaking forcefully out against the greed and excesses of the Catholic Church (key to which was the money collected by way of selling indulgences) and opposing papal authority, Hus was burned at the stake. A huge and quite striking statue of Hus dominates Old Town Square in the center of old Prague.

* The medieval astronomical clock adorns the Town Hall in Old Town Square. The clock attracts droves of tourists, who fill the square in front of the clock every hour when the clock strikes and the remarkable features mentioned in the poem—including the walk of the twelve apostles and the crowing of the golden cock—can be witnessed.

* Our Lady before Tyn is the name of a church on Old Town Square. The church contains the tomb of the legendary astronomer Tycho Brahe, whose observations were essential to Kepler's confirmation of heliocentrism.

* The Charles River is traversed by a bridge peopled with numerous stone sculpures. The Strahov Monastery includes two high-vaulted library rooms devoted, respectively, to theology and philosophy. St. Vitus Cathedral is one of the impressive buildings that is part of the Prague Castle complex that sits high above the town on the other side of the Charles from the Old Town and its square. Golden Lane, part of the castle complex, is a line of tiny abodes that initially housed the fusiliers who defended the castle and later was populated by goldsmiths. Rudolf II (1552–1612) was the king of Hungary, Croatia, and Bohemia and Holy Roman Emperor from 1576–1612. Rudolf possessed an intense interest in esoteric magic and science. During his reign, alchemists worked in hidden underground chambers because such magical arts were forbidden by the Church.

* The Jewish Cemetery in Prague features innumerable closely packed old gravestones, including those of at least one legendary figure: Rabbi Loew, a 16th-century scholar and Jewish occultist reputedly the creator of the Prague Golem. Rabbi Loew is the central figure in one of an early cycle of Rilke's poems called *Visions of Christ*. As a young man, Rilke harbored aspirations of becoming a playwright: then, as now, Café Slavia hosts theatergoers near the banks of the Charles.

* Staré Mêsto is the Old Town section of Prague, characterized by a tangle of labyrinthine streets.

* The peaceful Velvet Revolution in November 1989 ended decades of Communist rule of Czechoslavakia. In demonstrations during the latter part of November, hundreds of thousands of people gathered in protest on Wenceslas Square. The revolution culminated in the resignation and exit of Communist leaders and the election of the poet, playwright, and dissident Vaclav Havel as president on December 29, 1989.

* The end of the second stanza of the poem alludes to Yeats' poem, "Sailing to Byzantium." https://www.poetryfoundation.org/poems/43291/sailing-to-byzantium. The poem,

like the clock, contains a golden bird. The last line of postscript 2 is the first line of Yeats' poem; the last line of "Sailing" finds its way into "Prague."

* 30 miles north of Prague, Theresienstadt was a ghetto–transit camp established by the Nazis in World War II. Jews from Prague and surrounding German-held areas were held there pending deportation to concentration camps and labor or killing centers. The Nazis publicly portrayed Theresienstadt as a civilized place, but in reality conditions were harsh and dehumanizing. For most, it was a way station en route to an untimely death.

INDEX

Note: References followed by "n" refer to endnotes.